Radiopharmaceuticals - Current Research for Better Diagnosis and Therapy

Edited by Farid A. Badria

Published in London, United Kingdom

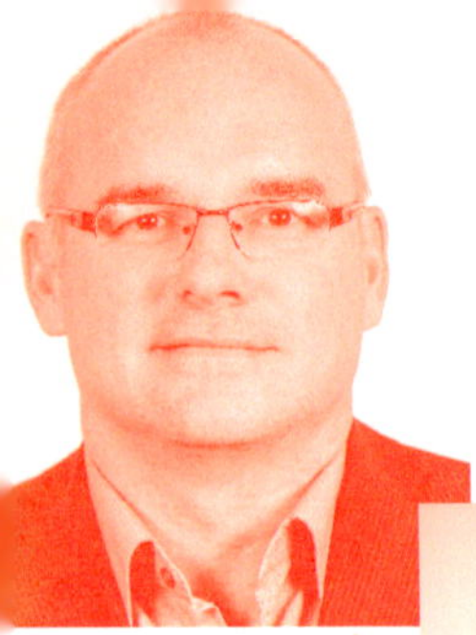
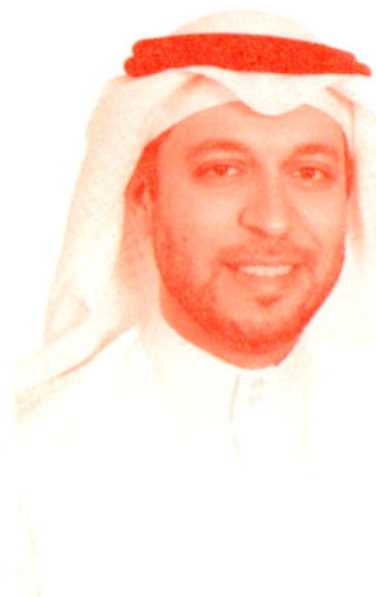
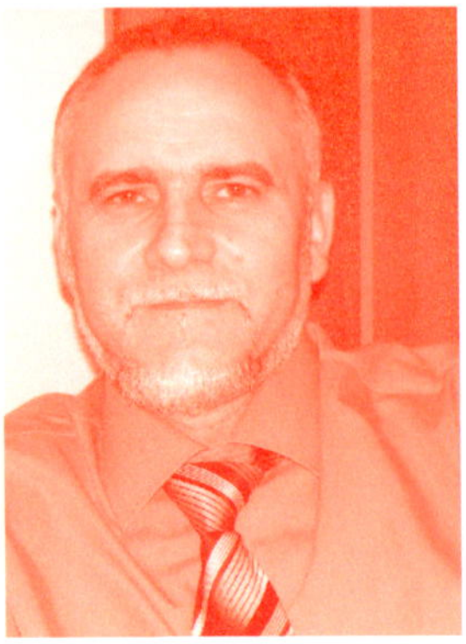
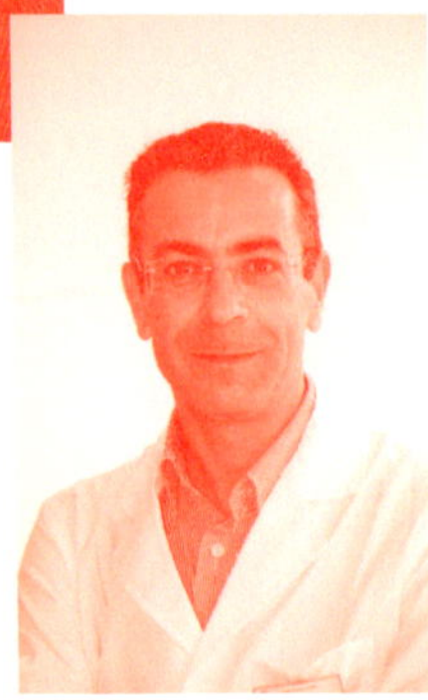
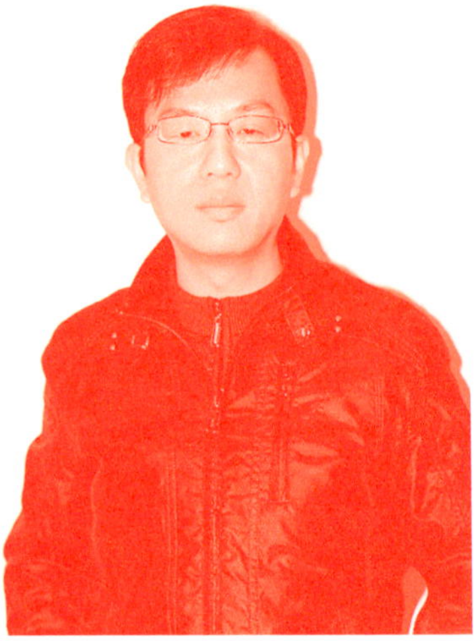
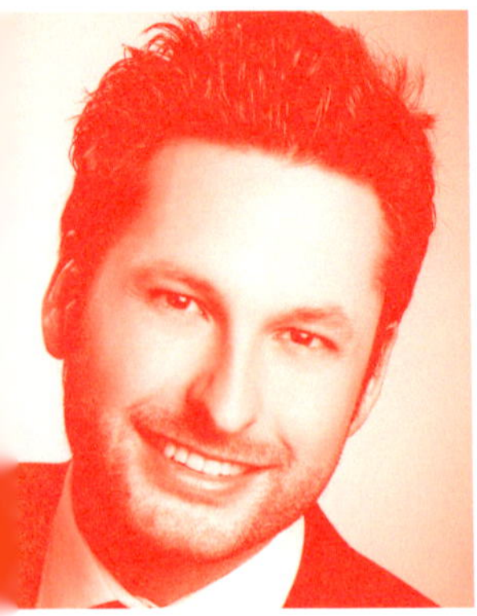
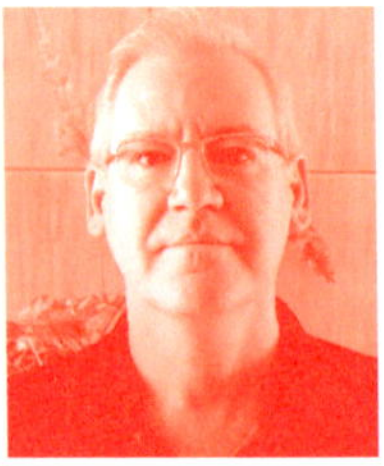

IntechOpen

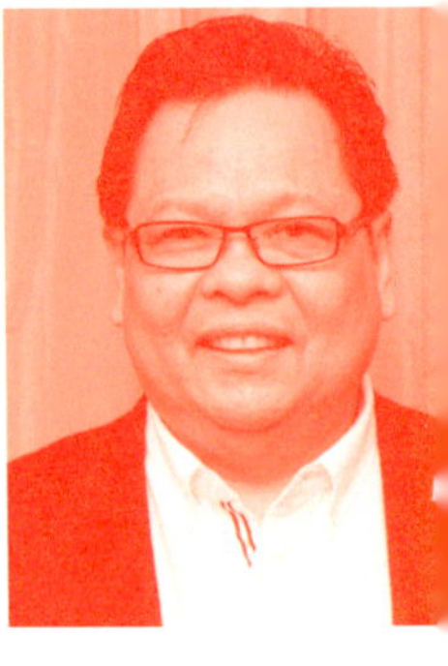
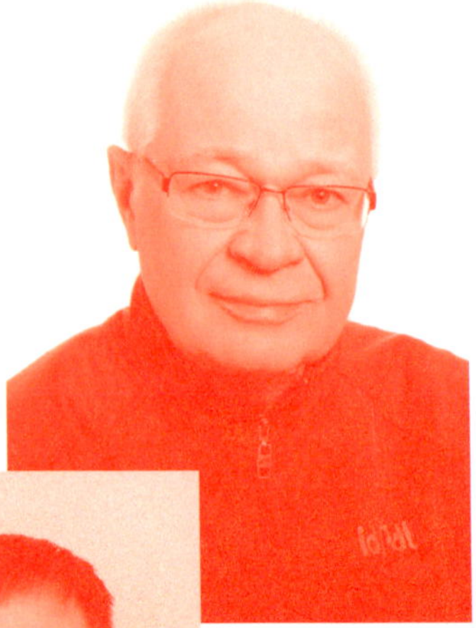
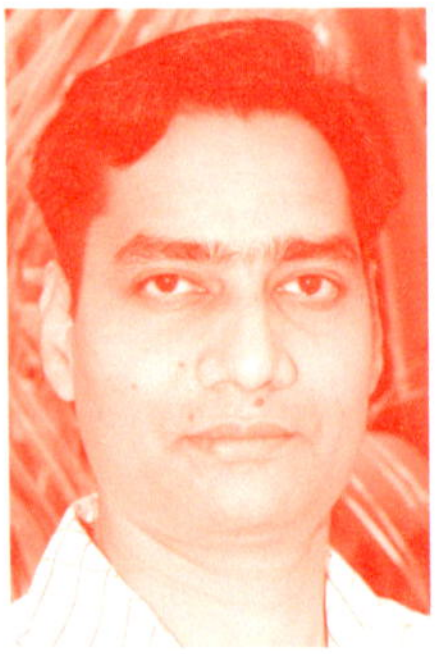
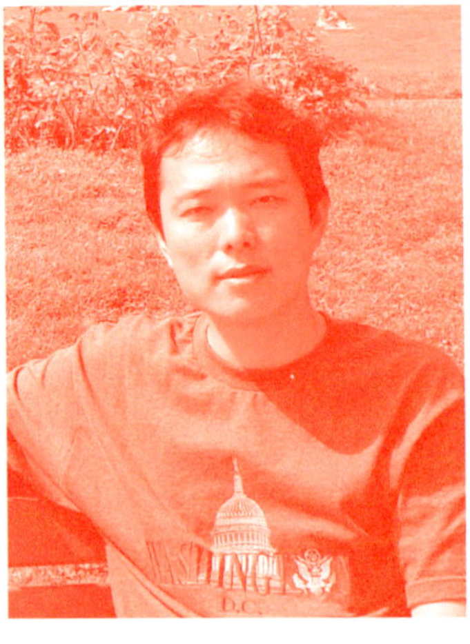
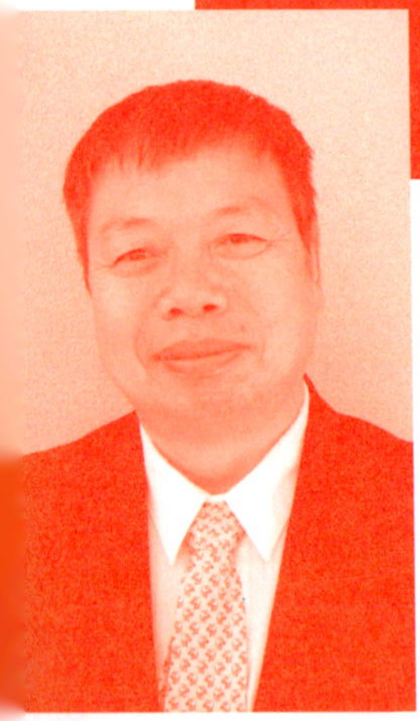
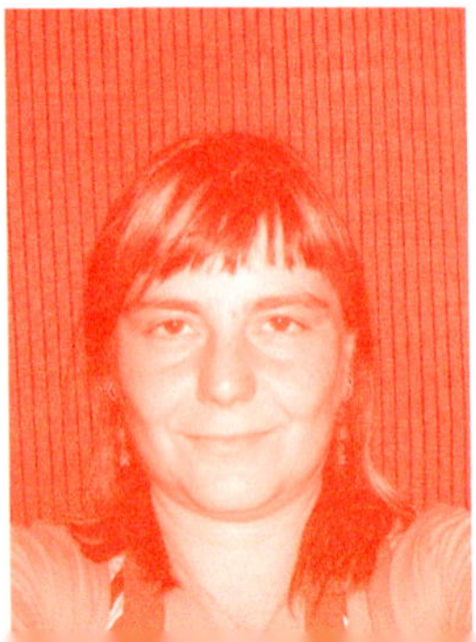

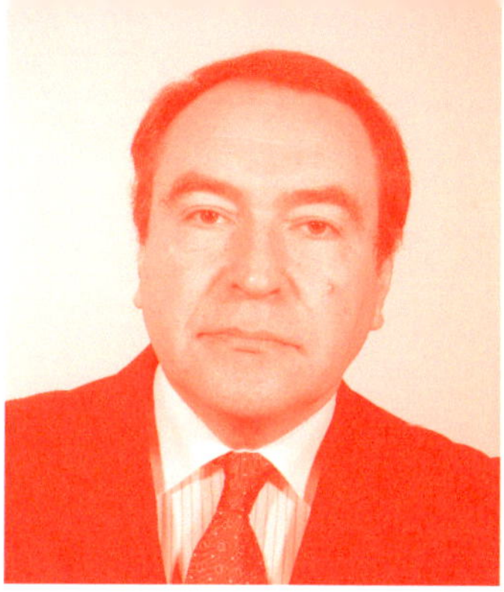

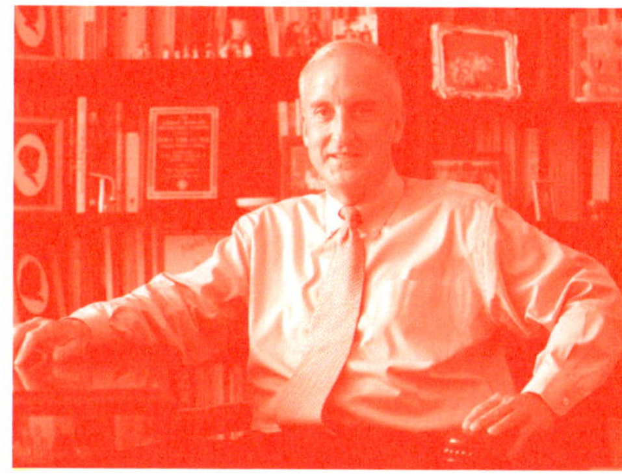

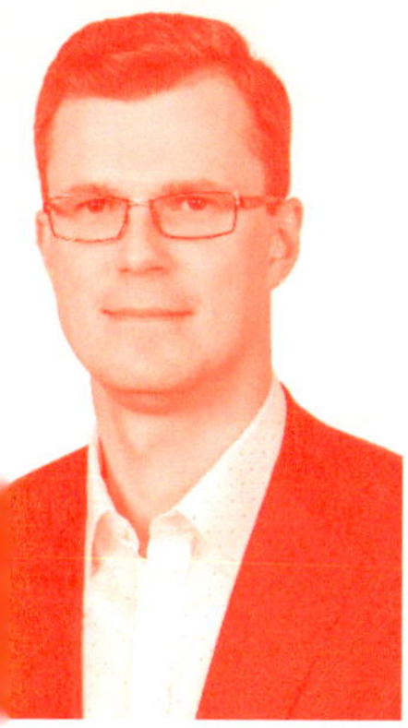

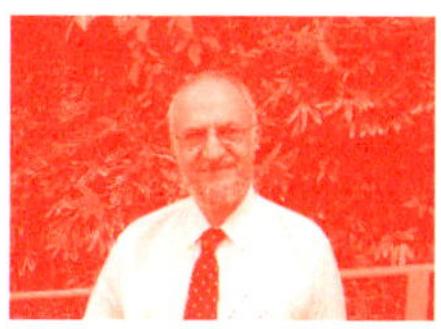

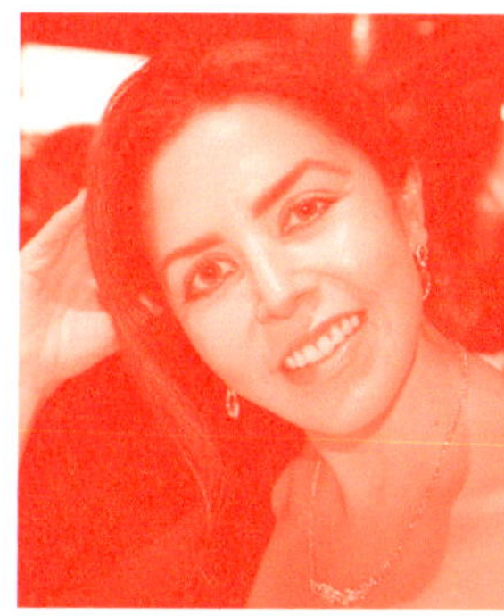

Supporting open minds since 2005

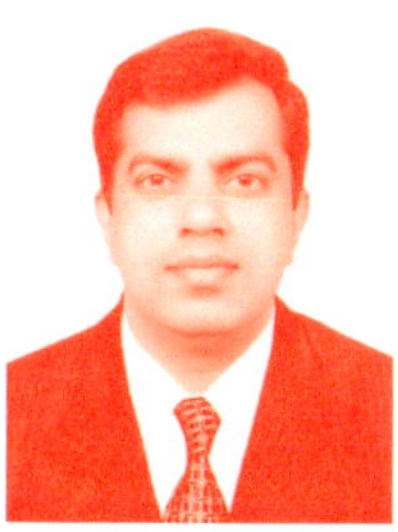

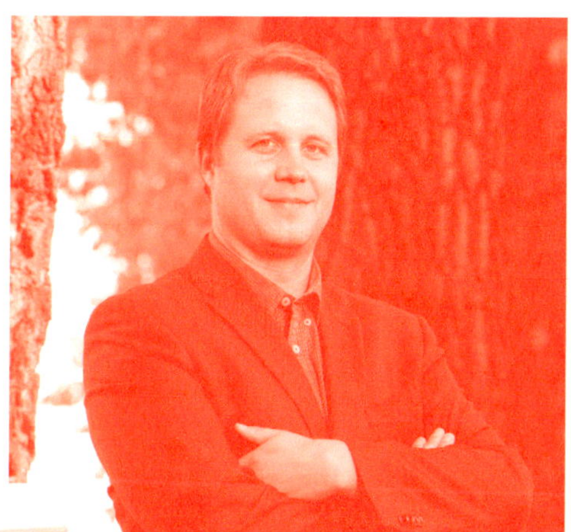

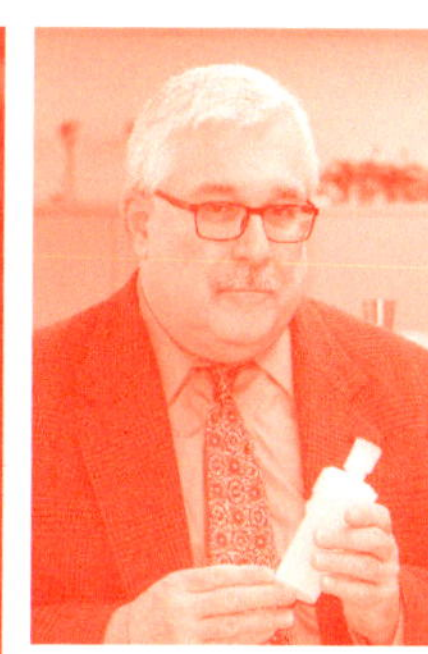

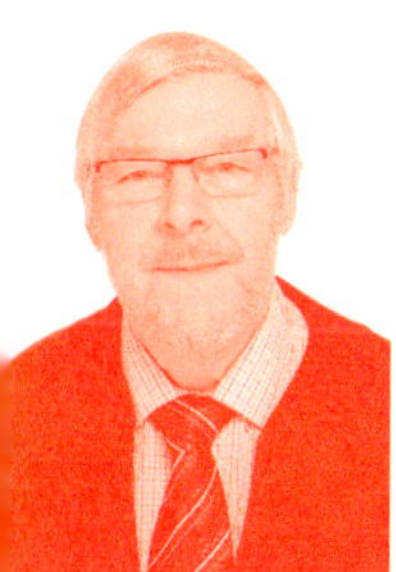

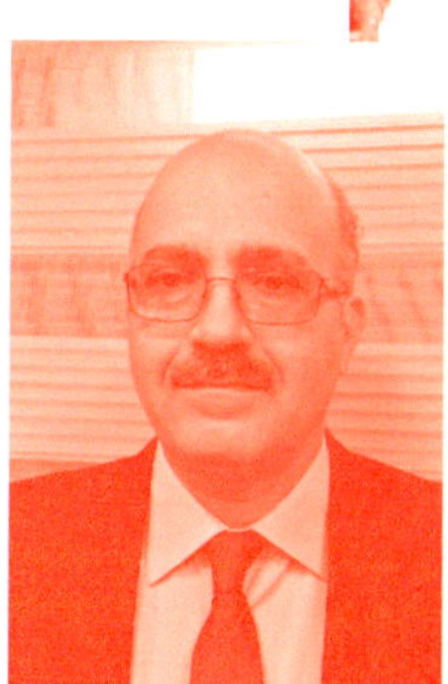

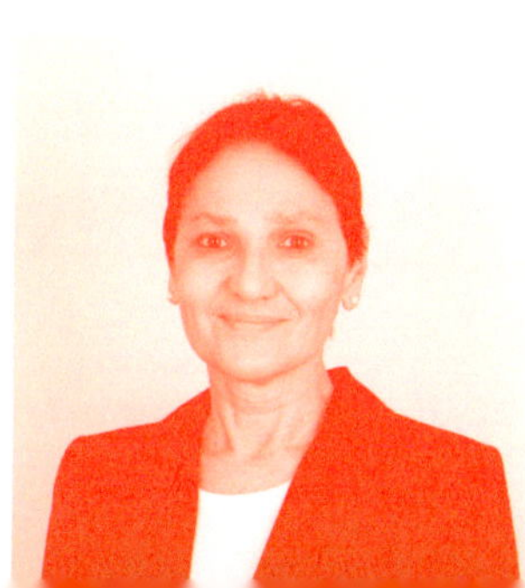

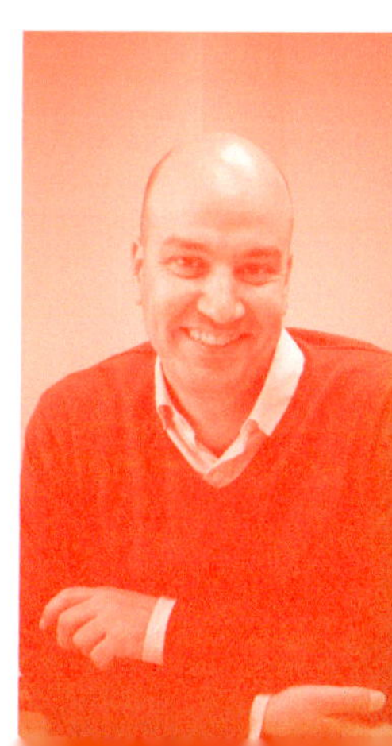

Radiopharmaceuticals - Current Research for Better Diagnosis and Therapy
http://dx.doi.org/10.5772/intechopen.95709
Edited by Farid A. Badria

Contributors
Donna E. Goldhawk, Farid A. Badria, Estrella Moya Sánchez, Akbar Abbasi, Hesham M. H. Zakaly, Fatemeh Mirekhtiary, Khaled Soliman, Ahmed Alenezi, Abdullah Alrushoud, Salman Altimyat, Mousa Bakkari, Hanna Alsheikh, Turki Alruwaili, Hasna Albander, Maisoon Ibrahim Aljalis, V. Sivasubramaniyan, K. Venkataramaniah, Aisyah Elliyanti, Santosh Kumar Gupta, Venkatesh Rangarajan, Ingrid Dijkgraaf, Stijn M. Agten, Matthias Bauwens, Tilman M. Hackeng, Carla Daruich De Souza, Jin Joo Kim, Jin Tae Hong, Carmen Alexandra Tuca, Ana Stochioiu

First published in London, United Kingdom, 2022 by IntechOpen
IntechOpen is the global imprint of INTECHOPEN LIMITED, registered in England and Wales, registration number: 11086078, 5 Princes Gate Court, London, SW7 2QJ, United Kingdom
Printed in Croatia

British Library Cataloguing-in-Publication Data
A catalogue record for this book is available from the British Library

Additional hard and PDF copies can be obtained from orders@intechopen.com

Radiopharmaceuticals - Current Research for Better Diagnosis and Therapy
Edited by Farid A. Badria
p. cm.
Print ISBN 978-1-83969-659-6
Online ISBN 978-1-83969-660-2
eBook (PDF) ISBN 978-1-83969-661-9

For EU product safety concerns:
IN TECH d.o.o., Prolaz Marije Krucifikse Kozulić 3, 51000 Rijeka, Croatia, info@intechopen.com or visit our website at intechopen.com.

Meet the editor

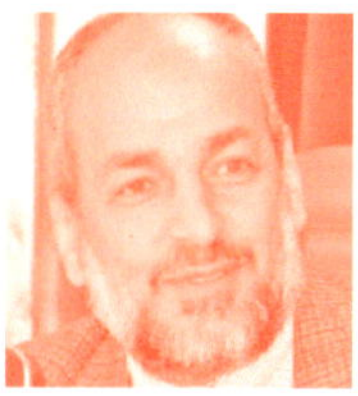

Farid A. Badria, Ph.D., is the recipient of several awards, including The World Academy of Sciences (TWAS) Prize for Public Understanding of Science; the World Intellectual Property Organization (WIPO) Gold Medal for best invention; Outstanding Arab Scholar, Kuwait; and the Khwarizmi International Award, Iran. He has 250 publications, 12 books, 20 patents, and several marketed pharmaceutical products to his credit. He continues to lead research projects on developing new therapies for liver, skin disorders, and cancer. Dr. Badria was listed among the world's top 2% of scientists in medicinal and biomolecular chemistry in 2019 and 2020. He is a member of the Arab Development Fund, Kuwait; International Cell Research Organization–United Nations Educational, Scientific and Cultural Organization (ICRO–UNESCO), Chile; and UNESCO Biotechnology France

Contents

Preface

A radiopharmaceutical is a pharmaceutical product or drug that may exert spontaneous degradation of unstable nuclei with nuclear particles or photon emission. Radiopharmaceuticals may be used for research, diagnosis, therapy, and environmental purposes. Moreover, radiopharmaceuticals act as radioactive tracers among patients via gamma-ray emissions. The best-known example of a therapeutic radiopharmaceutical is iodide^{131} for thyroid ablation in patients with hyperthyroidism. In addition to diagnosis and therapy, radiopharmaceuticals are used in research to investigate the metabolism, bio-distribution, pharmacodynamics, and pharmacokinetics of certain drugs in nonradioactive form.

This book examines the importance of radiopharmaceuticals as diagnostic agents to examine biochemical, molecular biology, physiological, or anatomical abnormalities in patients. Therapeutic radiopharmaceuticals may be administered internally for their selective effects on certain abnormal cells or organs. This book includes four chapters. Chapter 1 focuses on the fundamentals of radiopharmaceutical chemistry and preparation, and the environmental, pharmaceutical, diagnostic, therapeutic, and research applications of these products. Chapter 2 discusses fabrication, materials manipulation, and characterization of radiopharmaceuticals. Chapter 3 presents up-to-date applications of radiopharmaceuticals in preclinical studies Chapter 4 presents the most recent research in radiopharmaceutical applications in diagnosis and therapy, including molecular imaging with genetically programmed nanoparticles, radiopharmaceuticals in modern cancer therapy, and new trends in preparation, biodistribution, and pharmacokinetics of radiopharmaceuticals in diagnosis and research.

The figure below presents the diagnostic, therapeutic, environmental, and industrial applications of radiopharmaceuticals.

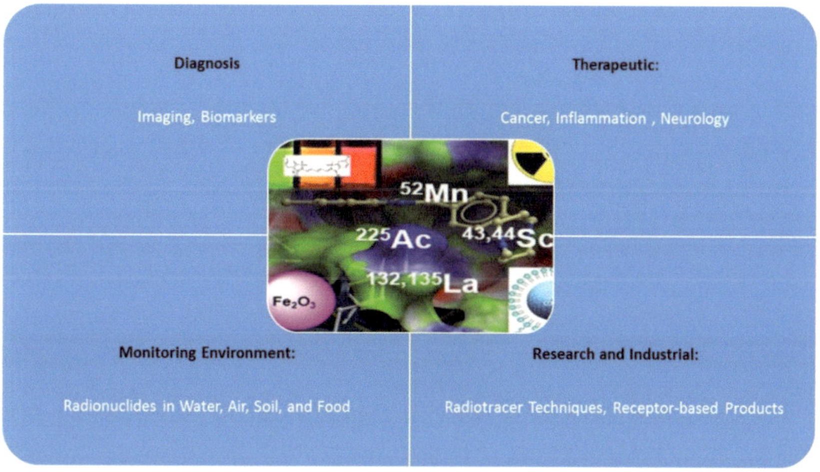

Section 1: This section composes of two chapters and focuses mainly on basic fundamentals of radiopharmaceutical chemistry, preparation, environmental, pharmaceutical, diagnostic, therapeutic, and research applications.

Section 2: This section composes of 5 chapters and presents Fabrication, Materials Manipulation, and Characterization of Radiopharmaceuticals

Section 3: This section composes of two chapters and presents the up-to-date applications of Radiopharmaceuticals in Preclinical Studies.

Section 4: This section composes of three chapters and presents the most recent research in Radiopharmaceuticals Applications in Diagnosis and Therapy including Molecular Imaging with Genetically Programmed Nanoparticles, Radiopharmaceuticals in Modern Cancer Therapy, and New Trends in Preparation, bio-distribution, and Pharmacokinetics of Radiopharmaceuticals in Diagnosis and Research

This book strikes a balance between developments in scientific research and the premises that researchers must be able to absorb and links scientific advances with clinical practice so that the management of diseases can be based on sound physiological concepts. It is a useful resource for students, clinicians, nutrition specialists, and researchers.

Farid A. Badria, Ph.D.
Liver Research Lab,
FAB-Lab,
Pharmacognosy Department,
Faculty of Pharmacy,
Mansoura University,
Mansoura, Egypt

Section 1

Radiopharmaceuticals: On-Going Research

Chapter 1

Radiopharmaceuticals: On-Going Research for Better Diagnosis, Therapy, Environmental, and Pharmaceutical Applications

Farid A. Badria

Abstract

Radiopharmaceutical material is a pharmaceutical product or drug that may exert spontaneous degradation of unstable nuclei with nuclear particles or photons emission. Radiopharmaceuticals may be used in research, diagnosis, therapy, and environmental purposes. Moreover, radiopharmaceuticals act as radioactive tracers among patients via gamma-ray emissions. Therefore, the uses of radiopharmaceuticals as diagnostic agents may be given to patients to examine any biochemical, molecular biology, physiological, or anatomical abnormalities. Therapeutic radiopharmaceutical may be administered internally for therapeutic purposes via selective effect on certain abnormal cells or organs. The best known example for therapeutic radiopharmaceuticala is iodide^{131} for thyroid ablation in among patients with hyperthyroid. A third class of radiopharmaceutical is drug labeling which mainly used in research by using small amount of radioactive substances not for diagnostic purposes, but to investigate the metabolism, bio-distribution, pharmakodynamic, and pharmakokinetic of certain drugs in a nonradioactive form. This chapter focuses mainly on basic fundamentals of radiopharmaceutical chemistry, preparation, environmental, pharmaceutical, diagnostic, therapeutic, and research applications.

Keywords: Radiopharmaceutical, Diagnosis, Environment, Research, Bio-evaluation

1. Introduction

Radiopharmaceuticals were first defined by the Federal Register of the USA as radioactive agents- potassium (^{40}K) and carbon (^{14}C) based natural compounds- or biological products contain unstable nuclei which may degrade spontaneously and emit photons or nuclear particles. These drugs might be prepared using nuclide generator or nonradioactive reagent [1].

Radiopharmaceuticals are categorized into 4 main classes: research, diagnostic, environmental and therapeutic pharmaceuticals as presented in **Figure 1**. Research radiopharmaceuticals are administrated to track metabolic reactions and kinetics including bio-distribution, bioavailability, pharmacokinetic, and pharmakodynamic of a drug that is intended to be used later as nonradioactive form [1].

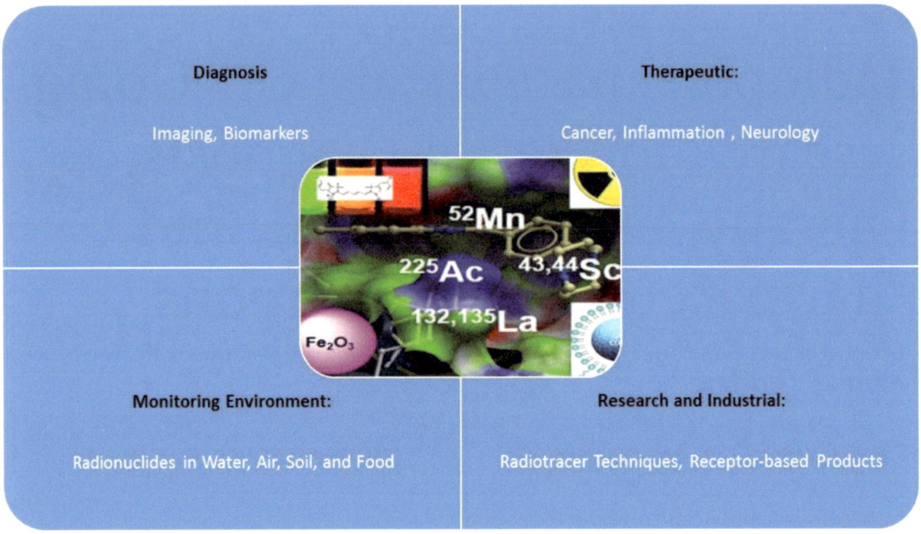

Figure 1.
Radiopharmaceutical applications in diagnosis, therapeutic, monitoring environment, and new trends in research.

Diagnostic radiopharmaceuticals Known as radioactive drugs/ompoundsc which used tracers for many diseases. Using gamma-ray emissions from radiopharmaceuticals drugs would help on broadcasting their positions inside the body. The concentrations of the radioactive materials could be deduced by observing these broadcasts in several organs. Images of different organs with low-resolution could be obtained using the signals [2].

The pharmacodynamics -the metabolism of the drug inside the body- and the kinetics could be studies by monitoring these broadcasts in a time-dependent manner. The device of monitoring is a collimated external gamma-ray detector. Therefore, in diagnosis purposes the radioactive materials are used to detect any sort of molecular, biochemical, physiological, and even anatomical abnormalities.

However, the diagnostic radioactive materials are not limited to gamma emitters types which allow their *in-situ* determination with noninvasive external radiation detectors. There are other types of radiopharmaceuticals that made of tritium, phosphorus 32, or carbon 14. Remarkably, these isotopes do not emit the same type of rays- gamma rays- therefore, it is impractical to monitor and examine their situation inside the body by external detectors. However, this type of isotypes could be applied in tracer diagnosis by analysis of samples. For instance, the administration of ^{14}C to glucose and monitoring the elimination of CO_2 (^{14}C) in the breathing as metabolic end-product and used as indication for the assimilation of the compound, its metabolism throughout the body.

There are many variant body samples and fluids could be considered as well such as urine, blood, and biopsies samples in specific conditions.

Therapeutic radiopharmaceuticals are radioactive substance which could help in delivering the radiation entirely of body tissues by administration to radioactive substances such as iodide I3I for thyroid removal in hyperthyroidism patients. The thyroid organ is irradiated entirely by radioactive iodine. Other different radiopharmaceutical materials could be used in treatment of cancer and known as radiotherapy [1].

2. History of Radiopharmacy

Although training on the use and management of labeled compounds is provided in various institutions, the demand for pharmacists who specialize in radiolabeled drugs has been determined, and radiopharmaceuticals have become the first specialty in the late 1960 in Pharmacy school at the U. of Southern California (USC), USA. The short-term research courses (usually 30 days for non-graduate students) and the radiopharmaceutical technician training program conducted from 1969 to 1986 enabled 201 pharmacists and other personnel to obtain a master's degree in radiopharmaceuticals, and 15 of them obtained technology Certificate, and more than 500 people have participated and provide such expert training elsewhere and completed its plan in 1986 [3].

Clinical needs can be in image performances which may have a vital role either in staging or prognosis of the disease. Long ago, several programs that are educational and anxious with radiopharmaceutical analysis have not addressed this question. The program is frequently specialize in labeling a particular compound and on its application without any thoughts for its potential application in future. Even once a specific biological target is being targeted, the question of whether or not it addresses a true clinical would like is usually not considered [4]. The usage of radiolabeled organism antibodies for imaging a neoplasm is taken into account a decent example. On the last decades, a great deal of studies were on developing programs based on aforesaid materials and this terminated and resulted in radiopharmaceuticals that may image cancer effectively and thought of as highly sensitive and specific methodology for imaging comparable or superior to other techniques.

3. Obstacles in academic research in radiopharmaceutical field

Most important modifications in health care in west were in the 1990's. At this time, many resources became unrestricted in conjunction with complete clinical freedom and open-ended budgets this led to high level of control for health-care requirements with limited budgets, established protocols, and internal markets. The development of drug has regulated as well. Radiopharmaceuticals considered as one of the regulators which regulate conventional drugs which in turn increase the costs for the development of these drugs.

The academic discoveries in commercial development of radiopharmaceuticals were limited due to limitation in radiopharmaceutical industry and many vicissitudes in the institutions carrying out development in this field.

National nuclear centers whole over the world faced a lot of obstacles such as being privatized or being overburdened to make commercial gains. Academic funding for scientific research has also been cut off for long periods at universities. The academic curiosity was one of many reasons for scientists to put radiopharmaceutical field in the scope of research. To gain success in this field, projects should be developed, more directed, productive, and focused than was required earlier. Particularly, developing the clinical application of the product must be taken in consideration combined with the overcoming the financial obstacles. Therefore, unique new radiopharmaceuticals must fulfill a clinical requirement [5].

4. Nuclear medicine: clinical uses

Many new therapies in clinical practice have other requirements, such as managed care plans and expensive restrictions. This represents both an opportunity and a challenge for new radiopharmaceuticals [6]. It is necessary to maintain a reputation for safety and efficacy, and to improve existing treatments for any new products. In such a restrictive environment, it will be difficult to find a place in the market for radioactive compounds of these new drugs in clinical practice. Another way to introduce new and expensive treatments is to determine the subset of patients most likely to benefit from that particular treatment. The unique advantage of medicine is that it has the ability to combine diagnostic and therapeutic radionuclides for the same purpose, and may remain unchanged. In the future, diagnostic and therapeutic radiopharmaceutical pairs will increasingly be used to perform this function [6]. At the scientific level, radiopharmaceutical research has undergone a process of substitution in recent years. This review of compounds which describes certain aspects of current radiopharmaceutical research that have appeared in recently published literature or have become the subject of conference presentations [7]. Some of these issues are also the subject of more detailed review. However, this chapter deliberately excludes certain subject areas, especially not trying to cover developments in the field of positron emission tomography [7].

Radiopharmaceuticals are the cornerstone of nuclear medicine. Although there are many types of drugs that can study the structure and function of many essential organs, there is still a need for radiopharmaceutical substitution to study the subtle mechanisms of human body function. Under this trend, 15O, 18F and 123I appeared in the throttle body. With the emergence of such radionuclide-labeled drugs, especially the most widely used 99mTc, people are also doing their best to translate this success into daily clinical practice. β-labeled drugs can also be used for targeted radiotherapy of various malignant tumors. In addition to laboratories in industrialized countries, some developing countries have also shown interest in these fields and participated in research projects [8].

Therapeutic radiopharmaceuticals have a critical effect on patient care specifically on medicine which have a promising role in the future. Many of latest therapies in clinical practice in need of different requirements like managed care programs, restrictions which are expensive. This symbolizes both a chance and a challenge for brand spanking new radiopharmaceuticals [6]. Efficacy and safety are among many others advantages to be added over the current treatments for any new product. Therefore, in such a restrictive environment there'll be an issue for these new medicinal radio compounds to urge their place within the routine of clinical practice. Though, another route to abide with the new protocols is to define which group of patients may benefit from this special treatment. The strength of nuclear medicine is its capability to merge the uses of radionuclides in both diagnostic and therapeutic purposes for matching targets in diagnostic and therapeutic radiopharmaceuticals [6].

This chapter describes, generally terms, some aspects of current radiopharmaceutical research which have appeared within the recent published literature or are the topic of conference presentations [7]. Several of these topics are also the subject of more detailed reviews during this publication. However, some specialized areas of labor are deliberately excluded from this chapter, especially, no attempt is formed to hide developments within the field of Positron Emitting Tomography [7].

5. Radiopharmaceuticals and its bodily functions

Radiopharmaceuticals form the cornerstone of nuclear medicine. While the existing range of radiopharmaceuticals permits study of the structure and function of many important organs, there is a need for new radiopharmaceuticals that could be used to explore more subtle mechanisms of bodily functions. Important progress has been achieved in this direction by the development of tracers labeled with cyclotron produced isotopes, including UC, 13 N, I5O, I8F and 123*I. major* efforts are also under way to translate this success into regular clinical practice by developing similar agents labeled with metallic radionuclides, particularly with the most widely used 99mTc. The agents labeled with beta emitting isotopes for potential use in the targeted radiotherapy of various malignancies is also being widely pursued. In addition to laboratories in advanced countries, several developing countries are also interested in these areas and have been participating in research programs organized by the IAEA. New advancement of Radiopharmaceuticals for therapy and Diagnosis will help speeding communication, and widespread knowledge for the better health of human being [8].

6. Current directions in radiopharmaceutical research

Nowadays, most of research in the area radiopharmaceutical is focusing on the tracers of receptor binding in biochemical reactions. The nature of these reactions may be Intra-extracellular in nature and may exhibit a good progress in tissue characterization using imaging technique in-vivo. Several of these agents are depending upon wide range of size; large MoAbs to tiny peptides (e.g. neuropeptide) which utilize bifunctional chelating agents to radiolabeling drugs/compounds. Radiopharmaceuticals of polypeptide may be in the brain whereas low molecular weight molecules retained high lipophilic characters to interact intercellular are highly needed (e.g. cell-surface receptors). Radiopharmaceutical chemists are facing many challenges to synthesis these compounds via one of two methods; namely integrated method or pendant method to utilize technetium coordination with interest on technetium (v) cores. Malignancy, neurology, inflammation, neurology, and infectious diseases are among many other health disorders which are in dire need of cytotoxic radionuclides in the area of radioimmunotherapy. This may prompt researchers to focus their research and the newly developed radiopharmaceuticals toward specific clinical and biological targets [9].

7. Therapeutic applications

Emerging MoAbs associated with radionuclide(s) to target selective Tumors (antigens) may considered as an early research took place using iodine radionuclides in cancer. Moreover, some of these drugs/compounds are targeting the outer surface of cells, others may interact with the inner surface of the targeted cells. There are many examples for applications of different radiopharmaceutical in diverse therapeutic applications, e.g. nucleosides and their analogues in modulation of both cell proliferation as well as mRNA transcription. Besides imaging of cell proliferation and mRNA transcription, a good advancement had been made to articulate a sort of tracers for imaging cell hypoxia. Interestingly, the progress in radiolabeled agents may exhibit remarkable benefits for speculating the resulted outcomes of tumors to radiotherapy beam which is greatly affected by the potential oxygen of the cell as in cardiac hypoxia. Discovery and search for new radiolpharmaceutical with new therapeutic applications revealed by chance non-nitroimidazole technetium-labeled molecule during a research program at Amersham International which is also trapped by reduction in hypoxic cells and this new agent is currently in the final stage of drug approval.. Several therapy applications are summarized in the next section [7].

7.1 Inflammation and infection

This area has provided a rich field for radiopharmaceutical research in last few years. Many of the newly developed radiopharmaceuticals products are derived from peptides, antibodies, cytokines, and polypeptides and very much similar to the ones which have been used in cancer [7].

The capability to image the indirect or direct inflammatory response to the infection is the key for clinical management with high selectivity, e.g. Antibiotic complex of Technetium (Ciprofloxacin = Tcinfecton "Tc") [8]. Tc is good for labeling leucocytes to hammer Tc-leucocytes to place of infection. Several other examples, Tc-HMPAO, Tc-ECD, Tc-citrate, and Tc-glutathione etc. All of these Tcs proved to be concentrated in some tumor and/or inflammatory sites. Moreover, other complexes for imaging inflammation, e.g. human immunoglobulin Gb and 99Tcm "HIgG-99Tcm" is an interesting serendipity drug developed from the reduction of disulphides (-S-S-) under very mild conditions to produce free –SH groups. The efficacy of the formed labeled chemotactic complexes act as substrate(s) for imaging infection *via* binding to receptors whereas WBC (leucocytes) are in high concentration at the location of infection [8, 10].

7.1.1 Tcm-Ciprofloxacin

HPLC analysis showed that the efficacy of the radiolabeled Tcm-Ciprofloxacin is over 95%. Meanwhile, *In vivo* bioavailability studies using mice showed that "Tcm-CIP is quickly bioavailable and distributed upon intravenous administration with a major renal clearance. In the infection inflammatory model on mice induced by turpentine oil, *S. aureus*, and *E. coli*, the radiopharmaceutical preparation was successful in localization of bacteria in the inflamed site [11].

7.2 Neurology and psychiatry

Molecular biology plays a crucial role in identifying many receptors and subtype receptors for neurotransmitters. Subsequently, this encourages radiopharmaceutical industry to conduct neuroreceptors brain imaging as is one of the major application of the radiopharmaceutical research [7].

7.3 Renal tubular function agents

A true replacement to hippuran-123I has been a challenging task in the development of technetium complexes, as no Tc compound is completely extracted and secreted into urine. It has, however, been possible to develop compounds which are handled by the renal tubules and actively secreted into urine. Structural feature requirements for recognition by renal tubules and for delivery by serum protein bound transport propounded way back by Despopoulos, [-C(=O)-NH-CH2-COOH], have been sought in the technetium complexes to achieve some degree of success. For most clinical purposes, a renogram agent based on renal tubular handling would be very much more useful, apart from being superior to purely GFR based agent such as 99Tcm -DTP A, and hence the intense research efforts. Tc-MAG3 complex contains the structure referred to above, while Tc-EC has a structural mimic, 3 oxygen atoms at 3–4 A0 to one another in Tc(=O)-NH-CH2-COOH, cf. -C(=O)-NH-CH2-COOH [9]. Both Tc-MAG3 and Tc-EC show less excretion than hippuran, but Tc-EC has relatively superior features. The room temperature formulation recipe of Tc-EC is another practical advantage. The early apprehensions of differences in the purity of kit formulated and chromatographically purified product were removed with refinements in kit formulation procedures. However, due to inherent nature of possible trace impurities in MAGS synthesis as well as different types of TcMAG3 complexes feasible, interference from hepatobiliary involvement during renography studies has not been ruled out. One study is in fact devoted to the anomalies in Tc-MAG3 behavior, Modifications to MAG3 ligands to overcome the drawbacks have been sought, replacing glycine by another amino acid, introduction of chiral center to influence the stereochemical role etc.; some superior results have been achieved, like 99Tcm -D-MAGAG. Tc-L, L-EC requires to be prepared at highly alkaline pH of 11–12 and it is consequently difficult to present in a reliable single component lyophilized kit form, though a commercial kit has been cited in literature. Detailed stringent protocol for kit formulation has been suggested. A multi-component kit recipe would be generally necessary, but advantage of ease of transchelation (using GHA) based kit has also been reported. As discussed earlier, the development of Tc-EC for renal tubular function, is an outcome based on the excretory pattern of Tc-ECD and the study of its metabolite(s) [12]. The attempts to utilize cysteine, cystine and analogues for complexing technetium for obtaining renal agents had shown mixed findings, but the same group from India has recently demonstrated a new product for renal tubular function imaging. 99Tcm complex of dimethyl ester of DTPA denoted as Tc-DMDTPA, has shown promising results including in human volunteers. Analogous to Tc-DTPA, the Tc-DMDTPA complex is anionic, but has predictably less (−50%) electrophoretic mobility. Ease of reliable, stable, single component lyophilized kit formulation, room temperature preparation of Tc-DMDTPA in high yield, purity and stability and similarity in biological behavior to hippuran- l j lI and Tc-MAG3 in both normal and probenecid (renal tubular transport inhibitor) treated mice are the salient advantages reported. A cationic pathway renal tubular agent has also been reported from UK involving the complex of 1,2-diaminocyclohexane (DACH). The product, [Tc(V)02(DACH)2]", is formulated using stannous tartrate reduction of pertechnetate and has shown utility for eliciting renal tubular function, when anionic pathway is not freely accessible due to high concentrations of circulating anions, like during chemotherapy [9, 12].

8. Research and Development

8.1 Milestones and concepts in the evolution of new products

In the genesis of the growth of 99Tcm compounds, the introduction of DTPA chelate of technetium, use of stannous tin for reduction of Tc (VTT) in pertechnetate and lyophilization of premixed stannous tin - ligand formulation would merit the first mention despite the passage of time. Suitable variation(s) in the functional groups on the ligand backbone to influence the pharmaco-kinetic behavior of the resultant technetium complexes, while retaining the same chelating environment for technetium, was a major development. This eventually led to introduction of the most preferred hepatobiliary tracer, 99Tcm-mebrofenin [2]. Such systematic investigations of structure - activity distribution relation (SADR) provided a fresh approach for the development of many other new products. The concept of bifunctional nature of ligands was also propounded after this work, for in LID As, IDA groups participate in complexing technetium, while the phenylcarbamoyl moiety bestows some of the required biological features. Although in the present sense of the term BCA, this may not be strictly correct, the way was paved for a new approach to develop "Tcm compounds [13].

8.2 Receptor-based products

99Tcm based receptor radiopharmaceuticals are not yet a clinical reality. The only successful case is that of 99Tcm - neogalactosyl glycoalbumin (NGA) for a bound receptor named hepatocyte binding protein (HBP) receptor, that binds galactose end glyco proteins. Tc-NGA would be useful for staging certain liver diseases (since HBP is implicated in liver malignancy) and for monitoring response to therapy [13]. The concept of BCA to attach receptor specific molecules with 99Tcm has been extensively investigated, but with limited success. Arduous chemical studies followed by receptor binding experiments have revealed poor specificity in most cases, like [Tc(V)O(DADS)-Progestin],[Tc(ra)(CO)(diethyldithiocarbamato-Spiperone)3], [Tc^-BATO-QNB] & [Tc(V)O(DADS)-QNB]. It appears that in all cases the complexation with technetium severely alters the bioactivity and precludes receptor binding. Attempts to overcome steric effects by increasing the distance between the essential functional groups have not been much successful. The important aspects to be reckoned with are molecular weight & size, lipophilicity changes, stereochemical effects and non-specific binding; two approaches called tridentate-monodentate (3 + 1) scheme (the former for facile chelation with Tc and the latter for presenting the receptor avid moiety) and pendant scheme have been pursued [13]. The novel concept of molecular mimics, i.e. Tc-chelate simulating a regular ring structure in a native receptor binding molecule, especially in a steroid (e.g. progesterone)/drug (e.g. morphine), is being pursued to target receptor sites for imaging using 99Tcm. Radiolabeled peptides have been recognized as the most likely successful candidates for imaging receptors (covered in another article in this Volume), based on the promising experience with mini labeled octreotide. The earlier stated problems in disguising and presenting technetium to the receptors persist, but scope for optimism is seen in this approach. In view of the importance of receptor imaging capability in health and disease, research efforts are continuing in more than one way [13, 14].

8.3 Computational chemistry of metal-based radiopharmaceuticals

Calculation of radiopharmaceutical doses is a very crucial process and considered one of the main task of radiopharmacist as illustrated later. It is noteworthy to mention that there is the method of prescription calculation is completely different from conventional organic drugs. The most common method of calculation or computational chemistry of metal-based radiopharmaceuticals [14]. Other factors must be considered and may have role in pharmacokinetic and biodistribution, e.g. molecule geometry, dipole moments, ionic charge [15].

8.4 Bioevaluation (biological assessment)

Eventhough methods of diagnosis and therapy are very important for both patients and physicians but bioevaluation or biological assessment protocol(s) are highly recommended [16–20]. The studies proved that some chelating agents (e.g. EDTA and DPTA) may chelate radionuclides to provide good images especially in cases of advanced cancer. For early diagnosis, Re-186(V) and Re-188(V)-DMSA are among drugs which will help in both diagnosis and monitoring cancer with good bio-distribution and pharmacokinetics properties [21]. This will enable specialist to understand if the radiopharmaceutical reached the appropriate location or site(s) (tumor for example). This also may enhance the delivery and improver the efficacy of drug [21]. Interestingly, measuring all three tumor space could be examined in vivo using drugs labeled with 95 mPt [22]. This protocol is valuable for cytotoxic drugs *via* the first pass phenomenon, e.g. cisplatin and 5-FU. However, other drugs that control tumor *via* a slow diffusion mechanism will behave differently. The use of radiopharmaceutical in meager quantity may help in calculating the number of locations/sites needed to attain the optimal delivery and bio-distribution to reach the best therapeutic activity [23–27].

Coupled with the ease of antibody production, these facts make 125 I-labeled immunoassays an ideal choice for many research activities [28, 29], especially in the medical field where radioisotopes are In short, even a cursory examination of the public health statistics of different countries on all continents shows the need for a simple, economic, and reliable analytical with this in mind, it is expected that [30].

8.5 Current status of radioactive signal immunoassays

The future development of radiolabeled immunoassays use reagents containing radioisotopes as indicators to monitor the distribution of free and bound antigens or free antibodies The distribution of free antibodies (free Immune radiological reagent analysis. (IRMA) [28, 29, 31–33].

8.6 Development of a simple immunofluorescence test method that uses AVIDIN to connect with general polystyrene spheres

Immunoradioassay (IRA) based on using beads of polystyrene as solid phase conjugated to avidin [34]. The commercially MoAbs is bio-tinylated with N-hydroxysuccinimide ester of biotin aminocaproate, and the detection Ab is I^{125}.

A simple assay composed mainly of two steps;, mixing 2 labeled Abs with either sample or positive control [35]. This method has been used for hormonal analysis; Lutinizing hormones (LH), Follicle Stimulating Hormones (FSH), and prolactin [36]. For example, theaccuracy in analysis of prolactin is 8 (μU/ml (0.3 ng/ml), FSH is 1 mlU/ml, and LH is 0.9 mlU/ml [37].

8.7 Magnetic particle separation technique

There are 5 classes of magnetic particles(MP) (with/or without –CHO, NH2-, and COOh groups) were used to conjugate the 1st or 2nd antibody(Ab) using three methods; immmunoaffinity, adsorption, and chemical coupling to form 4 different MPAbs [38]. The 2nd immobilized Ab on polyacrolein MPs through -CHO and also the 1st Abs immobilized on -COO polystyrene MPs through -COOH to use in RIAs and/or IRMAs [39]. Commercial MPS were immobilized on NH2- for "Streptavidin" to separating polymerase chain reaction product quantitatively for CMV (Cytomegalovirus) [40, 41].

There are over forty eight cyclotrons and forty two reactors to provide radioisotopesfor biomedical applications [42, 43].

Nuclear reactors have played a main role in production of radioisotopes required for medical, industrial, agricultural purposes, education within the nuclear sciences and research. Millions of people worldwide have benefited from the 99Mo - > 99mTc generator for diagnostic imaging, and 131I for the treatment of cancer. Advances in accelerator and medical imaging technology are driving the demand for radioisotopes and radiopharmaceuticals required by nuclear medicine [44]. Conditions like public perception arising from concern for the environment either from radiation accidents or future storage of nuclear waste, additionally because the operating and replacement costs for aging reactors are factors influencing the prospects of future availability of radioisotopes. This may well be often reflected in recent decisions taken to initiate the de-commissioning of some research TRIGA reactor(s) that were installed in hospitals during the 1960's [45].

8.8 Design of radiopharmaceuticals and gene transfer therapy

Gene transfer therapy among cancer patients require monitoring emission for better management during treatment as presented in **Figure 2** [46–49]. The first clinical experience employing gene therapy was gained in 1989. leukocytes were transduced with heterologous DNA to look at the biological in vivo properties of tumor-infiltrating lymphocytes, and thereby optimizing antitumour imrnuno-therapy strategies [50]. There are numerous approaches were undertaken to use powerful strategy of therapeutic gene transfer to the majority varieties of human diseases [51].

8.9 Radiopharmaceuticals for diagnosis and tumor therapy

For effective imaging in diagnosis and tumor therapy [52], three enzymes -which are not commonly expressed by normal/non-infected cells- encoded by viral gene are required [53]:

1. Nucleoside kinase: This enzyme can convert selectively the unnatural nucleosides to nucleotides in gene-transfected cells or in virus-infected cells does not act on normal cells as in case of thymidine kinase(TK), e.g. *Herpes simplex*-I (HSV-I TK) [54].

2. Tyrosinase: These enzyme can convert tyrosine amino acid to L-dopa, dopamine, dopaquinone and melanin via either neurotransmitter or pigmentation pathways, e.g. melanomas

3. Reductases: These enzyme are active mainly within the liver in hypoxic tissues. The process of bioreduction of active compounds may enhance the sensitivity of the hypoxic cells to the radiolabeled compound [55].

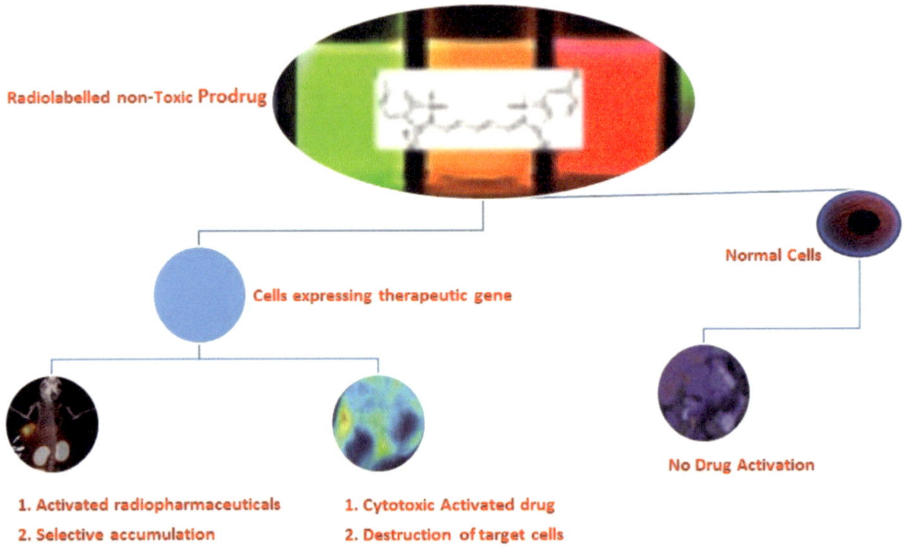

Figure 2.
Selective prodrug gene therapy.

9. Relation between Physcian in nuclear medicine and Radiopharmacist

Nuclear Pharmacy or Radiopharmacy is currently a very well recognized pharmaceutical specialty and a sort of cooperation is highly recommended to build a strong and clear relation between Physcian in nuclear medicine and radiopharmacist. The concept of this relation is presented in **Figure 3**. In 1970, radiopharmacy speciality was recognized by the American Board of Pharmaceutical specialties. Nowdays, radiopharmacy has implemented in many health care systems with official credential certificate. Meanwhile, each country has its own regulatory radiopharmacy products [56].

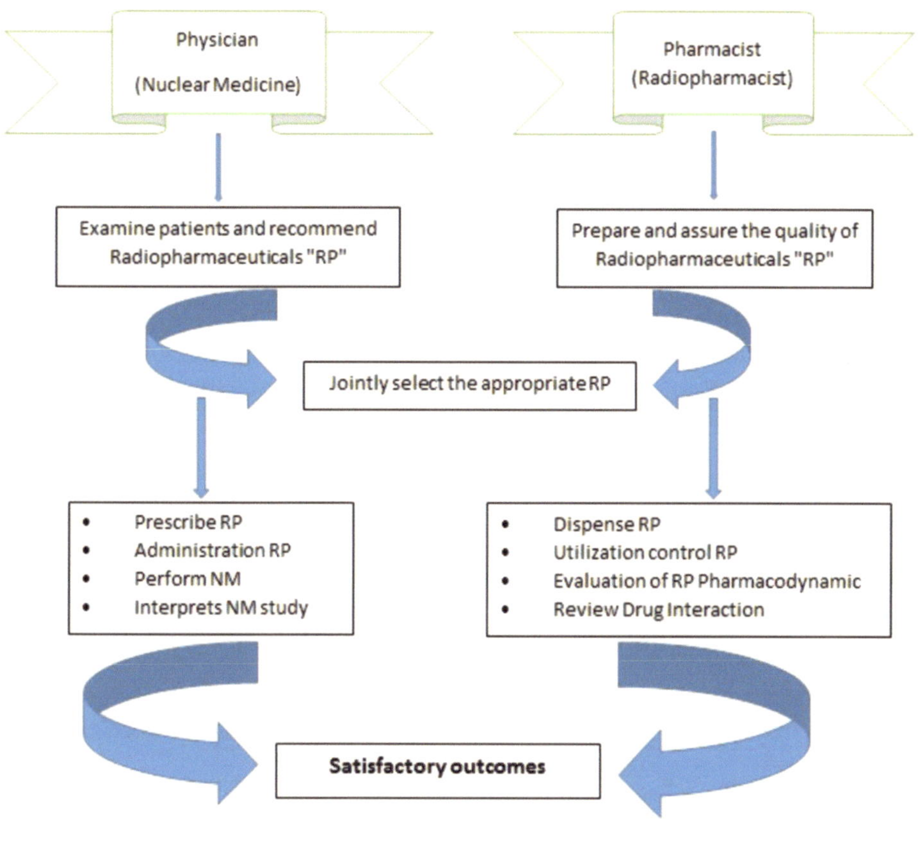

Figure 3.
Relation between Physcian in nuclear medicine and Radiopharmacist.

10. Conclusion

As the search continues for new products and newer areas of applications, 12jI compounds would provide the vital bridge between truly biological PET tracers based on nC/18F labeled compounds and the much more easily accessible SPECT tracers based on "Tcm and inIn products, thereby rendering a transition from PET to SPECT, that is from medical research to clinical utility, a reality. products would provide a fine complement to "Tcm compounds, especially for imaging process(es) involving slower kinetics of tracer and in the cases where conjugation of In-BCA with the bio-active substrate causes less alterations of the biological activity. Though the question "After 99Tcm, what next?" is posed time and again, the well-known attractive advantages of 99Tcm are not likely to be matched by any other tracer in the foreseeable future and consequently the impetus to develop 99Tcra based radiopharmaceuticals will continue. It could be safely predicted that the future of radiopharmaceuticals and in turn, clinical nuclear medicine, will continue to be dominated by "Tcm products, as has been the case in the past.

Conflict of interest

The authors declare no conflict of interest.

Abbreviations

- Radionuclides emitting Gamma-rays: γ e.g. Technetium-99m (^{99m}Tc)
- Iodine-123(123I): Iodine-123 (^{123}I)
- Galium-67 (67Ga): Gallium-67 (^{67}Ga)
- Radionuclides emitting positrons: e.g. Fluorine 18 (^{18}F), Oxygen-15 (^{15}O), Carbon-11(^{11}C), and Zirconium-89(^{89}Zr).
- Radionuclides emitting beta particles: e.g. Rhenium-186/Rhenium-188 (^{186}Re/^{188}Re), Strontium-89 (^{89}St), and Yttrium-90(^{90}Y), Bismuth213(^{213}Bi), and Astatine-211(^{211}At).

Author details

Farid A. Badria
Pharmacognosy Department, Liver Research Lab—FAB-Lab, Faculty of Pharmacy, Mansoura University, Mansoura, Egypt

*Address all correspondence to: badri002@mans.edu.eg

References

[1] Rhodes BA, Croft BY. Basics of Radiopharmacy: Mosby; 1978 1978///.

[2] Ercan MT, Caglar M. Therapeutic radiopharmaceuticals. Current pharmaceutical design. 2000;6(11):1085-1121.

[3] Wolf W, Kawada T, Shani J. The radiopharmacist as a professional speciality: past, present and future. International Atomic Energy Agency (IAEA): 1998 1011-4289 Contract No.: IAEA-TECDOC--1029.

[4] Silva ACQ, Vilela C, Santos HA, Silvestre AJD, Freire CSR. Recent trends on the development of systems for cancer diagnosis and treatment by microfluidic technology. Applied Materials Today. 2020;18:100450.

[5] Vermeulen K, Vandamme M, Bormans G, Cleeren F. Design and Challenges of Radiopharmaceuticals. Seminars in Nuclear Medicine. 2019.

[6] Cox PH, Mather SJ, Sampson CB, Lazarus CR. Progress in Radiopharmacy. Dordrecht, The Netherlands: Springer; 1986 1986///.

[7] Mather SJ. Current Directions in Radiopharmaceutical Research and Development. Dordrecht, The Netherlands: Springer; 1996 1996///.

[8] Boschi A, Uccelli L, Martini P. A Picture of Modern Tc-99m Radiopharmaceuticals: Production, Chemistry, and Applications in Molecular Imaging. Applied Sciences. 2019;9(12).

[9] Modern trends in radiopharmaceuticals for diagnosis and therapy1998; Lisbon, Portugal: INTERNATIONAL ATOMIC ENERGY AGENCY.

[10] Auletta S, Galli F, Lauri C, Martinelli D, Santino I, Signore A. Imaging bacteria with radiolabeled quinolones, cephalosporins and siderophores for imaging infection: a systematic review. Clinical and Translational Imaging. 2016;4(4):229-252.

[11] Naqvi SAR, Roohi S, Iqbal A, Sherazi TA, Zahoor AF, Imran M. Ciprofloxacin: from infection therapy to molecular imaging. Molecular biology reports. 2018;45(5):1457-1468.

[12] Verbruggen A, Nosco D, Nerom C, Bormans G, Adriaens P, Roo M. Technetium 99m L,L ethylenedicysteine: A renal imaging agent. I. Labeling and evaluation in animals. Journal of nuclear medicine : official publication, Society of Nuclear Medicine. 1992;33:551-557.

[13] Alberto R, Abram U. 99mTc: Labeling Chemistry and Labeled Compounds. In: Vértes A, Nagy S, Klencsár Z, Lovas RG, Rösch F, editors. Handbook of Nuclear Chemistry. Boston, MA: Springer US; 2011. p. 2073-2120.

[14] Rathmann S, Ahmad Z, Slikboer S, Bilton H, Snider D, Valliant J. The Radiopharmaceutical Chemistry of Technetium-99m. 2019. p. 311-333.

[15] Neves M, Fausto R. Computational chemistry and metal-based radiopharmaceuticals. International Atomic Energy Agency (IAEA): 1998 1011-4289 Contract No.: IAEA-TECDOC--1029.

[16] CASTELLINO, R.A., DELAPAZ, R.L., LARSON, S.M., "Imaging techniques in cancer", Cancer: Principles & Practice of Oncology (DeVITA, V:T:, Jr., HELLMAN, S:, ROSENBERG, S.A., Eds.), J.B. Lippincott Co., Philadelphia (1993) 507-531.

[17] LIOTTA, L.A., STETLER-STEVENSON, W.G., "Principles of

molecular cell biology of cancer: cancer metastases", Cancer: Principles & Practice of Oncology (DeVITA, V:T:, Jr., HELLMAN, S:, ROSENBERG, S.A., Eds.), J.B. Lippincott Co., Philadeplphia (1993) 134-149

[18] KARESH, S.M., "Principles of radiopharmacy", Nuclear Medicine (HENKIN, R.E., BOLES, M.A., DILLEHAY, G.L, HALAMA, J.R., KARESH, S.M., WAGNER, R.H., ZIMMER, A.M., Eds.), Mosby, St. Louis (1996) 334-349.

[19] BISCHOF DELALOYE, A., DELALOYE, B., Radiolabeled monoclonal antibodies in tumour imaging and therapy: out of fashion?, Eur. J. Nucl. Med. 22 (1995) 571-580

[20] MEREDITH, R.F., BUCHSBAUM, D.J., "Radioimmunotherapy of solid tumors", Nuclear Medicine (HENKIN, R.E., BOLES, M.A., DILLEHAY, G.L., HALAMA, J.R., KARESH, S.M., WAGNER, R.H., ZIMMER, A.M., Eds.), Mosby, St. Louis (1996) 601-608

[21] A new, semi-automated system for the micro-scale synthesis of 195mPt-cisplatin suitable for clinical studies. Deepak Anand and Walter Wolf, Appl. Radn. Isotop., 43, 809-814, 1992.

[22] M.H. Hanigan, H.F. Frierson, J.E. Brown, M.A. Lovell, and P.T. Taylor. Human ovarian tumors express gamma-glutamyl transpeptidase. Cancer Res. 54:286-290 (1994). The Effect of Anesthesia on the Biodistribution of Drugs in Rats: a Carboplatin Study.

[23] Alfredo R. Sancho, James A. Dowell and Walter Wolf. Cancer Chemotherapy and Pharmacology, 40: 521-525, 1997.

[24] R.J. Gillies, Z. Liu, and Z. Bhujwalla. 3IP-MRS measurements of extracellular pH of tumors using 3-aminopropylphosphonate. Am. J. Physiol. 267:C 195-C 203 (1994).

[25] PAL, N., YOJANA, S., KADWAD, V.B, JYOTSNA, N., SIVAPRASAD, N., Development of IRMA for human prolactin using antibody coated magnetisable cellulose, Ind. J. NucL Med., 10 (1995) 211.

[26] JYOTSNA, N., VUAY, K, SIVAPRASAD, N., NIRMALA,V., PAL, N., YOJANA, S., KARIR,T., VRINDA, C, SHALAKA, P. Evaluation of some magnetizable immunosorbents in Radioimmunoassays and immunoradiometeric assays of hormones. IAEA-TECDOC-914, (1996) 69-77. 357

[27] JYOTSNA, N., SHALAKA, N.P., VRINDA, P.C., SIVAPRASAD, N., Development of hFSH IRMA based on antibody coupled magnetisable cellulose, in Proc. Of XXIQ Annual Conference of the Association of Clinical Biochemists of India, (1996) 9

[28] Sufi, S.B., Micallef, R., Ahsan, W., Charoensiriwatana, W., Diaz-Sanchez, V.,Gonzalez-Suarez, R., Quiroga, S., Goncharov, N.P. (1992) Developments in Radioimmunoassay andrelatedpixxedures IAEA (Vienna) pp 167-176

[29] Zaheer, F., Mahmood, S., Akram, M., Shadid, M.A. (1992) Developments in Radioimmunoassay andrelatedprocedures'IAEA (Vienna) pp 187 - 196

[30] AKMAN, S., LEVENT, KL, TURKER, K. An Enzymeimmunoassay for total Thyroxine using avidin-biotin separation system and Thyroxine-Peroxidase conjugate. J.Immunoassay.,16 (1995) 325-341.

[31] Bartolini, P. (1992) Developments in Radioimmunoassay and related procedures IAEA (Vienna) pp 159-166

[32] Special Evaluation Review (1995) IAEA-SER-95/04 (Vienna)

[33] Edwards R. (1992) Applications of isotopes and radiation in conservation of the environment IAEA (Vienna)

[34] WILSON, C.B., SNOOK, D.E., DHOKIA, B., et al., Quantitative measurement of monoclonal antibody distribution and blood flow using positron emission tomography and 124lodine in patients with breast cancer. Int. J. Cancer 4 7 (1991) 344-347.

[35] FLOWER, M.A., AL-SAADI, A., HARMER, C.L., et al., Dose-response study on thyrotoxic patients undergoing positron emission tomography and radioiodine therapy. Eur. J. Nucl. Med. 2 1 (1994) 531-536.

[36] ROELCKE, U., BLASBERG, R., MISSIMER, J., et al., 1-124 lodode-oxyuridine (lUdR) retention in peritumoral edema of glioblastomas. J. Neuro-Oncol. 3 5 Suppl. 1 (1997) S38. (Abstract).

[37] STEPANEK, J., LARSSON, B., WEINREICH, R., Auger-electron spectra of radionuclides for therapy and diagnostics. Acta Oncol. 3 5 (1996) 863-868.

[38] SHEN RONGSEN, WANG RENZHI, XING RUIYUN, et al., Magnetic microparticle antibodies and their application to RIAs, J. Radioanal. Nucl. Chem., 206,2(1996)205-218.

[39] SHEN RONGSEN, SHEN DECUN, et al., Preparation and supply of magnetic particles for RIA and IRMA of hormones, Final Report of IAEA Technical Contract No. 8955/DPA, from 1996-02 - 1 5 to 1997-02-14 , Vienna, Austria, March 1997.

[40] Products Information, Paesel + Lorei GmbH & Co., P. O. Box 630347, 60353 Frankfurt/M, Germany, 1994.

[41] SHEN RONGSEN, LUO QINGLIANG, YU SHUI, et al., An external standard method for quantification of human cytomegalovirus by PCR using magnetic particle separation technique, Progress Report of IAEA Research Contract No. 8178/R2/RB, from 1996-11 - 01 to 1997-10 - 31, Vienna, Austria, November 1997.

[42] Stoecklin, G., V. Pike, V. (Eds.), "Radiopharmaceuticals for Positron Emission Tomography - Methodological Aspects", (1993), Kluwer Academic Publishers, Dordrecht, 178 pp.

[43] Mather, S. J., (Ed), "Current Directions in Radiopharmaceutical Research and Development", (1996), Kluwer Academic Publishers, Dordrecht, 237 pp.

[44] Lambrecht, R. M., "Biological Models in Radiopharmaceutical Development" (1996), Kluwer Academic Publishers, Dordrecht, 270 pp.

[45] Pagani, M., Stone-Elander, S., Larsson, S. A., "Alternative positron emission tomography with non-conventional positron emitters: effects of their physical properties on image quality and potential clinical applications", (1997), Eur. J. Nucl. Med. 24:1301-1327.

[46] Rosenberg, S. A., Aebersold, P., Cornetta, K.; Kasid, A., Morgan, R. A., Moen, R., Karson, E. M., Lotze, M. T., Yang, J. C, Topalian, S. L., Merino, M. J., Culver, J., Miller, M., Blase, R. M., and Anderson, W. F., " Gene transfer into humans - immunotherapy of patients with advanced melanoma using tumour-inflitrating lymphocytes modified by retroviral gene transduction". New England J. Med. (1990)323:570-578

[47] Larson S. M., Tjuvajev, J., and Blasberg, R. "Triumph over mischance; A role for nuclear medicine in gene therapy", (1997) J. Nucl. Med. 38: 1230-1233.

[48] Herschman, R., Sharfstein, S., Gambir, S. S., MaClaren, D., Cherry, S.,

Srinfasan, A., Satyamurthy, N., Barrio, J. R., and Phelps, M. E., "In vivo imaging of gene expression associated with cell replication", (1997), J. Nucl. Med. 38: 250P.

[49] Tjuvajev, J. G., Avril, N., Safer, M., Joshi, R., Oku, T., Sasajima, T., Miyagawa, T., Beattie, B., Daghigan, F., Augenson, F., Di Resta, G., J. Koutcher. J., Sweit, J., Finn, R., Larson, S. and Blasberg, R., "Quantitative PET imaging of HSKl-tk gene expression with 124I-FIAU" (1997), J. Nucl. Med. 38: 239P.

[50] Staehler, P., Spiegel, M., Wybranietz, W., Schenk, A., Gross, C, Oberdorfer, F., Gregor, M., Lauer, U., and Lambrecht, R. M. "Pilot study of a positron emitting radiopharmaceutical for in vivo monitoring of gene transfer therapy", Fortuene Colloquium, University of Tuebingen, October (1997).

[51] Bitzer, M., Lauer, U., Baumann, C, Spiegel, M., Gregor, M., and Neubert, W. J., "Sendai virus efficiently infects cellls via the asialoglycoprotein-receptor and requires the presence of cleaved FO precursor proteins for this alternative route of cell entry". J Virology (1997) 71: 5481-5486.

[52] Giovacchini G, Giovannini E, Riondato M, Ciarmiello A. Radiopharmaceuticals for the Diagnosis and Therapy of Neuroendocrine Differentiated Prostate Cancer. Curr Radiopharm. 2017;10(1):6-15

[53] Morin, K.W., Atrazheva, E.D., Knaus, E.E. and Wiebe, L.I. Synthesis and cellular uptake of 2′-substituted analogues of (E)-5-(2-[13H]iodovinyl)-2′-deoxyuridine in tumor cells transduced with the herpes simplex type-1 thymidine kinase gene: evaluation as probes for monitoring gene therapy. J. Med. Chem. 140, 2184-2190 (1997).

[54] Giovacchini G, Giovannini E, Riondato M, Ciarmiello A. Radiopharmaceuticals for the Diagnosis and Therapy of Neuroendocrine Differentiated Prostate Cancer. Curr Radiopharm. 2017;10(1):6-15

[55] Morin, K.W., Atrazheva, E.D., Knaus, E.E. and Wiebe, L.I. Synthesis and cellular uptake of 2'-substituted analogues of (E)-5-(2-[13H]iodovinyl)-2'-deoxyuridine in tumor cells transduced with the herpes simplex type-1 thymidine kinase gene: evaluation as probes for monitoring gene therapy. J. Med. Chem. 140, 2184-2190 (1997).

[56] Benefits of certification for pharmacy specialists. J.P. McArtor and K.L. Rascati, J. Am. Pharm. Assoc. NS36(2): 128-34, 1996

Chapter 2

Start Here When Performing Radiochemical Reactions

Carla Daruich de Souza, Jin Joo Kim and Jin Tae Hong

Abstract

Radiation products are present in several fields of knowledge. From the energy field, with nuclear reactors and nuclear batteries, to the medical field, with nuclear medicine and radiation therapy (brachytherapy). Although chemistry works in the same way for radioactive and non-radioactive chemicals, an extra layer of problems is present in the radiochemical counter-part. Reactions can be unpredictable due to several factors. For example, iodine-125 in deposited in a silver wire to create the core of a medical radioactive seed. This core is the sealed forming a radioactive seed that are placed inside the cancer. Several aspects can be discussed in regards to radiation chemistry. For example: are there any competing ions? Each way my reaction is going? Each reaction is more likely to occur? Those are important questions, because, in the case of iodine, a volatile product can be formed causing contamination of laboratory, equipment, personal, and environment. This chapter attempts to create a guideline on how to safely proceed when a new radioactive chemical reaction. It discusses the steps by giving practical examples. The focus is in protecting the operator and the environment. The result can be achieved safely and be reliable contribution to science and society.

Keywords: Radiation chemistry, radioactive material manipulation, radiation sources fabrication

1. Introduction

Radiation products are present in several fields of knowledge. From the energy field, with nuclear reactors and nuclear batteries, to the medical field, with nuclear medicine and radiation therapy.

Although chemistry works in the same way for radioactive and non-radioactive chemicals, an extra layer of problems is present in the radiochemical counter-part. Reactions can be unpredictable due to several factors.

According with Neeb, radiation chemistry is a branch of chemistry, but is possible to identify in its context characteristics of an autonomous discipline. Usually, the incredibly high radiation solutions can be manufactured that actually correspond to a low concentration of chemicals. An example is several fission products with extremely high radioactivity with an actual concentration of 10^{-9} mol/L measured in nuclear spend fuel. With so small masses, is possible that expected reaction simply will not occur and a more "secondary" reaction becomes primary [1, 2].

This chapter attempts to create a guideline on how to safely proceed when a new radioactive chemical reaction is being investigated. It discusses the steps by giving practical examples.

2. Why is harder to predict radioactive chemical reactants

To answer the question, the manufacturing route for radioisotopes must be explained. Isotopes can basically be manufactured in 3 different ways (**Figure 1**).

In **Figure 1**, presented in pink, is the nuclear activation form. A thorough study of irradiation must be performed followed by purification essays. An example for promethium-147, used in pacemaker nuclear batteries, by Broderick et al. [3] is shown. Presented in green in the natural decay mode. Radioisotopes are obtained by purification of decay products or concentrated from natural radioactive isotopes. Examples are the Marie and Pierre Curie work in discovering Polonium and Radium and the Uranium-235 enrichment process. In yellow, the spent nuclear fuel reprocessing route is presented. If the isotope is a by-product of fission, then it can be recovered from the nuclear fuel that has already been used. Many isotopes are only found/fabricated through reprocessing. This process is known to be the most dangerous chemical process invented in human history [12]. The chemical process is relatively simple, but the byproducts are sometimes instable, highly radioactive, long lasting, even being able to reach criticality (nuclear chain reaction) [18]. For example, strontium-90 used in nuclear medicine and in nuclear batteries and plutonium-238 used in most RTG (Radioisotope Thermoelectric Generator) are

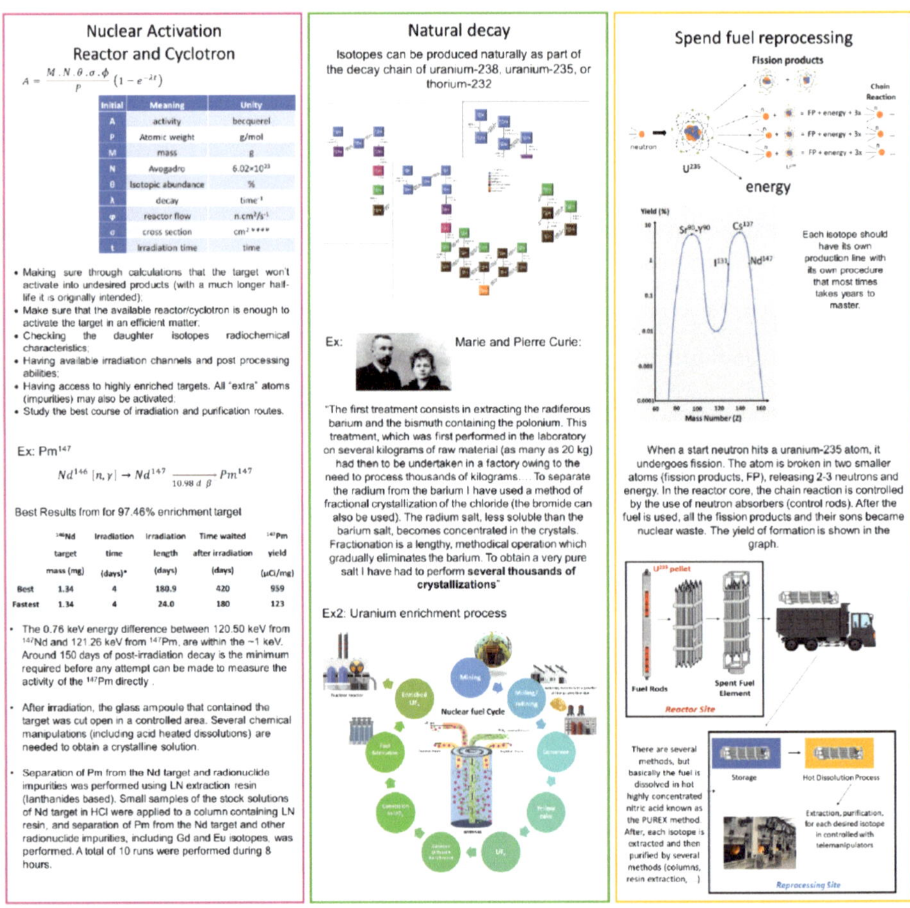

Figure 1.

Modes of radioisotope production: Nuclear activation [3, 4], natural decay [5–11] and spend fuel reprocessing [12–17].

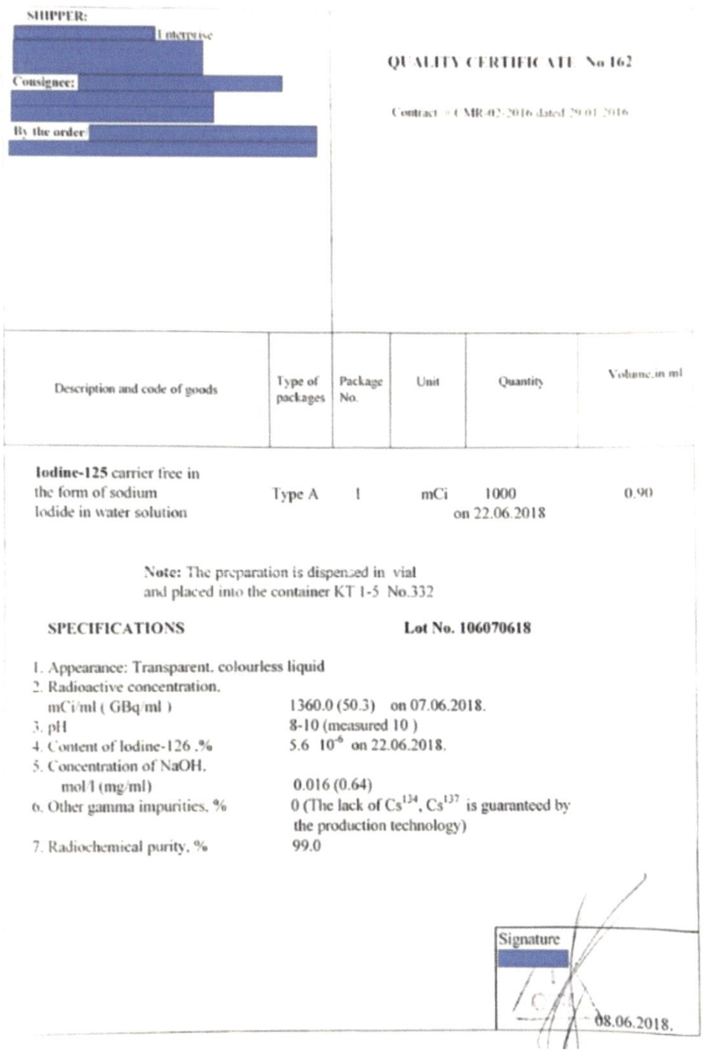

SHIPPER:
[redacted]
Consignee: [redacted]
By the order [redacted]

QUALITY CERTIFICATE No 162

Contract № CMR-02-2016 dated 29.01.2016

Description and code of goods	Type of packages	Package No.	Unit	Quantity	Volume, in ml
Iodine-125 carrier free in the form of sodium Iodide in water solution	Type A	1	mCi	1000 on 22.06.2018	0.90

Note: The preparation is dispensed in vial and placed into the container KT 1-5 No.332

SPECIFICATIONS **Lot No. 106070618**

1. Appearance: Transparent, colourless liquid	
2. Radioactive concentration, mCi/ml (GBq/ml)	1360.0 (50.3) on 07.06.2018.
3. pH	8-10 (measured 10)
4. Content of Iodine-126 ,%	5.6 10^{-6} on 22.06.2018.
5. Concentration of NaOH, mol/l (mg/ml)	0.016 (0.64)
6. Other gamma impurities, %	0 (The lack of Cs^{134}, Cs^{137} is guaranteed by the production technology)
7. Radiochemical purity, %	99.0

Signature
[redacted]
08.06.2018.

Figure 2.
Iodine-125 fact sheet.

produced by reprocessing. Besides that, many stable fission products are high cost and in high demand elements such as rubidium, palladium, and ruthenium.

Performing chemical analysis that would allow to identify contaminant most of the times are impossible. Isotopes with high half-life, may contaminate and permanently disable equipments. For example, Tritium, used in nuclear batteries, have 12.32-year half-life. It means that in 12.32 years the Tritium mass will emits half of its radioactive material. If an equipment such as an EDS would be used, even supposing that one half-life would yield background level radioactivity, the equipment would be contaminated and unusable for 12 years! In large productions centers, each isotope has its own production line containing exclusive equipment for analysis.

Besides that, a radiochemical fact sheet contains very little information. **Figure 2** shows an example of iodine-125, used in radiation therapy.

The issue of not having more information arises when the following comparison is done. For example, in a thyroid cancer treatment with iodine-131, the activity of 5.55–7.40 GBq (150–200 mCi) is administered. Converting:

$$\lambda = \frac{\ln 2}{T_{\frac{1}{2}}} = \frac{\ln 2}{8.02d\ x\ 24h\ x\ 3600} = 10^{-6}s^{-1} \quad (1)$$

$$A = \lambda.N \rightarrow N = \frac{A}{\lambda} = \frac{7.40\ x\ 10^9}{10^{-6}} = 7.40\ x\ 10^{15} atoms \quad (2)$$

$$mass_{sample}(g) = \frac{MW\ x\ N}{N_a} = \frac{131\ x\ 7.40\ x\ 10^{15}}{6.02\ x\ 10^{23}} = 1.61.10^{-6}g \quad (3)$$

were: $T_{\frac{1}{2}}$ = Half-life (s), A = Activity in Bq (decays/second), λ = decay constant (s^{-1}), MW = atomic mass, N_a = Avogadro Number ≈ 6.02 x 1023.

The small mass calculated indicate that great chemical purity must exist in the entire course of a methodology/product development. For example, 1% impurity in 1 g of solution results in 0.01 g, an amount that is probably much greater than the total radioactive iodine. If the manufacturer changes significantly, for example, purification steps, new contaminants might be introduced and old expected results might not be achievable.

Ultimately, the best way to achieve the best results in radiation chemistry is to understand how reactions take place, and to recognize the various factors that influence their course.

3. Chemistry background

It is helpful to identify some general features of a reaction and then study the related topics. Some of the most important of these are [19]:

- Energetics: The potential energy of a reacting system changes as the reaction progresses. The reaction might release energy (exothermic) or need energy to occur (endothermic), plus the activation energy requirement. Always the reaction that needs less energy to occur will have preference;

- Electronic Effects: The distribution of electrons at the reaction sites is a particularly important factor. Electron deficient species or groups (electrophiles), which may or may not be positively charged, are attracted to electron rich species or groups (nucleophiles), which may or may not be negatively charged. The charge distribution in a molecule is usually discussed with respect to two interacting effects. The first is an inductive effect, that relates to electronegativity differences that exist between atoms (and groups). The second is a resonance effect, in which electrons move in a discontinuous fashion between parts of a molecule.

- Steric Effects: Atoms occupy space. When they are crowded together, van der Waals repulsions produce an unfavorable steric hindrance. Steric effects are nonbonding interactions that influence the shape (conformation) and reactivity of ions and molecules (destabilization of transition states) may be influenced by steric hindrance (the slowing of chemical reactions due to steric bulk).

- Stereoelectronic Effects: In many reactions atomic or molecular orbitals interact in a manner that has an optimal configurational or geometrical alignment. Departure from this alignment inhibits the reaction. It explains a particular molecular property or reactivity by invoking stabilizing or destabilizing interactions that depend on the relative orientations of electrons (bonding or non-bonding) in space.

- Solvent Effects: Most reactions are conducted in solution, not in a gaseous state. The solvent selected for a given reaction may exert a strong influence on its course. Remember, solvents are chemicals, and most undergo chemical reaction under the right conditions.

Next, the basic concepts will be explained with radiochemistry examples.

3.1 Reactivity

Reactivity is a concept used for many things in chemistry [20, 21]. In this paper, the focus will be if a determined reaction can occur or not, or if a "secondary" reaction can take place instead of the expected one.

Reactivity encompasses both thermodynamic factors and kinetic factors. For example, it is commonly stated that the reactivity of alkali metals (group one metals) (Na, K, etc.) increases down the group in the periodic table [20, 21]. The behavior is shown in the periodic table in **Figure 3**.

Reactivity is related to the rate at which a chemical substance tends to undergo a chemical reaction in time. In pure compounds, reactivity is regulated by the physical properties of the sample. For instance, grinding a sample to a higher specific surface area increases its reactivity. In impure compounds, the reactivity is affected by the inclusion of contaminants [22].

In double-replacement reaction (most common in the fabrication of medical radioactive sources), if one of the products isn't aqueous, by rule of thumb the reaction is possible [22].

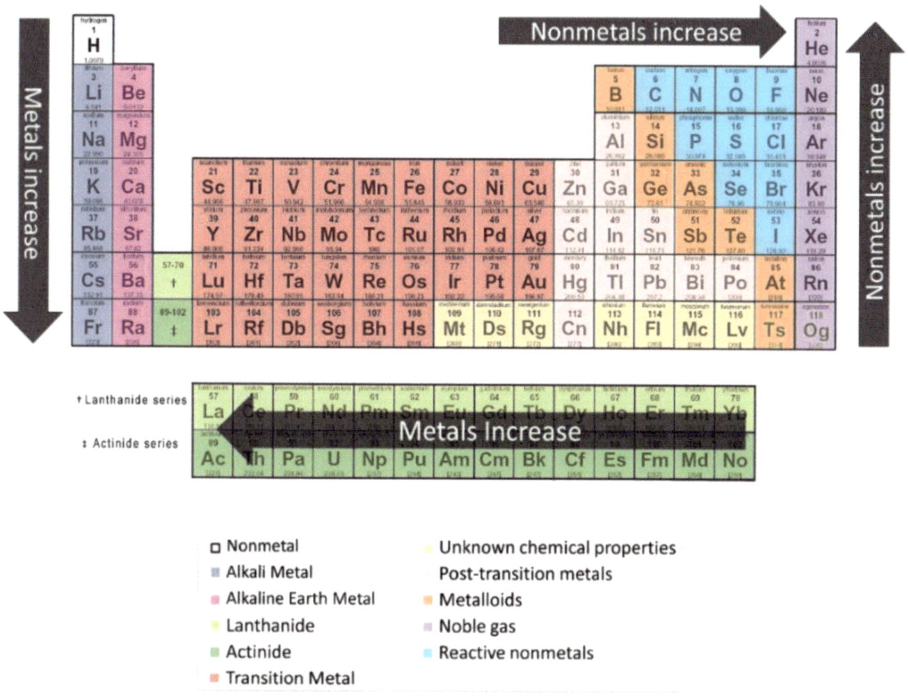

Figure 3.
Reactivity shown in the periodic table.

$$AB + CD \rightarrow AD + CB \quad (4)$$

In this reaction, A and C are positively-charged cations, while B and D are negatively-charged anions. Double-replacement reactions generally occur between substances in aqueous solution. In order for a reaction to occur, one of the products is usually a solid precipitate, a gas, or a molecular compound such as water [19].

For example, the 1982 patent (US Pat. n. 4.323.055), filed by the Minnesota Mining and Manufacturing Company [23], describes a method of impregnating Ag rods with iodine-125, forming the core of a brachytherapy seed. The silver rods previously reacted to for a layer of silver nitrate. That modified rod reacted with the radioactive NaI^{125} solution. The reaction will be:

$$AgNO_3 + NaI^{125} \rightarrow AgI^{125} + NaNO_3 \quad (5)$$

Accordingly with **Table 1** (explained ahead):

$$AgNO_{3\,(aq)} + NaI^{125}{}_{(aq)} \rightarrow AgI^{125}{}_{(s)} + NaNO_{3(aq)} \quad (6)$$

Because there is a solid product, theoretically the reaction will occur.

For example, if the silver rod wasn't pure silver and had contained potassium in high proportions, KI^{125} will form more favorably than AgI^{125} because potassium is more reactive than sodium.

3.2 Electronegativity

Electronegativity is a measure of the tendency of an atom to attract a bonding pair of electrons. Large electronegativity values indicate a stronger attraction for electrons than small values. Electronegativities increase from left to right across the periodic table (**Figure 4**). Elements on the left of the periodic table have low electronegativities and are frequently called electropositive elements [24].

If an atom B is more electron negative than A, the electron pair is dragged right over to B's end of the bond (Eq. (7)). A has lost control of its electron, and B has

Ions that form soluble compounds	Exceptions	Ions that form soluble compounds	Exceptions
Group 1 ions (Li^+, Na^+, K^+, ...)	—	Carbonate (CO_3^{2-})	When combined with group 1 ions or ammonium (NH_4^+)
Ammonium (NH_4^+)	—	Chromate (CrO_4^{2-})	When combined with group 1 ions, Ca^{2+}, Mg2+, or ammonium (NH_4^+)
Nitrate (NO_3^-)	—	Phosphate (PO_4^{3-})	When combined with group 1 ions or ammonium (NH_4^+)
Acetate ($C_2H_3O_2^-$ or CH_3COO^-)	—	Sulfide (S^{2-})	When combined with group 1 ions or ammonium (NH_4^+)
Hydrogen Carbonate (HCO_3^-)	—	Hydroxide (OH^-)	When combined with group 1 ions, Ca^{2+}, Ba^{2+}, Sr^{2+} or ammonium (NH_4^+)
Chlorate (ClO_3^-)	—	Sulfates (SO_4^{2-})	When combined with Ag^+, Ca^{2+}, Sr^{2+}, Ba^{2+}, and Pb^{2+}
Perchlorate (ClO_4^-)	—	Halides (Cl^-, Br^-, I^-)	When combined with Ag^+, Pb^{2+}, and Hg_2^{2+}

Table 1.
Solubility guidelines for Aqueous Solutions.

DOI: http://dx.doi.org/10.5772/intechopen.98766

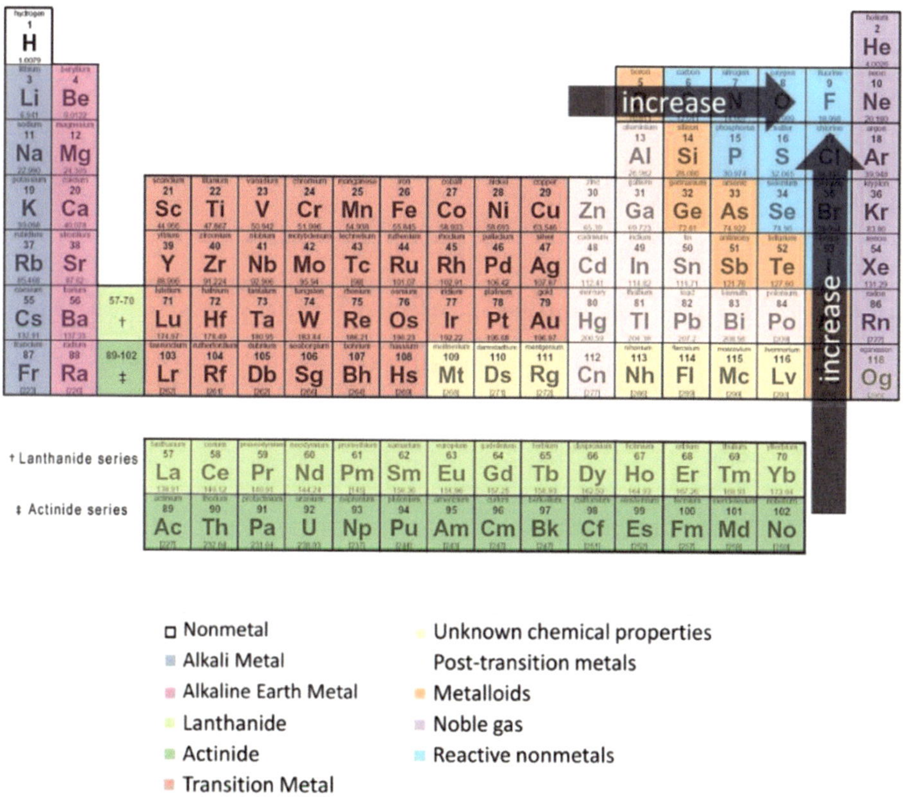

Figure 4.
Electronegativity shown in the periodic table.

complete control over both electrons, forming an ion pair [25]. Electronegativity series follow **Figure 4**.

$$A^{+}\overset{\circ}{\underset{\circ}{-}}B^{+} \tag{7}$$

When a situation with two possible outcomes is present, it is interesting to evaluate electronegativity. For example, the paper by Lee et al. [26] mixes pre-treated silver rods with iodine-125, forming the core of a brachytherapy seed. Usually the radioactive iodine-125 solution is in the form of NaI^{125}. Let's suppose that there is excess of Cl^{-} as a contaminant in the mixture. **Figure 5** explain the possible outcome.

3.3 Gibbs free energy

In chemistry, a spontaneous process is one that occurs without the addition of external energy. A spontaneous process may take place rapidly or slowly, because spontaneity is not related to kinetics or reaction rate. According to the second law of thermodynamics, any spontaneous process must increase the entropy in the universe [27, 28]. This can be expressed mathematically as follows:

$$\Delta S_{universe} = \Delta S_{system} + \Delta S_{surroundings} > 0 \tag{8}$$

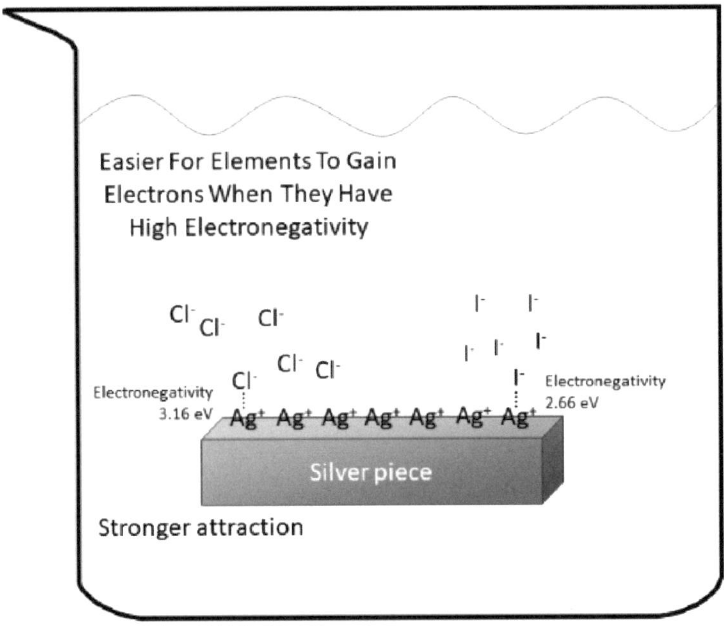

Figure 5.
Scheme of what happens when two anions, Cl^- and I^-, with two different electronegativities compete for the same cation, Ag^+. AgCl will form in a higher rate than AgI. Since silver iodide is the desired product, the reaction yield is impaired.

Measuring the entropy change in the universe is not practical and the real interest is to observe the desired system (chemical reaction). When a process occurs at constant temperature T and pressure P, the second law of thermodynamics can be rearranged and define a new quantity known as Gibbs free energy (**Figure 6**). In other words, Gibbs free energy is a thermodynamic potential used to calculate the maximum reversible work that may be performed by a thermodynamic system at a constant temperature and pressure. The Gibbs energy, G, represents also the thermodynamic potential that is minimized when a system reaches chemical equilibrium [27, 28].

The Gibbs free energy of a system at any moment in time is defined as the enthalpy of the system minus the product of the temperature times the entropy of the system [27, 28].

$$\textit{Gibbs free energy} \rightarrow G = H - TS \tag{9}$$

The change in the Gibbs free energy of the system that occurs during a chemical reaction is therefore equal to:

$$\Delta G = \Delta H - \Delta(TS) \tag{10}$$

If temperature is constant:

$$\Delta G = \Delta H - T\Delta S \tag{11}$$

The change in the free energy of a system that occurs during a reaction can be measured under any set of conditions. If the data are collected under standard conditions, the result is the standard-state free energy of reaction (ΔG^o) [27, 28].

$$\Delta G^0 = \Delta H^0 - T\Delta S^0 \tag{12}$$

- Favorable or spontaneous reactions: $\Delta G^0 < 0$
- Unfavorable or non-spontaneous reactions: $\Delta G^0 > 0$
- equilibrium: $\Delta G^0 = 0$
- exothermic reactions: $\Delta H < 0$
- endothermic reactions: $\Delta H > 0$
- Favorable or spontaneous reactions: $\Delta H^0 < 0, \Delta S^0 > 0$
- Unfavorable or non-spontaneous reactions: $\Delta H^0 > 0, \Delta S^0 < 0$
- Unfavorable or non-spontaneous reactions at low temperatures: $\Delta H^0 < 0, \Delta S^0 < 0$
- Favorable, or spontaneous reactions at high temperatures: $\Delta H^0 > 0, \Delta S^0 > 0$

Reference [30] has a 25-page list of Gibbs Free Energy values.

Continuing to use the paper by Lee et al. [26] as an example, one of the methods is to pre-coat the silver rod with PO_4^{-3} forming Ag_3PO_4 following:

$$Ag_3PO_{4\,(s)} + 3NaI^{125}{}_{(aq)} \rightarrow 3AgI^{125}{}_{(s)} + Na_3PO_{4(s)} \tag{13}$$

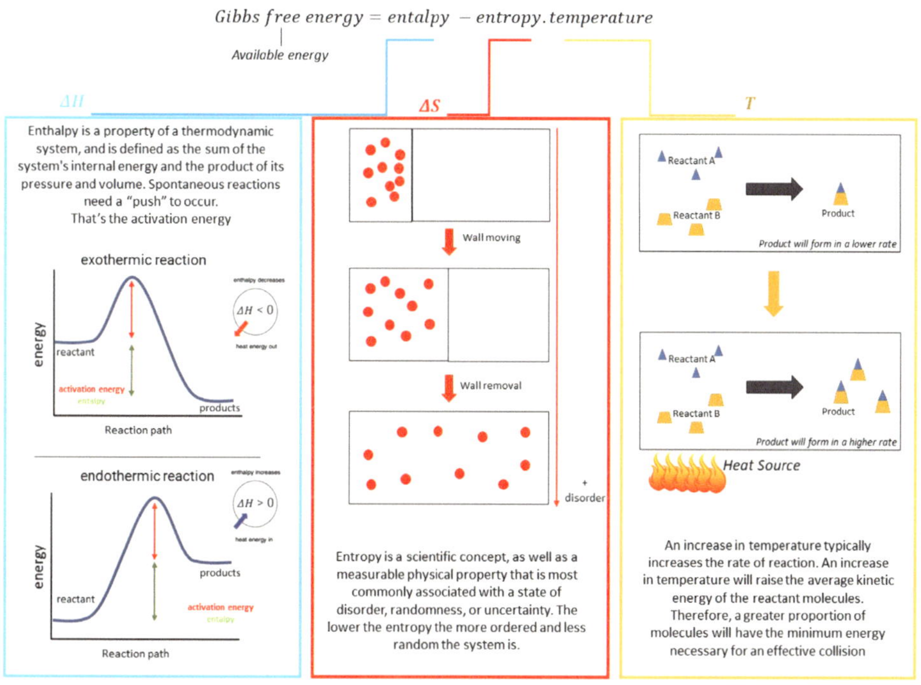

Figure 6.
*Explanation of the Gibbs Free Energy equation indexes. *activation energy is the minimum amount of energy that must be provided to compounds to result in a chemical reaction [27–29].*

Gibbs free energy for the equation is:

$Ag_3PO_{4\,(s)}$	+	$3NaI^{125}{}_{(aq)}$	→	$3AgI^{125}{}_{(s)}$	+	$Na_3PO_{4(s)}$
Reactants				Products		
$\Delta G^0 Ag_3PO_4$		3 x $\Delta G^0 NaI^{125}$		3 x $\Delta G^0 AgI^{125}$		$\Delta G^0\ Na_3PO_{4(s)}$
87 kJ/mol		3 x(−284.512) kJ/mol		3 x (−66.19) kJ/mol		−1819 kJ/mol
−766.536 kJ/mol				−2017.57 kJ/mol		

$$\boldsymbol{\Delta G^0} = \boldsymbol{\Delta G^0}_{\boldsymbol{products}} - \boldsymbol{\Delta G^0}_{\textbf{reactants}} \tag{14}$$

$\boldsymbol{\Delta G^0}$ = -2017.57+ 766.536 = −1251.034 kJ/mol.

$\boldsymbol{\Delta G^0} < 0$ = Favorable, or spontaneous reactions.

To correlate between 2 reactions, it is more practical to investigate activation energy. A reaction with lower activation energy will be preferable, thus preferable to occur. **Figure** 7 explains it.

For example, for the AgI^{125} source fabrication, ions such as Cl^- and Br^- might be present. Activation energies are for AgBr 0.34 eV, AgI 0.48 eV, and 0.53 eV for AgCl. In a reaction when Br- and I- are present, is more likely that AgBr will form more easily than AgI. And, in a reaction when Cl^- and I^- are present, is more likely that AgI^{125} will form more easily than AgCl. This contradicts the previous electronegativity statement. All of these influences are occurring at the same time, possibly influencing the final result [31–33].

3.4 Solubility

Solubility is the capability of a solid, liquid, or gaseous substance (named solute) to dissolve in solvent (usually a liquid) and form a solution. The solubility of a chemical is dependent on the solvent used, temperature, and pressure. Solubility does not depend on particle size (even large particles will eventually dissolve given enough time). It is measured by the concentration of the saturated solution. A saturated solution is a solution that contains the maximum amount of solute that is capable of being dissolved. In other words, adding additional solute no longer

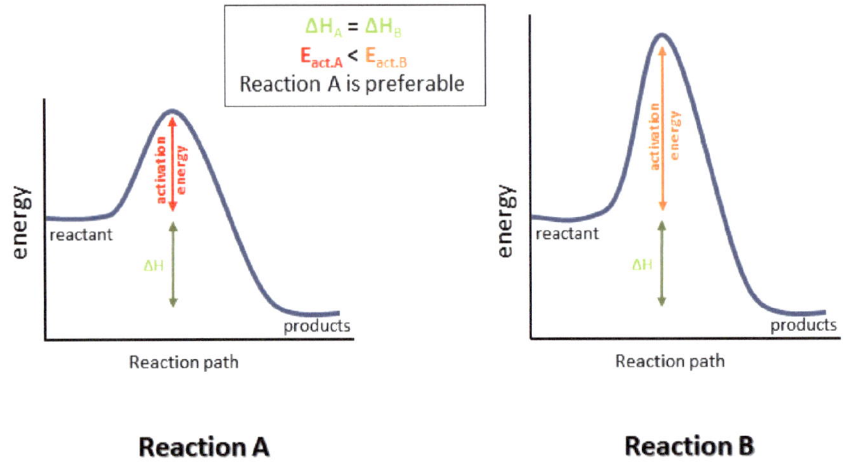

Figure 7.
Two reactions with different activation energies.

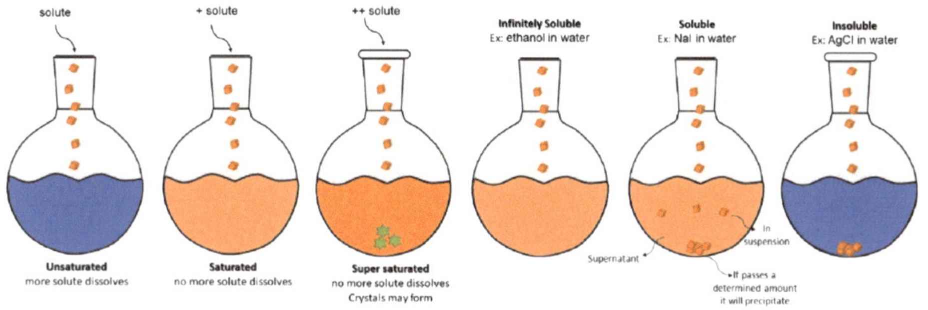

Figure 8.
Solubility. The degree of solubility ranges broadly depending on the substances, from infinitely soluble to poorly soluble (insoluble). Under certain conditions, the equilibrium solubility can be exceeded, yielding a supersaturated solution.

increases the concentration of the solution. **Figure 8** explains solubility classifications.

To evaluate a desired reaction, **Table 1** can be used [22].

Solubility is important because is directly impacts the amount of radioisotope available for the reaction. It may affect distribution in the radiation source resulting in dosimetry issues. For example, in Benega et al. [34] a phosphorus-32 radioactive source for spinal cancer treatment was developed by mixing the radioisotope with a catalyst solution. This solution is then added to an epoxy resin. Both solutions need to result in a homogenous product. This won't be achievable if the isotope doesn't properly mix with the catalyst solution (water based).

The solubility product constant, Ksp, is the equilibrium constant for a solid substance dissolving in an aqueous solution. It represents the level at which a solute dissolve in solution. Eq. (16) shows the correlation.

$$aA_{(s)} \leftrightarrow bB_{(aq)} + cC_{(aq)} \tag{15}$$

$$K_{sp} = [C]^c[D]^d \tag{16}$$

If two competing ions are present, solubility and quantity play an important role in each reaction will be preferable. For example, in the iodine-125 seed manufacture, NaOH is used in pH control. NaOH is soluble in water, resulting in ionic completion for the silver biding sites. It maybe would be better to use $Fe(OH)_3$ that is insoluble. For instance, let's use the information in **Figure 2**. Iodine-125 solution has 50.3 GBq/mL and pH 10 (pOH 4). Calculating the amount of OH- and I-:

OH^-

pOH = 4 = 10^4 mol/L
MW_{OH-} = 17 g/mol

For 1 mL
10^4 mol --------- 1000 mL
x --------- 1 mL
x= 10^1 mol/mL

17 g --------- 1 mol
y --------- 10^1 mol/mL
y= 170 g

170 g x $6.02x10^{23}$ atoms = $1,02x10^{26}\ OH^-\ ions$

I^-

50,3 GBq/mL

$$A = \lambda . N \Rightarrow A = \frac{\ln 2}{T_{\frac{1}{2}}} N$$

$$\Rightarrow 50.3x10^9 = \frac{\ln 2}{59.407x24x3600} N$$

$$\Rightarrow 3.724x10^{17}\ I^-\ atoms/mL$$

$2.7\ x10^8$ *more* OH^- *ions then* I^- *atoms*

3.5 Characteristic of the isotope and other problems (pH, reaction volume, vial type)

Characteristics of the isotope being used needs to be extensively investigated. Several problems may be present such as toxic decay atoms to a high possibility of contamination and volatilization. For example, Gold-198 used in colloid or nanoparticles for cancer treatment decays to the highly toxic mercury, demanding that a through toxicity study be done [35].

In another example, iodine salts and solutions are advised to be stored in dark bottles due to the fact that iodine reacts with light and undergo a photo decomposition reaction [36]. Even though performing a radioactive reaction in the absence of light is impractical, with this information the researcher can avoid light as much as possible.

In most cases, errors can be originated by unpredicted places. Eight different storage vials were tested by Kennedy et al. [37] in regards to its ability to contain iodine-131, used in thyroid cancer treatment, during 24 hours. Glass yielded the best results, with 10% loss and polyethylene the worse with >50% loss. He et al. [38] evaluate the iodine-125 activity intake on silver cores by varying the value of pH. They have found that the intake in the silver cores were higher at a low pH. The authors affirm that if pH is kept high, the $Na^{125}I$ solution will remain stable not releasing the $^{125}I^{-}$ for silver binding. Both of these issues were confirmed by Daruich de Souza et al. [39].

Isotopes are being replaced for others or adapted in different fields all the time. For example, cobalt-60 teletherapy machines were the first developed. In the 1950's they were widely used, by producing a beam of gamma rays which was directed into the patient's body to kill tumor tissue. Cobalt-60 is produced by neutron irradiation of ordinary cobalt metal in a nuclear reactor. It is a high energy gamma ray emitter, 1.17 and 1.33 MeV, with specific activity of 44 TBq/g (≈1100 Ci/g). Because of its longer half-life, 5.27 years, cobalt-60 was widely used in radiation therapy. Nevertheless, this half-life still requires sources to be replaced every 5 years. As technology advanced, these machines were replaced by linear accelerators, that doesn't contain radiation sources [40, 41]. In recent years, the technology was revised, now in a new machine called gamma knife, were cobalt-60 sources are mounted [42]. Applications for Gamma Knife surgery include the treatment of cerebral vascular malformations, head tumors, certain pain conditions such as trigeminal neuralgia, along with the treatment of some movement and psychiatric disorders [42].

4. Mock trials and radiation safety

4.1 How to set up mock trials

The steps to set up mock trials are in **Figure 9**.

The first step is to analyze all possible reactions accordingly with item 3 of this chapter. After that, the reaction set up is investigated. Three important observations are:

1. Avoid heating: heating makes molecules more reactive and can cause secondary reactions, for example, the formation of a volaille product.

2. Add traps: the more enclosed the set-up is, the better it will retain possible radiation leakage;

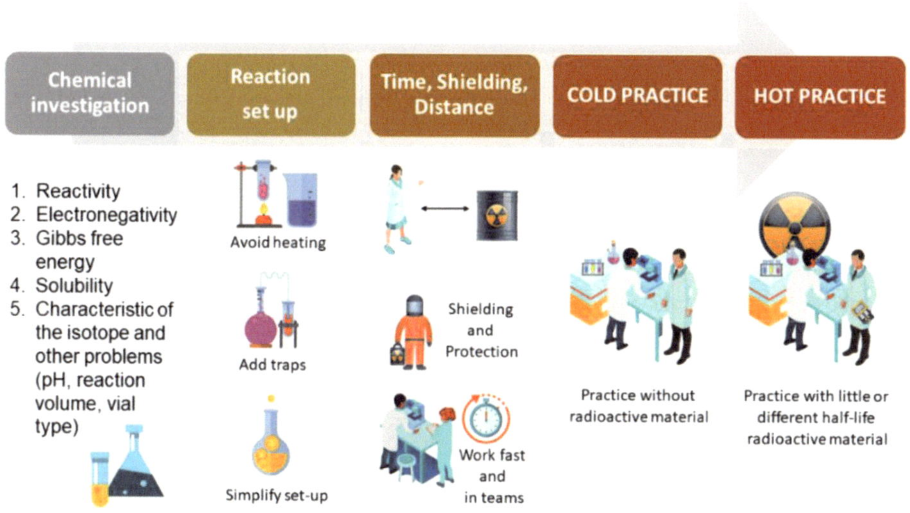

Figure 9.
Steps to set up mock trials [9, 43–45].

3. Simplify set-up: less material usage result in less radioactive waste.

The third step is to follow the 3 radiation principles: distance, shielding, and time.

1. Distance: A greater distance from the radiation source can reduce radiation exposure. The amount of radiation exposure is inversely proportional to the square of the distance. Using extension tweezers and moving away stock radioactive solutions will diminish radiation exposure;

2. Shielding: There are many shielding devices such as caps, lead glasses (**Figure 10**), thyroid protectors, aprons, even radiation reducing gloves. Shielding follows the attenuation rule being:

3. Radiation exposure can be accumulated over the time of exposure. The longer the exposure time, the more radiation exposure to the operator. For reducing laboratory time, the operator has to improve his skill by practicing thus acquiring more experience.

The fourth step is about setting up cold mock trials, meaning, the test of expected reaction and set-up with no radioactive material. Pay special attention to:

- optimizing results;
- simplifying set-ups;
- having easy access to necessary solutions;
- check for availability of all materials and equipment that will be use;
- having easy access to protective equipment;

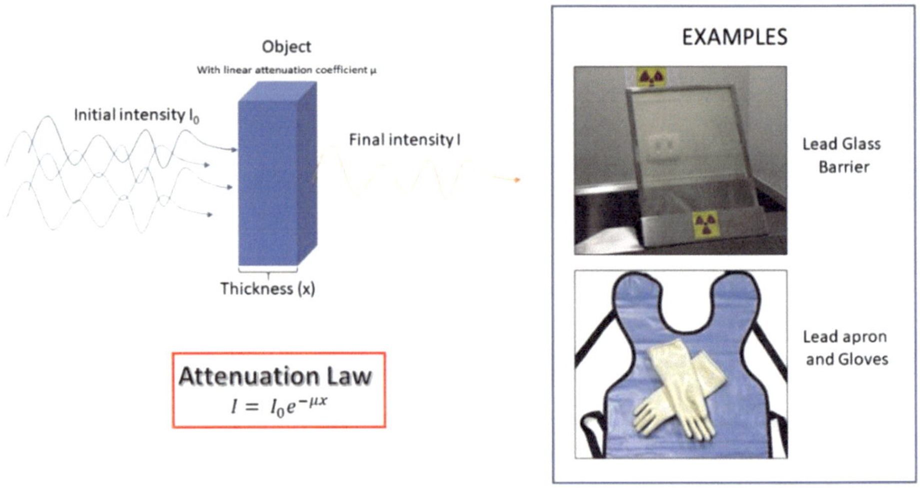

Figure 10.
Attenuation Law and examples of shielding materials (apron and gloves from [46]).

- installing protection were needed;
- make sure all detectors used in contamination assessment are working properly;
- perform the reaction several times to gain speed and experience;
- determined individuals' tasks: person that will perform the experiment, radiation protection team member that will give support, and person that will write in the lab book during the experiment. Make certain that a support person that can take over in case of an emergency are informed of the experiments schedule;
- use multiple pairs of gloves and change them numerous times during experiment to diminish radiation contamination on the experiment location;
- verify that exhaustion in the experiment location is working properly;
- and select the place that radioactive waste will go.

In Daruich de Souza PhD thesis [2] the set-up in **Figure 11** was used to handle iodine-125.

In Silva et al. [47] the cold fabrication of a phosphorous-32 radioactive source to be used in CNS cancer using epoxy resin was described. MCNP simulation was used to evaluate the radiation dose. Special attention was given to factors that can impact dose distribution such as source thickness and thickness variance. Two molds, Teflon and Silicon were used. The epoxy plaque fabricated with Teflon mold presented better agreement. MCNP for this plaque resulted in an average dose of 8.54 ± 0.01% cGy/s. It was also found that, differences of less than 0.01 cm in thickness within the plaque lead to alterations of up to 25% in the dose rate. This work now set up the foundation to the hot tests.

It is also possible to access possible yields by using different equipment and procedure. In Uhm et al. [48] a nickel-63 betavoltaic battery using a three-dimensional single trenched p-n transduction was designed. The optimum thickness

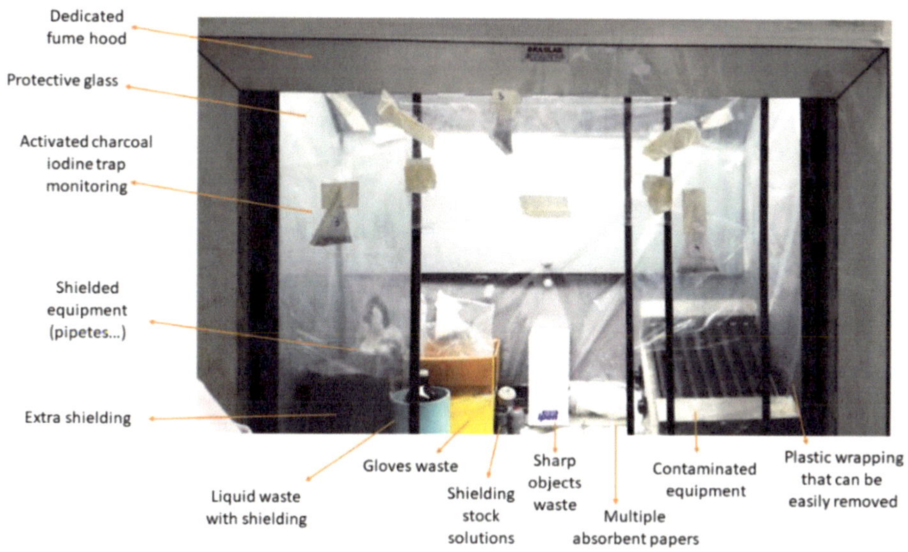

Figure 11.
Set-up was used to handle iodine-125 [2].

of the niquel-63 layer was determined to be approximately 2 μm, considering the minimum self-shielding effect of beta particles. The experiments to evaluate the P-N junction were first carried out by electron beam induced current technique employed to experimentally simulate beta emission from nickel-63 and to estimate the total device current. The open-circuit voltage was found to be 0.29 V and the short-circuit current was 3.3 A. The power output was found to be 66.5 W/cm^2. From the e-beam test, the good operation of the P-N absorber was confirmed before a radioactive source was fabricated.

The fifth step is to use less radioactive material or a different radioisotope to practice. This will ensure that the expected reaction is working and that the radiation protection measuring methods are efficient. For example, the AgI^{125} reaction can be performed by using AgI^{131} initially. Iodine-131 has a half-life of 8.04 days (59.43 for iodine-125) with energy 364.49 keV gamma and 191.58 keV beta (29 keV average gamma for iodine-125). This has the advantage of:

- the lower half-life allows contaminations to end faster. As a rule of thumb, 10 half-lifes are counted to consider a material not contaminated (except for living animals – the biological half-life is also considered in this case). For iodine-125 that would be roughly 2 years and for iodine-131, less than 2 months;

- since iodine-131 has a much higher gamma emission, it can be easily detected by radiation detectors. This is convenient to access each reaction step is more contaminant, when to change gloves, and the overall radiation exposure;

- being easy to detect also makes it useful to access experiment yields. If 0.5 mCi (18.4 MBq) is used and 0.4 (14.8) is measured, that is equal to an 80% fixation efficiency.

But it has the disadvantages of:

- a higher gamma emission results in higher radiation exposure to the operator;

- one mCi (370 MBq) of each isotope result in a different number of atoms. The results obtained might not be representative of the real reaction:

To iodine-131:	To iodine-125:
Half-life: 8.04 days	Half-life: 59.43 days
$A = \lambda \cdot N$	$A = \lambda \cdot N$
$10^{-3} \cdot 3.7 \cdot 10^{10} = \frac{\ln 2}{8.04 \cdot 24 \cdot 60 \cdot 60} \cdot N$	$10^{-3} \cdot 3.7 \cdot 10^{10} = \frac{\ln 2}{59.43 \cdot 24 \cdot 60 \cdot 60} \cdot N$
$N = 3.70 \cdot 10^{13}\ atoms\ in\ 1\ mCi$	$N = 2.70 \cdot 10^{14}\ atoms\ in\ 1\ mCi$
$m = 8.06 \cdot 10^{-9}\ g\ in\ 1\ mCi$	$m = 5.75 \cdot 10^{-8}\ g\ in\ 1\ mCi$

4.2 Radiation safety

The guiding principle of radiation safety is “ALARA”. ALARA stands for “as low as reasonably achievable”. This principle means that even if it is a small dose, if receiving that dose has no direct benefit, it should be avoided. To achieve this:

- the three basic protective measures in radiation safety already discussed can be used: time, distance, and shielding;
- use the three basic principles of radiation protection: justification, optimization, and dose limitation [49].

The International Commission on Radiological Protection (ICRP) system of radiological protection is a fundamental outline for dealing with any exposure situation in a systematic and coherent manner. At its core, the system relies on the three principles of justification, optimization and dose limitation. The principle of justification ensures that any decision that alters the radiation exposure should do better than harm. The outcome needs to be beneficial to society and the environment. The principle of optimization is for application in situations for which the implementation of protection strategies has been justified. Optimization of the protection strategy ensures that the likelihood of incurring exposures, the numbers of people exposed and the magnitude of their individual doses should be kept as low as reasonably achievable, taking into account societal and economic factors. This means that the level of protection should be the best under the prevailing circumstances, maximizing benefit over harm. Reference levels are adopted as an indicator of the level of exposure considered tolerable. This guideline help liming the dose for workers and public (**Table 2**) [51–53]. Specific environmental discharge of radioisotopes can be found in Ref. [54].

The basic requirements for achieving the highest standard in radiation safety are:

- Dose limits for radiation workers and members of the public;
- Monitoring and labeling radioactive materials;
- Using personal dosimeter and accurate monitoring detectors;
- Posting signs in and around radiation areas;
- Reporting the theft or loss of radioactive material;
- Having a trained radiation protection team available;
- Managing radioactive waste correctly.

4.3 Leakage tests

Radioactive sources that are used for medical treatments, industrial radiography, and nuclear batteries are routinely leak tested at the time of manufacture and, in some cases, during the lifetime of the sources. The various leak test procedures are designed to detect the presence of leak paths in the containment walls of sources through which radioactive material might escape to the surroundings. Shielding harboring liquid radioisotopes, such as Mo^{99}/Tc^{99m} generators are also leak tested. There are several requirements for the tests and they are presented in the ISO 2919 [55] and ISO 9978 [56].

A series of classification steps must be performed so a classification code can be emitted. Each of the tests (temperature, pressure, impact, vibration, and punching) corresponds to a specific digit in the product classification code, and can assume different values (1 to 6), according to the required performance level. The classification result will be an alphanumeric code that characterizes the product according

Categories of exposure (Publications)	1990 Recommendations and subsequent publications	Present Recommendations
Occupational exposure including recovery operations	20 mSv/year average over defined periods of 5 years*	20 mSv/year average over defined periods of 5 years
Eye lens	150 mSv/year	150 mSv/year
Skin	500 mSv/year	500 mSv/year
Hands and feet	500 mSv/year	500 mSv/year
Pregnant women, remainder of pregnancy	2 mSv to the surface of abdomen or 1 mSv from intake of radionuclides	1 mSv to the embryo/fetus
Public exposure	1 mSv in a year	1 mSv in a year
eye lens	15 mSv/year	15 mSv/year
skin	50 mSv/year	50 mSv/year

**With the further provision that the effective dose should not exceed 50 mSv in any one year.*

Table 2.
Acceptable dose limits separated by ICRP's publications [50].

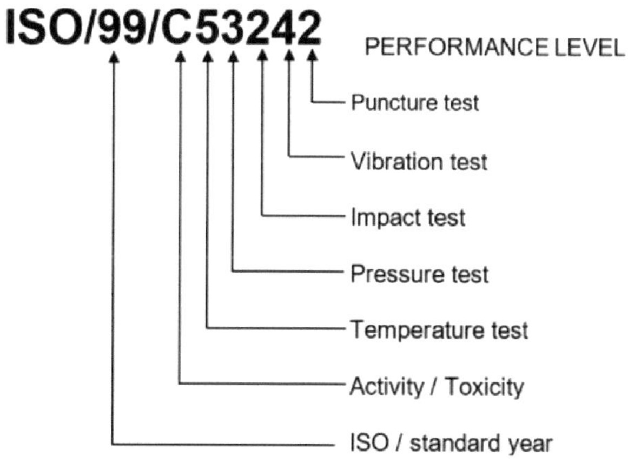

Figure 12.
Sealed source classification accordingly with the ISO 2919 standard. The numbers are the classification obtained.

	Source type	Tests for production sources		Tests to establish classification of source	
A	Sealed sources containing radioactive material	Immersion (5.1)	Wipe (5.3)	Immersion (5.1)	Wipe (5.3)
A1	Thin single integral window, e.g. smoke detectors				
A2	Low-activity reference sources, e.g. encapsulated in plastic				
A3	Single or double encapsulated sources (excluding H^3, Ra^{226}) for gauging, radiography and brachytherapy	Immersion (5.1) Helium (6.1)	Bubble (6.2)	Immersion (5.1) Helium (6.1)	Bubble (6.2)
A4	Single or double encapsulated Ra^{226} and other gaseous sources	Gaseous emanation (5.2)	Immersion (5.1)	Gaseous emanation (5.2)	Immersion (5.1)
A5	Double encapsulated sources for teletherapy and high activity irradiation sources	Helium (6.1)	Wipe (5.3.2)	Immersion (5.1) Helium (6.1)	Bubble (6.2)
B	Simulated sealed sources of Types A3, A4 and A5			Immersion (5.1) Helium (6.1)	Bubble (6.2)
C	Dummy sealed sources			Helium (6.1)	Bubble (6.2)

Table 3.
All recommended leakage tests. Numbers in () refers to the standard subtitles where the test description can be found.

to the ISO 2919 standard. **Figure 12** shows an example of a sealed source classification.

The ISO 9978 standard establishes the conditions and procedures for carrying out leakage tests on sealed radioactive sources, presenting various methods for inspecting these sources. Appendix A presents a guide for choosing the type of test, depending on the type of source to be controlled. Basically, they are (**Table 3**).

The test choice and performance level depend on the source being evaluated and its use. A source is considered leak thigh if less than 185 Bq (5nCi) is detected.

5. Conclusion and future perspective

The future perspective is that research in the different fields will increase. In the medical field new forms of treatment are being developed. Two new of interest are the lutetium-177 radiopharmaceuticals and nanobrachytherapy. Accordingly with Banerjee et al. [57] research with ^{177}Lu-based radiopharmaceuticals has demonstrated spectacular growth in recent years. ^{177}Lu Radiolabeling was performed with monoclonal antibodies, peptides, phosphonate ligands, particulates, steroids, and other small molecules. High success was achieved on treating neuroendocrine tumors with ^{177}Lu-labeled DOTA-Tyr^3-octreotate (DOTA-TATE). Nanobrachytherapy is a new form of brachytherapy that uses radioactive nanoparticles. The major advance is the small size makes it possible to penetrate tumor vascularity and cell barrier, delivering the treatment directly into the target

[35]. Works with gold-198, palladium-103, indium-111, and lutetium-177 are currently being investigated. In industrial applications, one major area that can be highlighted is nuclear power systems, more specifically, nuclear batteries. Withing this, Radioisotope Thermoelectric Generator and betavoltaic batteries. The first mode converts the decay heat to power by using the seebeck effect. Efforts are being made in several countries such as South Korea using strontium-90 for space exploration, Brazil using strontium-90 for oil extraction, and Europe using americium-241 for space exploration. The second mode uses beta decay (electron) to generate power directly. They are used in micro sensors and random number generators. Betavoltaic batteries using diamond are being developed in Russia and the UK. In South Korea, a p-i-n diode Nickel-63 beta battery is under development.

With research increasing at a fast pace, new students are starting in radiation chemistry, more collaborations are being signed, and the field is becoming more multidisciplinary in nature. This chapter created a guide by summarizing the basic chemistry, concepts, and steps to be consider to achieved the expected results when performing a radioactive reaction. The focus is, through knowledge and practical examples, in achieving high degree of success, protecting the operator, and the environment.

Author details

Carla Daruich de Souza*, Jin Joo Kim and Jin Tae Hong
Korea Atomic Energy Research Institute, Daejeon, South Korea

*Address all correspondence to: carla@kaeri.re.kr; carladdsouza@yahoo.com.br

References

[1] Neeb KH. The Radiochemistry of Nuclear Power Plants with Light Water Reactors. Berlin: Walter de Gruyter; 1997.

[2] Daruich de Souza C. Parâmetros para produção de fontes de iodo-125 utilizadas em Braquiterapia [Doctorate, PhD] . IPEN-CNEN/SP, São Paulo: Instituto de Pesquisas Energéticas e Nucleares; 2016.

[3] Broderick K, Lusk R, Hinderer J, Griswold J, Boll R, Garland M, et al. Reactor production of promethium-147. Applied Radiation and Isotopes. 2019; 144:54-63.

[4] Meyerhof WE. Elements of Nuclear Physics. New York: McGraw-Hill Book Company; 1989.

[5] Marie Curie Charity. Marie Curie the scientist [2021] . Available from: https://www.mariecurie.org.uk/who/our-history/marie-curie-the-scientist. Access in: 2021, May 17.

[6] Nobel. Nobel Lectures: Marie Curie Biographical. , Amsterdam. https://www.nobelprize.org/prizes/physics/1903/marie-curie/biographical/: Elsevier Publishing Company; 1967.

[7] Macrovector. Gold vector created by macrovector [2021] . Available from: https://www.freepik.com/vectors/gold. Access in: 2021, May 17.

[8] Macrovector. Buildings factory vector created by macrovector [2021] . Available from: https://www.freepik.com/vectors/design. Access in: 2021, May 17.

[9] Macrovector. Nuclear Energy Icons Vector Created by Macrovector [2021] . Available from: https://www.freepik.com/vectors/background. Access in: 2021, May 17.

[10] Macrovector. Technology vector created by macrovector [2021]. Available from: https://www.freepik.com/vectors/technology. Access in: 2021, May 17.

[11] PCH.VECTOR. Circle vector created by pch.vector [2021] . Available from: https://www.freepik.com/vectors/circle. Access in: 2021, May 17.

[12] Centro de Tecnologia das Radiações - IPEN, Daruich de Souza C. Reprocessamento. Instituto de Pesquisas Energéticas e Nucleares; 2020.

[13] brgfx. Car vector created by brgfx [2021]. Available from: https://www.freepik.com/vectors/car. Access in: 2021, May 10.

[14] Sul UFdRGd. Usina Nuclear [2021] . Available from: http://www.if.ufrgs.br/tex/fis01043/20041/Moacir/usina_arquivos/usinanuclear.html. Access in: 2021, May 10.

[15] Laboratory AN. The Alpha-Gamma Hot Cell Facility: used to perform nuclear materials experiments and examinations for over 40 years [2019] . Available from: https://www1.anl.gov/images/ARRA_AGHCF-200.JPG. Access in: 2020, 24 abr.

[16] Fomin VV, Shevchenko VB, Zemlyanukhin VI, Chugreev NS, Shmidt VS, Kondrat'ev AN, et al. Fundamental Problems of The Reprocessing of Spent Fuel Elements. At Energ [Sov J At Energy]. 1977;43(6): 481-6.

[17] Maher CJ. Reprocessing and Recycling of Spent Nuclear Fuel (Woodhead Publishing Series in Energy Book 79): Current headend technologies and future developments in the reprocessing of spent nuclear fuels Taylor R, editor: Woodhead Publishing, Elsevier; 2015.

[18] NAYLOR A, BAXTER W, DUNCAN A, SCOTT AFD. A Miniature Pilot Plant

For The Reprocessing Of Nuclear Fuels Part I-Description And Operation. Journal of Nuclear Energy Parts 1964;18:14.

[19] Reusch W. Virtual Textbook of Organic Chemistry: Chemical Reactivity [2020]. Available from: Michigan State University, http://www.cem.msu.edu/~reusch/VirtualText/intro1.htm. Access in: 2021, May 18.

[20] Foltz RD. CRC Handbook of Chemistry and Physics: A Ready-Reference Book of Chemical and Physical Data. 4 ed: CRC Press Inc; 2000. 133 p.

[21] Mellor JW. A comprehensive treatise on inorganic and theoretical chemistry. Londres: Longmans, Green and CO; 1965.

[22] Miessler GL, Fischer PJ, Tarr DA. Inorganic Chemistry. EUA: Prentice Hall; 2013.

[23] Kubiatowicz DO, inventor; Minnesota Mining and Manufacturing Company, assignee. Radioactive iodine seed1982.

[24] Ouellette RJ, Rawn JD. 1 - Structure of Organic Compounds. In: Ouellette RJ, Rawn JD, editors. Principles of Organic Chemistry. Boston: Elsevier; 2015. p. 1-32.

[25] Clark J. https://www.chemguide.co.uk/atoms/bonding/electroneg.html [2013] . Available from: https://www.chemguide.co.uk/atoms/bonding/electroneg.html. Access in: 2021, May 20.

[26] Lee J-B, Park U, Son K, Choi K, Yu K. Mass Production of Source Core for Iodine-125 Seed. Bull Korean Chem Soc. 2014;35:2172-4.

[27] Morowitz HJ. CHAPTER XIII - Applications of the Gibbs Free Energy and the Gibbs Chemical Potential. In: Morowitz HJ, editor. Entropy for Biologists: Academic Press; 1970. p. 145-56.

[28] Schmitz KS. Chapter 3 - Gibbs Free Energy, Work, and Equilibrium. In: Schmitz KS, editor. Physical Chemistry. Boston: Elsevier; 2017. p. 99-157.

[29] Daněk V. Chapter 4 - Enthalpy. In: Daněk V, editor. Physico-Chemical Analysis of Molten Electrolytes. Amsterdam: Elsevier Science; 2006. p. 221-53.

[30] University of Central Oklahoma, Jezercak M. Standard Thermodynamic Values [2021] . Available from: https://www.drjez.com/uco/ChemTools/Standard%20Thermodynamic%20Values.pdf. Access in: 2021, May 21.

[31] Mudrak I. Ionic conductivity and interfacial interaction in penton/AgI composites. Ionics. 2014;20(1):83-8.

[32] Tani T, Mifune H, Yamashita S, Aiba S, Ohzeki T, Yamane K. Ionic and Electronic Properties of Silver Iodide Grains. Journal of Imaging Science and Technology - J IMAGING SCI TECHNOL. 2007;51(3).

[33] Shukla AK, Ramdas S, Rao CNR. Mechanism of ion movement in AgCl and AgBr. J Solid State Chem. 1973;8(2):120-5.

[34] Benega MG, Nagatomi H,s Rostelato MECM, Peleias Junior FDS, Tiezzi R, Souza CD, et al., editors. Development of radioactive sources fixated in epoxy matrix to verificate nuclear medicine equipments. ENC; 2014; Marselha.

[35] Daruich de Souza C, Zeituni CA, Arcos Rosero WA, Nogueira BR, Rostelato MECM. New gold-198 nanoparticle synthesis to be used in cancer treatment. Brazilian Journal of Radiation Sciences. 2021;09(01-A):18.

[36] Royal Chemical Society. Iodine [2015] . Available from: Access in: 2015, 30 out.

[37] Kennedy JA, Besses GS. Comparison of Adsorption of Iodine-131-Thyroxine to Glass and Plastic Containers. J Nucl Med. 1967;**8**:226-228

[38] He JH, Jiang L, Xingliang L, Wenbin Z, Jing W, Zongping M, et al. Preparation of the radioactive source core of iodine-125 seed. Nucl Sci Tech. 2009;**20**(4):231-234

[39] Daruich de Souza C, Alberto Zeituni C, Feher A, Augusto Moura J, Luiz da Costa O, Angelocci LV, et al. New core configuration for the fabrication of 125I radioactive sources for cancer treatment. Applied Radiation and Isotopes. 2020;165:109307.

[40] Podgorsak EB. Radiation Oncology Physics: A Handbook For Teachers And Students. Viena2005.

[41] Weinberg RAW, Robert A. The Biology of Cancer. 1st edition ed: Taylor & Francis; 2006.

[42] Lindquist *C. gamma* knife radiosurgery. Semin Radiat Oncol. 1995; 5(3):197-202.

[43] Katemangostar. Business vector created by katemangostar [2021] . Available from: https://www.freepik.com/vectors/business. Access in: 2021, May 25.

[44] Macrovector. Online medicine elements vector created by macrovector [2021] . Available from: https://www.freepik.com/vectors/design. Access in: 2021, May 25.

[45] Macrovector. Fast customer support technical assistance vector created by macrovector_official [2021] . Available from: https://www.freepik.com/vectors/business. Access in: 2021, May 27.

[46] Nuclead. Lead Safety Products, Lead Safety Clothing & Garments [2021]. Available from: https://www.nuclead.com/safety-2/. Access in: 2021, May 25.

[47] Silva JT. Distribuição da atividade de Fósforo-32 e o revestimento com silicone em placas poliméricas para tratamento de câncer paraespinhal e intracranial.: Instituto de Pesquisas Energéticas e Nucleares; 2020. Contract No.: Seminário de Área- 02/2020.

[48] Uhm YR, Choi BG, Kim JB, Jeong D-H, Son KJ. Study of a Betavoltaic Battery Using Electroplated Nickel-63 on Nickel Foil as a Power Source. Nuclear Engineering and Technology. 2016;48 (3):773-7.

[49] Shapiro J. Radiation protection. United States: Harvard University Press; 1990.

[50] International Commission on Radiological Protection. The 2007 Recommendations of the International Commission on Radiological Protection. https://www.icrp.org/publication.asp?id=ICRP%20Publication%20103: International Commission on Radiological Protection,; 2207. Contract No.: ICRP Publication 103.

[51] Protection ICoR. ICRP 60: Occupational radiological protection in interventional procedures. https://www.icrp.org/publication.asp?id=icrp%20publication%2060: International Commission on Radiological Protection. ICRP Publication 21; 1991.

[52] Lopez PO, Dauer LT, Loose R, Martin CJ, Miller DL, Vaño E, et al. Occupational radiological protection in interventional procedures. https://www.icrp.org/publication.asp?id=ICRP%20Publication%20139: International Commission on Radiological Protection. ICRP Publication 139; 2018.

[53] Nisbet A. Justification, Optimisation and Dose Limitation Following Nuclear Accidents – An ICRP Perspective.

European ALARA Network Workshop n°17; Lisbon; 2017.

[54] International Atomic Energy Agency. Clearance Levels for Radionuclides in Solid Materials: Application of Exemption Principles. https://www-pub.iaea.org/MTCD/Publications/PDF/te_855_web.pdf, Vienna: International Atomic Energy Agency,; 1996. Report No.: IAEA-TECDOC-8S5 Contract No.: IAEA-TECDOC-8S5.

[55] International Standard Organization. Radiological protection - Sealed radioactive sources - General requirements and classification. https://www.iso.org/standard/54441.html: International Standard Organization; 2012. p. 19.

[56] International Standard Organization. Radiation protection - Sealed radioactive sources - Leakage test methods. https://www.iso.org/standard/70598.html: International Standard Organization; 2020.

[57] Banerjee S, Pillai MRA, Knapp FF. Lutetium-177 Therapeutic Radiopharmaceuticals: Linking Chemistry, Radiochemistry, and Practical Applications. Chem Rev. 2015; 115(8):2934-74.

Section 2

Fabrication, Materials, Manipulation and Characterization of Radiopharmaceuticals

Chapter 3

Radiopharmaceutical Biodistribution and Dosimetry

Santosh Kumar Gupta and Venkatesh Rangarajan

Abstract

Nuclear medicine is a medical specialty, where diagnostic and or therapeutic radioisotopes are used to study the physiology of organs and the metabolism of various types of tumors. Pharmaceuticals labeled with radionuclides (radiopharmaceuticals) are studied at pre-clinical level before being used in humans. Animals (Rodents) are generally used to study the biokinetics of tracer in a group of predefined organs. The extrapolation of the results of these studies from animals to humans provides an estimate of the behavior of the radiopharmaceuticals and the irradiation delivered clinically. Nuclear Medicine is fundamentally based on Radiopharmaceuticals whose biodistribution in disease and healthy organ result in either images that are diagnostically useful or local irradiation of tissue that is therapeutically beneficial for treatment of tumors. In result, in most procedures the biodistribution is primarily dependent on clearance of the radiopharmaceuticals from the blood into organs, tissues or lesions. Radiation is harmful for living beings and hence radiation toxicity is required to assess for new radiopharmaceutical which can be calculated by following the methodology of Internal dose calculation. Basic principle of Internal dosimetry and calculation methodology are explained in this chapter.

Keywords: biodistribution of radiopharmaceuticals, radiopharmaceutical dosimetry, internal dosimetry

1. Introduction

It has been well known that ionizing radiation is harmful to humans or living beings since the era of X-ray discovery by WC Roentgen in 1985. Application of ionizing radiation should minimize and or optimize according to its requirement while allowing its beneficial application. In 1924, radioactive materials as biological tracers' were used by Georg de Hevesy and colleagues for radiotracer studies of the kinetics of Lead-210 (^{210}Pb) and Bismuth-210 (^{210}Bi) in animals. Iodine-131 (^{131}I) and Technetium-99m (^{99m}Tc) are the predominant radionuclides currently in diagnostic and therapeutic nuclear medicine studies [1]. Application of radiopharmaceuticals inside the human body that emit radiation photons which is detected by detectors available outside of the body to investigate the movements of body parts and help in finding functional information is interesting and revolutionary achievement of nuclear medicine technique. Nuclear Medicine procedures can be diagnostic; that is, studying structures and processes to diagnose diseases/tumors and guide medical response to potential human health issues. Almost 95% of Nuclear Medicine procedures are Diagnostic procedures, but radiopharmaceuticals used in nuclear medicine may also be used for the treatment of tumors as therapeutic procedures; that is, administering higher amounts of radiation doses with the aim of using radiation to kill tunours tissues in the body. From last one decade, use of therapeutic radiopharmaceuticals increased for the treatment of various tumors as many new therapeutic radiopharmaceuticals such as ^{177}Lu-DOTATATE, ^{177}Lu-PSMA617, ^{177}Lu-Rituximab etc. are innovated.

Incidence of thyroid cancer were high in the 1940s and 1950s in pediatric patients treated immediately after birth for thymus enlargement [2]. In a similar time period, higher amounts of radiation doses were given to patients suffering from spondylitis; the treatment was effective for treatment of spondylitis, but there was a radiation side effects which was associated with a high rate of leukemia. It was also observed that Radiologists and radiation therapists operating in the early years of radiation medicine suffered high rates of leukemia and pernicious anemia because of radiation awareness. In the early years, ^{226}Ra was the principal radionuclide used in radiation therapy in which high-activity sources were placed on or near tumors to attempt to treat them. Modern external radiation therapy still employs a number of brachytherapy techniques involving different radionuclides and radiation-producing machines that deliver high doses of radiation to malignant tissues while minimizing dose to healthy body tissues. Therapeutic radiopharmaceuticals are generally administered intravenously or orally and are intended to deliver cytotoxic levels of radiation selectively to tumor sites. Specific targeted delivery is generally achieved with the use of a targeting moiety, such as a peptide or an antibody (^{177}Lu-DOTATATE, ^{177}Lu-Rituximab etc). Organ seeking radionuclides are naturally directed to a particular organ, reaching a desired organ without a ligand such as ^{131}I for thyroid cancer and ^{153}Sm for bone palliation.

2. Radiopharmaceuticals

Radiopharmaceuticals contain radioisotopes and biological molecules where radioisotopes bound to biological molecules that are target specific organs, tissues or cells within the human body. These radioactive drugs can be used for the diagnosis and, increasingly, for the therapy of diseases. In nuclear medicine, more than 95% of the radiopharmaceuticals are used for diagnostic purposes, while the rest are used for therapeutic treatment. Radiopharmaceuticals should have minimal pharmacologic effect, because in most cases they are used in tracer quantities. Radiopharmaceuticals should be sterile and pyrogen free, and should undergo all quality control measures required of a conventional drug as they are administered to humans. A radiopharmaceutical may be a radioactive element such as ^{133}Xe, or a labeled compound such as ^{177}Lu-DOTATATE, ^{131}I-iodinated proteins and ^{99m}Tc-labeled compounds. Although the term radiopharmaceutical is most commonly used, other terms such as radiotracer, radio-diagnostic agent or radio-therapeutic agent, and tracer have been used by various groups. In the 1920s George de Hevesy coined the term radio-indicator or radiotracer, which introduced the tracer principle in biomedical sciences. A radiopharmaceutical term refers two terms and these are, a radionuclide and a pharmaceutical. Characteristics of these two terms radionuclide and pharmaceutical direct the use of radiopharmaceuticals. For designing a radiopharmaceutical, a pharmaceutical is first chosen on the basis of its preferential localization in a given organ or its participation in the physiologic function of the organ and this is verified by biodistribution of their pharmaceutical in concern organ or tissues or diseases. Then a suitable radionuclide either diagnostic or therapeutic radionuclide is tagged onto the selected pharmaceutical such that after administration of the radiopharmaceutical, radiations emitted from it are detected by a radiation detector of Gamma Camera or PET. The selection of pharmaceutical should be safe and nontoxic for human administration. Radiations from the radionuclide of choice should be easily detected by nuclear instruments, and the radiation dose to the patient should be minimal. Radiopharmaceutical must also be sterile, pyrogen free, safe for human use, and efficacious for a specific indication.

Radiopharmaceutical is a backbone of nuclear medicine, and its advances have the potential to affect imaging and radionuclide therapy developments and application protocols. Nuclear Medicine is fundamentally based on Radiopharmaceuticals whose biodistribution in organ, tissue or disease result in either images that are diagnostically useful or local irradiation of tissue that is therapeutically beneficial. All nuclear medicine procedures are dependent on the optimal biodistribution of radiopharmaceuticals in either for obtaining metabolic information from the images in diagnostic studies or for delivering maximally tolerated therapeutic doses of radiation to tumors in therapeutic studies. Hence, the biodistribution is primarily dependent on clearance of the radiopharmaceuticals from the blood into organs, tissues or lesions and it impact the overall efficacy Nuclear Medicine procedures.

Although several problems are associated with the clinical use of radiopharmaceuticals, important factors affecting the biodistribution of radiopharmaceuticals are:

a. Preparation and formulation of radiopharmaceutical.

b. Radiopharmaceutical administration techniques and procedures;

c. Pathophysiological and Biochemical changes;

d. factors caused by medical procedures; and.

e. factors associated with drug therapy or drug interaction.

In recent years, radiopharmaceuticals are re-emerging as attractive anticancer agents. To validate a radiopharmaceutical, it is desirous for the radiopharmaceutical to be target specific, very selective, and deliverable against tumors of a given, molecularly defined cancer for which it is intended to treat.

Development of new radiopharmaceuticals for clinical use typically follow complex drug-development sequences that expend considerable resources and time. Most of them are molecularly targeted radiopharmaceuticals for either diagnostic or therapeutic, and therefore, might only benefit a subgroup of cancer patients whose tumors express specific targets. Conventional drug-development sequences, which focus on preclinical in vitro and in vivo studies justifying early-phase I or II trials, and then if warranted, late-phase III trials without assessment of the target expression, are suboptimal in the clinical evaluation of radiopharmaceuticals. Radiopharmaceutical drug-development sequences therefore might benefit from 'enrichment' approaches that more reliably reduce patient resources and shorten trial timelines. Radiopharmaceutical validation might be considered one of those enrichment approaches.

Validation of radiopharmaceutical is basically a fundamental process whereby preclinical or clinical investigations demonstrate agent performance as being suitable for its intended clinical use. Successful validation improves efficiency in the drug-development sequence by increasing predictive power and by shortening timelines in which a treatment effect would be expected to be reasonably large.

It is well known that radiation can cause deleterious effects in living beings. It is therefore essential to assess these effects in humans for a given nuclear medicine procedure. The damaging effects arise from the absorption of energy in tissues and depend on a number of factors: these are-.

1. the activity of the administered radiopharmaceutical during nuclear medicine procedures.

2. the physical half-lives, biological half-lives and effective half-lives of the used radiopharmaceutical,

3. the spatial distribution of radiopharmaceutical and their metabolic fate in the subject,

4. the fraction of energy released per disintegration of radionuclide of radiopharmaceuticals from a source organ that is absorbed in the particular target volume of organ, and.

5. the shape of organ, composition of organ, and location of the source and target organs.

The physical characteristics of a radionuclide are well known and established which is available in tabular form. Biological information which depends on physiology of subjects can be obtained from various experimental studies in humans and animals or phantom model studies.

The ultimate test of the quality of a radiopharmaceutical is its biodistribution. Often the first indication that something might be wrong with a radiopharmaceutical is an unexpected pattern of biodistribution found during an imaging procedure.

Animal biodistribution studies are always performed during the development of a novel radiopharmaceutical before it is first administered to human for clinical trial. These studies may be done in animals with normal phenotypes but more increasingly are being performed in transgenic animals which have certain characteristics which mirror those of the ultimate human recipients of the tracer.

Biodistribution studies in animals may be performed by manufacturers of licensed radiopharmaceuticals as part of their Quality Assurance procedure before preparing a batch of kits for human applications.

Now a days, biodistribution studies mostly performed by imaging the animals on micro SPECT or PET imaging devices which avoid the killing of animals at certain times after administration of the radiopharmaceutical and measuring the distribution of the radioactivity in tissues by counting or autoradiographic techniques as used in conventional biodistribution studies. Once a radiopharmaceutical agent is administered to a patient, the biodistribution process occurs. This process consists of the substance's absorption, distribution, metabolism and excretion. When the normal biodistribution pattern of a substance is known, any irregular pattern may suggest the presence of disease.

3. Internal dose calculation

Radiation dosimetry is the calculation of the absorbed dose in matter and tissue resulting from the exposure to ionizing radiation. It is broadly classified as external dosimetry and internal dosimetry. External dosimetry is the measurement of radiation dose from exposure of external sources of radiation which is used in external beam radiotherapy whereas internal dosimetry deals with the determination of the amount and spatial and temporal distribution of radiation energy deposited in tissue by radionuclides within the body. Internal dosimetry has been applied to the determination of tissue doses and related quantities for occupational exposures in radiation protection, and, diagnostic and therapeutic exposures in nuclear medicine.

Internal Radiation dose estimates are performed via calculations, not measurements. Usually, they are based on standardized models of the human body and often on standardized models of radiopharmaceutical behavior in the body as well. Internal dose calculations are basically depending on two components: biology components (refers the biodistribution and retention of the radiopharmaceuticals), quite complex and require special phantoms and models and physics components basically physical part (refers the energy transport and their deposition within the body), are typically well known and stored in look-up tables. In early ages, printed paper tables, look-up tables were used for dosimetry calculation which was quite tedious work. But now a days, dosimetry software such as OLINDA/EXM, DOSISOFT, NUKDOS etc. are developed where all the physical parameters are integrated in the software. The quantification of data from human or animal studies and treatment of it by a kinetic model, the analysis of which ultimately yields the numbers of disintegrations that have occurred in all significant source organs within the body are important and needed to collect these data for dosimetry calculation. Combination of these values with dose factors from the standardized phantoms (which give the dose to target regions per disintegration occurring in a source region) that yields the dose estimates that are of interest.

Preclinical studies from animal model for radiation dose estimation always required for dosimetry correction but dose estimation based on human data are almost necessarily preferred, even though human based data are associated with some uncertainties. Data collection-based animal data is an essential and first step for new radiopharmaceuticals for their dose evaluation and must be followed by carefully designed and executed human studies that better establish the dose estimates. Collection of data is a very important overview document on data gathering and quantification for dosimetry. To determine the activity-time profile of the radioactivity in source regions, the following question should be solved which are-.

1. What are the source organs? (Identification of source organs).

2. How fast does the radiopharmaceuticals accumulate in these source organs? (Uptake of Radiopharmaceuticals).

3. How long does the radiopharmaceuticals remain in the source organs?

4. How much activity of radiopharmaceutical is in the source organs?

The above mention first question locate and identify the source organs, while the second and third questions relate to the appropriate number of imaging time points to be made in the source regions as well as the timing of these measurements. The fourth question explain quantification of images and/or sampling of tissues and excreta. Each source organ must be identified and its uptake and retention of radiopharmaceuticals as a function of time must be calculated. This provides the data required to calculate cumulated activity or residence time in all source organs. Each organ exhibiting significant radionuclide uptake should be evaluated directly where possible. The remainder of the body (total body minus the source organs) must usually be considered as a potential source as well. Mathematical models that describe the kinetic processes of a particular agent may be used to predict its behavior in organs where direct measurements are not possible, but where sufficient independent knowledge about the physiology of the organ is available to specify its interrelationship with the organs or tissues whose uptake and retention can be measured directly.

4. Clinical radiopharmaceutical dosimetry

Both diagnostic or therapeutic radiopharmaceuticals need to be estimated their dosimetry before their clinical use in humans to assess the radiation toxicity and overall effectiveness for the diagnosis or treatment of disease. The medical decision in order to treat a patient will depend on tumors and the organs at risk.

According to the article 56.1, of the Council Directive 2013/59/Euratom (The Council of the European Union, 2014), "For all medical exposure of patients for radiotherapeutic purposes, exposures of target volumes shall be individually planned and their delivery appropriately verified taking into account that doses to non-target volumes and tissues shall be as low as reasonably achievable and consistent with the intended radiotherapeutic purpose of the exposure". In the article 56.6, the same document mentioned "Member States shall ensure that in the case of a patient undergoing treatment or diagnosis with radionuclides, the practitioner or the undertaking, as specified by Member States, provides the patient or their representative with information on the risks of ionizing radiation and appropriate instructions with a view to restricting doses to persons in contact with the patient as far as reasonably achievable.

Dosimetry information will also help to modulate the therapeutic activity, which means that depending on the dosimetry results the physician will prescribe more or less activity. This is called "personalized medicine", where every patient is given what he or she required keeping in mind to protect critical organ and threshold radiation dose for critical organ. There are two types of situation where physician recommend the radionuclide therapy such as one cycle or single treatment and subsequent cycles.

when the radionuclide therapy consists in only one cycle of treatment and when cycles of treatment are repeated and close enough so that the results obtained on one cycle can be used to plan subsequent cycles.

In the one cycle of treatment, patient may follow a preparation process. Then, a low amount of activity will be administered to the patient to proceed with the dosimetry measurements. In the case of thyroid cancer cell, a saturation effect, called stunning is well known, then tracer activities as low as 35 MBq can be used to perform a pre-therapeutic dosimetry study.

For the subsequent cycle treatment situation, Nuclear Medicine Physicist will estimate absorbed doses to certain organ at risk for the first therapy cycle. Under the assumption that organs at risk will have same biokinetics among all treatment cycles, a dosimetry extrapolation can be done in order to calculate the activity that can safely be administered for subsequent cycles. This administration scheme could be implemented for PRRT patients. However now a day's patients receive the fixed activity for each cycle of treatment (7.4 GBq per cycle, five cycles of treatment subject to follow maximum cumulated absorbed dose delivered of 23 Gy to Kidney for stopping radionuclide therapy) [3].

Clinical dosimetry is an evolving area in which different patient pathologies are explained and the treatment is optimized during the time due to new equipment, new radiopharmaceuticals, more professional staff, dosimetry software availability (to acquire, to reconstruct, to correct images), new regulations, etc. In fact, implementing clinical dosimetry in practice is quite a demanding task. This is why different dosimetry approaches have been proposed, using mostly academic software as research tools, even though commercial software is becoming increasingly available.

The most famous and accepted radiopharmaceutical calculation scheme was proposed by the Medical Internal Radiation Dose (MIRD) Committee.

4.1 MIRD schema for absorbed dose determination

MIRD committee is part of the Society of Nuclear Medicine & Molecular Imaging (SNMMI). It develops standard methods, models, assumptions, and mathematical schemas for assessing internal dosimetry from administrated radiopharmaceuticals.

The Medical Internal Radiation Dose (MIRD) Committee started its publications in 1968 with the MIRD Pamphlet No. 1: Schema for absorbed-dose calculation for biologically distributed radionuclides. This first document was revised in 1975 and further publications published in 1988 and 1991 containing examples. In 2009, the MIRD Pamphlet No. 21 [4] proposed a new nomenclature, intended to conciliate MIRD and ICRP terminology. The main aims of the MIRD committee is to propose means to compute absorbed doses, several publications are intended to explain the complexity of nuclear medicine imaging quantification. In 1999 the MIRD Pamphlet No. 16 [5] showed quantification of images using planar images. In the same year the MIRD No. 17 [6] showed dosimetry calculation methodology for non-uniform activity distributions at voxel level. In 2012 the MIRD Pamphlet No. 23 [7] explained the quantification of SPECT images targeting for patient-specific 3D-dosimetry. In 2016 the MIRD Pamphlet No. 26 [8] was published, a joint document between the EANM and MIRD Committee and explained SPECT quantification for ^{177}Lu radionuclide.

4.2 Theoretical concept of absorbed dose and biokinetics of radiopharmaceuticals

Absorbed dose (D) is the energy (E) absorbed in a particular mass of tissue, divided by the tissue mass (m):

$$D = \frac{E}{m} \tag{1}$$

In radionuclide therapy:

E = number of radionuclide disintegrations in a particular volume × energy emitted per disintegration of the radionuclide × fraction of emitted energy that is absorbed by a particular (target) mass.

Number of radionuclide disintegrations in a particular volume for E depends on the half-life of the radionuclide and its spatial and temporal distribution. Number of radionuclide disintegrations is analogous to Cumulated Activity (Ã) which is the amount of activity in the source organ and the time over which it presents in source organ. Distribution of radionuclides is typically obtained by imaging or sampling. Images collected at different times after injection of the radionuclides/radiopharmaceuticals are used to estimate the amount or concentration of radioactivity in a specific region. The level of activity obtained at different times after injection, plotted against time, gives a time-activity curve for a particular organ. The integral of this curve gives the total number of disintegrations or the cumulated activity (Ã) for the region.

Energy emitted per disintegration of the radionuclide is the total energy (e.g., gamma, beta particle, Auger electron, or alpha particle) emitted per disintegration of the radionuclide. This is a characteristic of the radionuclide and is independent of all other factors involved in calculating absorbed dose.

Fraction of emitted energy that is absorbed by a particular target volume depends on the emission type of radiation, energy of radiation photons, and also the geometry and characteristics of the source and target organs which provide a net factor and this factor used to converts the total energy emitted in a particular source organs to that absorbed in the organs or in other organs. This absorbed fraction factor is conventionally calculated using the anthropomorphic phantom studies but it is determined generally by Monte Carlo calculation. The spectrum of emission types will determine the fraction of energy emitted by a particular radionuclide that is absorbed by a particular target mass. Radionuclide emissions may be broadly categorized according to their absorption properties. Particulate emissions, such as beta or alpha particles are generally absorbed within the tissue of origin because of short range. Photons, depending on their energy, will deposit energy in both the source tissue and other adjacent and nonadjacent tissues. Various methods are used for calculation of internal dose.

5. MIRD committee schema

Internal dose calculation in nuclear medicine (NM) is normally used the techniques, equations, and resources provided by the Medical Internal Radiation Dose Committee of the society of NM. To yield the absorbed dose to the target, the absorbed energy (E) is divided by the mass of the target which is symbolically expressed in the form of following Eq. (2).

$$D_{T\leftarrow S} = \frac{\tilde{A}_S \times \Delta \times \varphi_{T\leftarrow S}}{M_T} \tag{2}$$

Where $\tilde{A}_S$ cumulated activity in source region S; Δ energy emitted by the radionuclide per disintegration; $\varphi_{T\leftarrow S}$ fraction of energy emitted by the radionuclide in source region S that is absorbed in the target region, T; and M_T mass of region T.

The Eq. (2) is the starting point for most current approaches to absorbed dose estimation. This equation describes the dose contribution to a target region from a single region. The derivation as well as the conceptual framework used to arrive at this expression is attributed to the early work of the MIRD Committee, which also established the most commonly used practical approach for estimating absorbed dose. The MIRD Committee reduced Eq. (1) into a product, the cumulated activity in a source region and S, the absorbed dose to a target region per unit cumulated activity in the sources given by single Eq. (3).

$$D = \tilde{A} \times S = A_0 \times \tau \times S \tag{3}$$

τ is the residence time which is simply equal to $\tilde{A}/A_0$ and S is given by-.

$$S = \frac{k \sum_i n_i E_i \phi_i}{m} \tag{4}$$

There are various anthropomorphic body models which have been used for determination of absorption fraction or S-value. Current generation of anthropomorphic phantoms began with the development of the Fisher-Snyder phantom which employed a combination of geometric shapes e.g. spheres, cylinders, cones, etc. to create a reasonably accurate representation of the body [6, 9–15]. Monte Carlo computer programs is used to simulate the creation and transport of photons through these various structures in the body [13]. Cristy and Eckerman modified the adult male model and developed models for a series of individuals of different size and age [16–20].

A generalized expression for calculating internal dose, which may describe the equations shown in publications by different authors especially in OLINDA dosimetry software, can be calculated by the following equation:

$$D = N \times DF \tag{5}$$

N is the number of nuclear transitions that occur in source region S analogous to $\tilde{A}_S$, and DF is a "dose factor" analogous to S factor.

6. Implementation of clinical dosimetry

The dosimetry calculation steps or dosimetry chain is related with the phases that are associated to analyze all images and data in a Gamma Camera or SPECT/CT or PET/CT system, where nuclear medicine physicist can calculate the absorbed dose for a specific organ/tissue. The dosimetry calculation chain is addressed collection of data, arranging the data and analyzing the data for dose calculation. There is few software that has been created for this purpose, some are open-source software, other from commercial companies. The graphical view of dosimetry calculation chain is shown in **Figure 1**.

In general, the following steps required to be considered for dose calculation in almost all the dosimetry software.

6.1 System calibration factor

Calibration factor is a most important parameter that needs to be considered for absolute quantification. The calibration factor can be derived from the sensitivity of the SPECT/CT system.

The system calibration factor must be measured at some time before or after radiopharmaceutical administration in a separate experiment. The count rate per unit activity (in units of, e.g., cpm/MBq) represents the calibration factor.

A standard of known activity of the same radionuclide to be used for administration to subjects, usually a few tens of MBq in a suitable container. The standard should be counted in air for a fixed time (e.g., 5 minutes) at a source-to-collimator

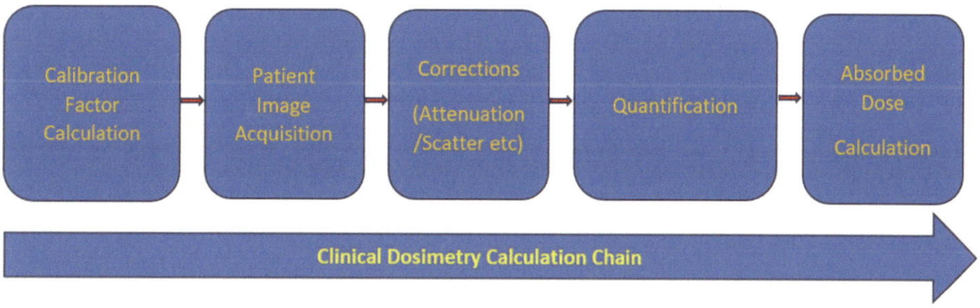

Figure 1.
Clinical dosimetric chain.

distance that approximates that of the patient midline distance used for the imaging study.

In principle the acquisition for calibration factor should be done using the same protocol used for patient imaging. Normally a phantom is used for that purpose. The calibration factor basically used to relate the number of counts within the image per voxel with the quantified activity per voxel.

Patient image acquisition: Depending on the availability of system, software and dosimetry protocol, images are acquired which must include section of the patient body, where critical organs and/or tumors are present. Normally several times point measurements are needed. At least three imaging time points over the physical half-life of radionuclide/radiopharmaceuticals are recommended to acquire for the best curve-fitting.

Corrections: Corrections like attenuation, scatter and partial volume corrections are implemented on every time points imaging to improve the counts. These corrections improve the quantitative accuracy in internal dosimetry which impact the dosimetry calculation.

6.2 Dead time correction

This correction must be done when high-count rates are present. Gamma camera is a para-lizable system, a second event occurring within the dead time due to the first event will not be recorded but will also initiate a pile-up effect. This means that not only will be recorded counting rate be less than the true counting rate but that, at high sample activities, the recorded counting rate will begin to decrease. Two source method proposed by Cherry [21–23] is used to correct the dead time correction.

6.3 Background correction

Background count is one which is originated from activity in the subject's body that is outside of desired source region on image, it might be scattered radiation from region of interest. Thus, scaling factor may be needed to correct the number of counts in background ROI. Alternatively, one may simply subtract the number of counts per pixel in Background ROI from the number of counts per pixel in the source ROI.

6.4 Organ overlapping correction

Organ overlapping can occurs for some organs or tumors, and this is the major drawback for planar quantification. For example, right kidney and liver are frequently partially superimposed on planar images.

M. Stabins propose the two approximation approaches. One approximation: for pairs organs, such as kidneys and lungs, is to quantify the activity in one of the organs in which there is no overlap, then double the number of counts obtained in this organ to estimate the counts in the two organs. The second approximation: is to draw an ROI over the organ region in scans where there is overlap, count the number of pixels and record the count per pixel, then use a ROI from another image in which there is no overlap; record the number of pixel from this new image, then multiply the count rate per pixel from the first image by the number of pixels in the second image.

6.5 Scatter correction

Scatter correction can be done by either using scatter correction technique such as dual or triple energy window methods during acquisition of images. It can also be corrected by using processing software after acquisition of images.

DOI: http://dx.doi.org/10.5772/intechopen.104917

Scatter correction must be applied to determine the amount of scatter photons included into the main energy window at its contribution to the total amount of counts within this energy window. The scatter counts will degrade the quality of the acquired image and it will affect the quantification.

In Energy window method one, two or more energy windows additionally to the main photo-peak energy window are implemented. Hence, one can estimate either the complete energy spectrum of scatter counts, or at least the integral of that spectrum from the lower energy cut-off of the photo-peak window to the upper-energy cut-off of that window, subtraction of the scattered counts, pixel by pixel, is required to correct it [6].

The dual-energy window (DEW), using just one energy window below the main, both with the same width. An assumption is made, considering that the number of scattered photons in the "low energy" window is proportional to the number of scattered photons in the main energy window. The number of primary photons is given by:

$$C_{Primary} = C_{Total} - \kappa.C_{scatter} \tag{6}$$

Where κ is a constant value, found to be 0.5 for ^{99m}Tc.

Triple Energy Window (TEW) method employs two energy windows close to the main energy window. The number of scattered photons can be determined as follows:

$$C_{Scatter} \cong \left(\frac{C_{left}}{W_S} + \frac{C_{Right}}{W_s}\right).\frac{W_m}{2} \tag{7}$$

Where C_{left} and C_{Right} are the acquired count from the two energy windows W_s, placed above and under the main energy window W_m. Then the amount of scatter counts can be estimated from the trapezoidal region having a left height of $\frac{C_{left}}{W_S}$, a right height of $\frac{C_{Right}}{W_s}$, and a base of W_m. **Figure 2** shows an illustration of this trapezoidal correction.

Therefore, using the result from Eq. (6), the count of primary photons is given by:

$$C_{Primary} = C_{Total} - \kappa.C_{scatter} \tag{8}$$

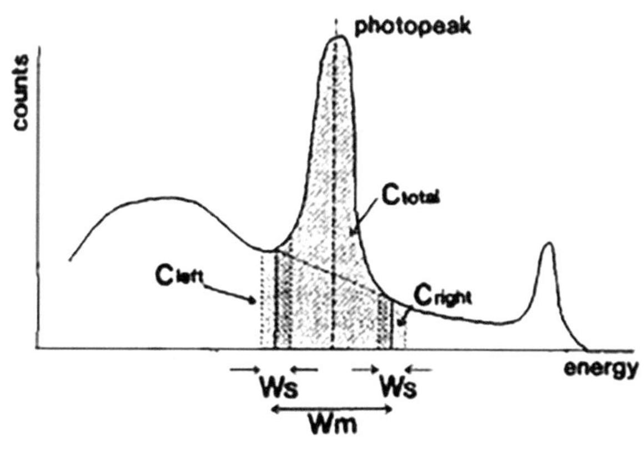

Figure 2.
The graphical representation of trapezoidal correction.

6.6 Attenuation correction (transmission method)

Attenuation compensation is required to maintain the intensity of photon which were lost during interaction of photons with tissues in body which impair the detection. Quantification from images are influenced by attenuation of photons.

In the conjugate view, the attenuation correction can be done by using a transmission factor (T_f). The attenuation is measured by acquisition of a separate *transmission scan* sometimes using a ^{57}Co sheet source, or flood phantoms (using ^{99m}Tc or ideally the isotope used for emission image acquisitions.

The transmission factor T_f can be expressed as follows:

$$T_f = \frac{\left[\frac{dN}{dt}\right]_{Roi,object}}{\left[\frac{dN}{dt}\right]_{Roi,no-object}} \quad (9)$$

Region of interest (ROI) is drawn on images acquired with object and without object.

In a whole-body scan, keep same bed speed for both scans.

If the isotope for transmission and isotope for emission images are different then a correction must be applied due to differences in linear attenuation coefficients between radionuclides with their energies. In this case, the transmission factor can be scaled and corrected as mention in below Eq. (10).

$$T_f = e^{\left(\frac{\mu}{\mu_{Measured}} \ln\left(T_{Measured}\right)\right)} \quad (10)$$

Where μ is the linear attenuation coefficient associated to the injected radionuclide, $\mu_{measured}$ and $T_{measured}$ are the attenuation coefficient and the transmission factor of the radionuclide used for the transmission scan, respectively.

Chang method which is an analytical method assuming homogeneous density and using a fixed linear attenuation coefficient to correct attenuation may be used. Chang method is applied after reconstruction, considering each pixel of the image, however, this method is assuming a constant attenuation coefficient. This method is not used nowadays, because of the hybrid SPECT/CT technology available in the nuclear medicine departments. The impact of Chang method in attenuation correction can be seen in **Figure 3**.

In SPECT/CT where inbuilt CT images used for attenuation correction, attenuation map is generated from CT images of patient. Because of heterogeneity in tissue composition in the human body, the estimation of an accurate and patient-specific attenuation map for nonuniform attenuation compensation is necessary. Attenuation map is a voxel-by-voxel representation of the linear attenuation coefficients at the SPECT photon energy. Generally, these maps have lower noise, better spatial

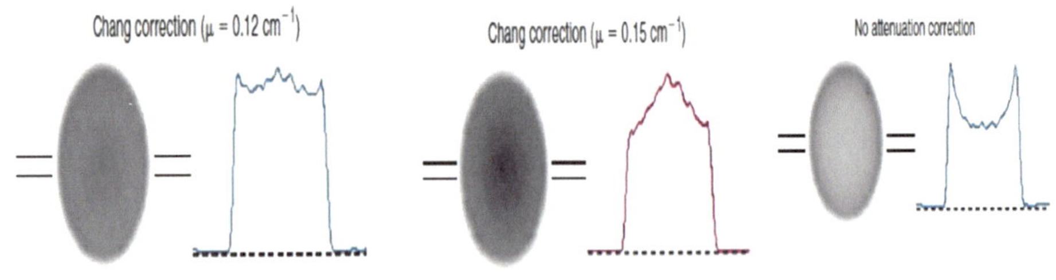

Figure 3.
Effect of Chang attenuation correction on SPECT images of a 20-cm diameter cylinder.

resolution, better contrast and are faster and easier to acquire [7, 22]. The attenuation map is expressed by the matrix of CT numbers associated with each pixel in a tomographic slice in CT images. The CT number can be defined as it is shown in Eq. (11).

$$CT\# = \left(\frac{\mu}{\mu_{H_2O}} - 1\right) * 1000 \tag{11}$$

Where μ is the linear attenuation coefficient of the medium and $\mu_{H2O}$is the linear attenuation coefficient of water. CT number units are Hounsfield Units (HU). Because linear attenuation coefficients are energy-dependent, the CT numbers at the x-ray energy must be scaled to the energy of the radioisotopes used for images.

The International Atomic Energy Agency (IAEA) in their book dedicated to Nuclear Medicine teachers and students [22–26] proposed to generated the attenuation map $\mu(h)$ considering the attenuation coefficients for water and bone as follows (h = Hounsfield units):

$$\mu(h) = \frac{1000 + h}{1000}\ \mu_{water} for\ h \le 0$$

$$\mu(h) = \mu_{water} + \frac{h}{h_{bone}}\ (\mu_{bone} - \mu_{water}) for\ 0 < h < h_{bone}$$

$$\mu(h) = \frac{h}{h_{bone}}\ \mu_{bone} for\ h < h_{bone}$$

6.7 Kinetic analysis

The bio-kinetics of a radiopharmaceutical can be addressed knowing the relationship of the activity (or number of counts) per time point. By plotting this relationship among all pairs (time, activity), a time activity curve (TAC) can be generated. **Figure 4** shows a theoretical representation of a TAC. Estimating the area under the TAC will produce the time-integrated activity (TIA), which was also known as cumulated activity, in units (Bq.S). Essentially this is a measure of the total number of disintegrations occurring in an organ source containing the radiopharmaceutical.

After gathering a series of whole-body scans or SPECT images at various time points based on selected radiopharmaceuticals that estimate uptake, retention,

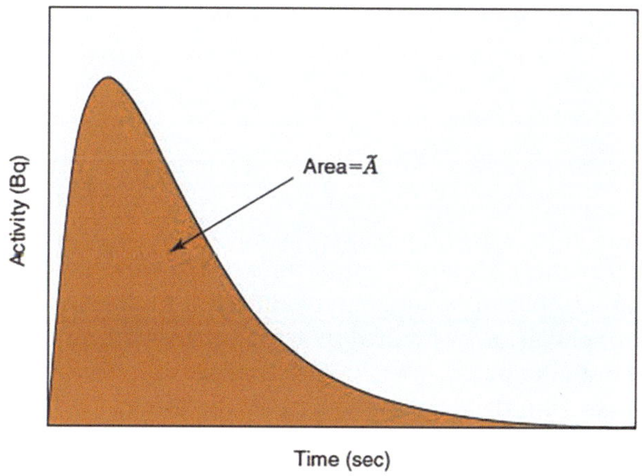

Figure 4.
A theoretical representation of a TAC.

and/or excretion of radiopharmaceuticals, the next step is to interpret these measurements in such a way as to design a kinetic model that can be used to estimate the number of disintegrations occurring in source organ. In general, three types analysis can take place depending of complexity of data-

A. Direct-Integration Method

Direct integration in which directly integrate under the actual measured values by a number of methods. It does not give very much information but it does allow to calculate the number of disintegrations rather easily. The most common method used is the trapezoidal method, simply approximating the area by a series of trapezoids.

B. Least-square Analysis

An alternative to direct integration of a data set is to attempt to fit curves of a given shape to the data. The curves are represented by mathematical expressions that can be directly integrated. The most common approach is to attempt to characterize a set of data by a series of exponential terms, as many systems are well represented by this form, and exponential terms are easy to integrate. In general, the approach is to minimize the sum of the squared distance of the data points from the fitted curve. The curve will have the form:

$$A_t = a_1 e^{-b_1 t} + a_2 e^{-b_2 t} + \ldots \quad (12)$$

The difference of the square between each point and the result of the fitted curve at that point and minimizing this quantity by taking the derivative of this expression with respect to each of the unknowns, a_i and b_i, and setting it equal to zero. Once the ideal estimates of a_i and b_i are obtained, the integration of A(t) from zero to infinity is expressed as:

$$\int_0^\infty A(t)d(t) = \frac{a_1}{b_1} + \frac{a_2}{b_2} + \ldots \quad (13)$$

Here the units of coefficients a_i are the same as the units of activity and the integration of it is the cumulated activity and the units of the b_i are time^{-1}. If the coefficients are the fractions of the administered activity or radiopharmaceuticals, then the area under the curve represents the normalized cumulated activity (e.g. Bq-h/Bq).

C. Compartmental Analysis

Biological system where a group of compartments interconnected through transfer rate coefficient. Cumulated activity of the various compartments requires a system of coupled differential equations expressing transfer of the radiopharmaceutical between compartments and elimination from the system. The result to the time-activity curve for each compartment will be a sum of exponentials, not obtained by least-squares fitting each compartment separately, but obtained by varying the transfer rate coefficients between compartments until the data are well fit by the model.

Absorbed dose calculation: There are several ways to calculate absorbed dose, for instance, the analytical, local energy deposition, dose point kernel, dose voxel kernels, Monte Carlo and Tabular approaches. All these methods will produce different types of outputs, average absorbed dose, absorbed dose maps and voxel-based absorbed dose in which absorbed dose volume histogram can be generated.

6.8 Activity quantification

Activity quantification is very important and this should be determined for a particular ROI/VOI/Structure before Time Activity Curve estimations can generated.

7. Planar imaging

Nowadays, most nuclear medicine department have a single- or dual-head imaging system. These systems can be used to image one section of the patient-body or the patient whole-body. Static, dynamic images or whole-body images can be acquired with these systems. Also, in the case of whole-body images an auto-contour can be activated to generate images as close as possible of the patient.

According to MIRD Pamphlet 16, "this method will be greatest for radiopharmaceuticals distributed in a single region or isolated regions that do not overlap (non-superimposed) in the planar projection". **Figure 5** shows an illustration to introduce the quantification situation.

In the conjugate view, an object with thickness τ is placed at depth δ. Here, it is assuming of no activity in the medium surrounding the object is considered, and also the medium and the object have same physical properties and no scatter radiation is presented. A differential slice of activity dA, with thickness dr is placed at distance r. Then, this differential of activity is expressed as-.

$$dA = C_A dt \tag{14}$$

The amount of activity per unit thickness in the object is:

$$C_A = \frac{A}{\tau} \tag{15}$$

The rate of photons detected from this differential thickness in the anterior and posterior views are:

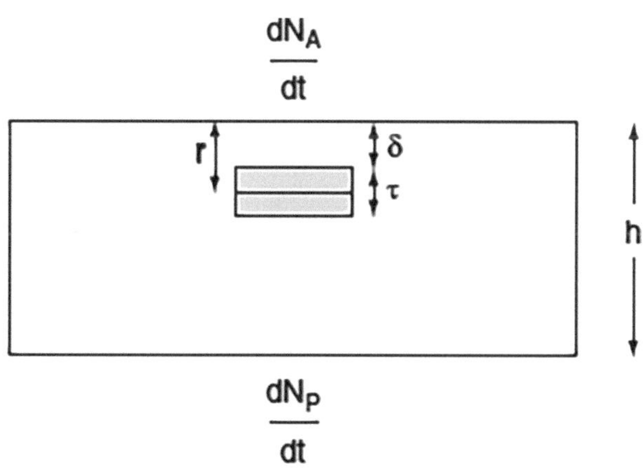

Figure 5.
Quantification scenario in planar imaging.

$$\text{Anterior, } \frac{d^2N_A}{d_t d_r} = \kappa C_A e^{-ur} \Longrightarrow \frac{dN_A}{dt} = \kappa C_A \int_{\delta}^{\delta+\tau} e^{-ur} dr \tag{16}$$

$$\text{Posterior, } \frac{d^2N_P}{d_t d_r} = \kappa C_A e^{-ur} \Longrightarrow \frac{dN_P}{dt} = \kappa C_A \int_{\delta}^{\delta+\tau} e^{-ur} dr \tag{17}$$

Where ξ is the planar calibration factor of the gamma-camera system, μ is the linear attenuation coefficient. Then the geometric mean of the two count rates is.

$$\left(\frac{dN}{dt}\right)_{geom} = \sqrt{\frac{dN_A}{dt}\frac{dN_P}{dt}} = \mathbf{K}\, A \frac{\sinh\left(\frac{\mu\tau}{2}\right)}{\left(\frac{\mu\tau}{2}\right)} \sqrt{\mathfrak{H}} \tag{18}$$

The attenuation of the emitted photons ($\mathfrak{H}$) through the entire thickness of the medium is given by:

$$\mathfrak{H} = e^{-\mu h} \tag{19}$$

Finally, for the object, the activity can be expressed as follows:

$$A = \frac{1}{\kappa\sqrt{\mathfrak{H}}}\left(\frac{dN}{dt}\right)_{geom}\left(\frac{\frac{\mu\tau}{2}}{\sinh\left(\frac{\mu\tau}{2}\right)}\right) = \frac{1}{\kappa\sqrt{\mathfrak{H}}}\left(\frac{dN}{dt}\right)_{geom} \tag{20}$$

Where ξ is called the self-attenuation factor of the activity contained in the object.

Now, considering a situation in which many overlaying source regions are presented, such as the case demonstrated in **Figure 6**, the activity for a source region jth A_j, is given by the general expression.

$$A_j = \frac{1}{\kappa\sqrt{\mathfrak{H}}}\left(\frac{dN}{dt}\right)_{geom}\left(\frac{\frac{\mu_j\tau_j}{2}}{\sinh\left(\frac{\mu_j\tau_j}{2}\right)}\right) \tag{21}$$

The **Figures 5** and **6** are ideal case, most of the time patient images are degraded by different physical effects, for example, dead time, background, organ overlapping, scatter and attenuation.

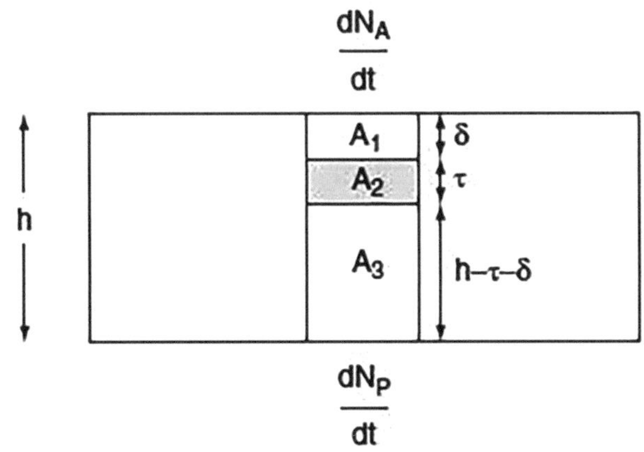

Figure 6.
An overlaying source region in planar imaging.

8. Absorbed dose calculation approaches

In radiopharmaceutical dosimetry, the absorbed dose can be calculated using S-values from a reference phantom model.

In targeted radionuclide therapy, the objective is to assess patient-specific dosimetry. Patients are different from reference models used in phantom in terms of total-body weight and size, organs masses, etc. Also, depending on the emission that is within the source, the radiation transport algorithm implemented for absorbed dose calculation may differ. Therefore, considerations regarding the size of the source and targets vs. radiation range are key aspects for the selection of absorbed dose calculation algorithms. Targeted radionuclide Therapeutic patient data sets are represented in 2D (pixel maps) or 3D (voxel maps) images in which the provided information will vary according to the biokinetics of the radiopharmaceutical product inside an organ.

9. Case studies: dose calculation using OLINDA/EXM software

Radiation absorbed dose of organs will be calculated with the help of series (minimum three series) of post therapy whole Body planar images acquired. **Figure** 7 Shows the Anterior and Posterior Images of post therapy scan with ^{177}Lu-DOTATATE. A Region of Interest (ROI) could be drawn over the Kidneys, liver, spleen and tumors and counts were extracted.

An important consideration in the extracting of counts from planar images is the drawing of appropriate background ROIs for organs. ROI is drawn outside the body images and subtracted its counts from outside the body is relatively easy (comparison with drawing ROIs for internal body structures). Background ROIs are just small circular or elliptical regions that are placed in an area that seems "reasonable" in representing counts that are underlying the image at all imaging time points where the ROI for the organ or whole body is drawn. Any reasonable placement of the background ROI in the image field will give an estimate of this background count rate.

Numerical values of counts from ROIs drawn over organs in post therapy images were extracted with the help of The ImageJ software (Open-source software). The ImageJ software displayed the counts of ROI over organs as the images at various times can be loaded into the software where the below given formulae was implemented [25, 26]. The source activity A_j is given as:

$$A_j = \sqrt{\frac{I_A.I_P}{e^{-\mu_e t}}}\left(\frac{f_j}{C}\right)$$

$$f_j = \frac{\mu_j t_j/2}{\sin\left(\frac{\mu_j.t_j}{2}\right)}$$

Where I_A and I_P are the counts over a given time for a given ROI in the anterior and posterior images, t is the patients thickness over the ROI, μ_e is the effective linear attenuation coefficient for the selected radionuclide/radiopharmaceuticals, camera, and the collimator (LEAP), C is the system calibration factor (counts/time per unit activity), and the factor f represents a correction for the source region attenuation coefficient (μ_j) and source thickness (t_j) (i.e., source self-attenuation correction).

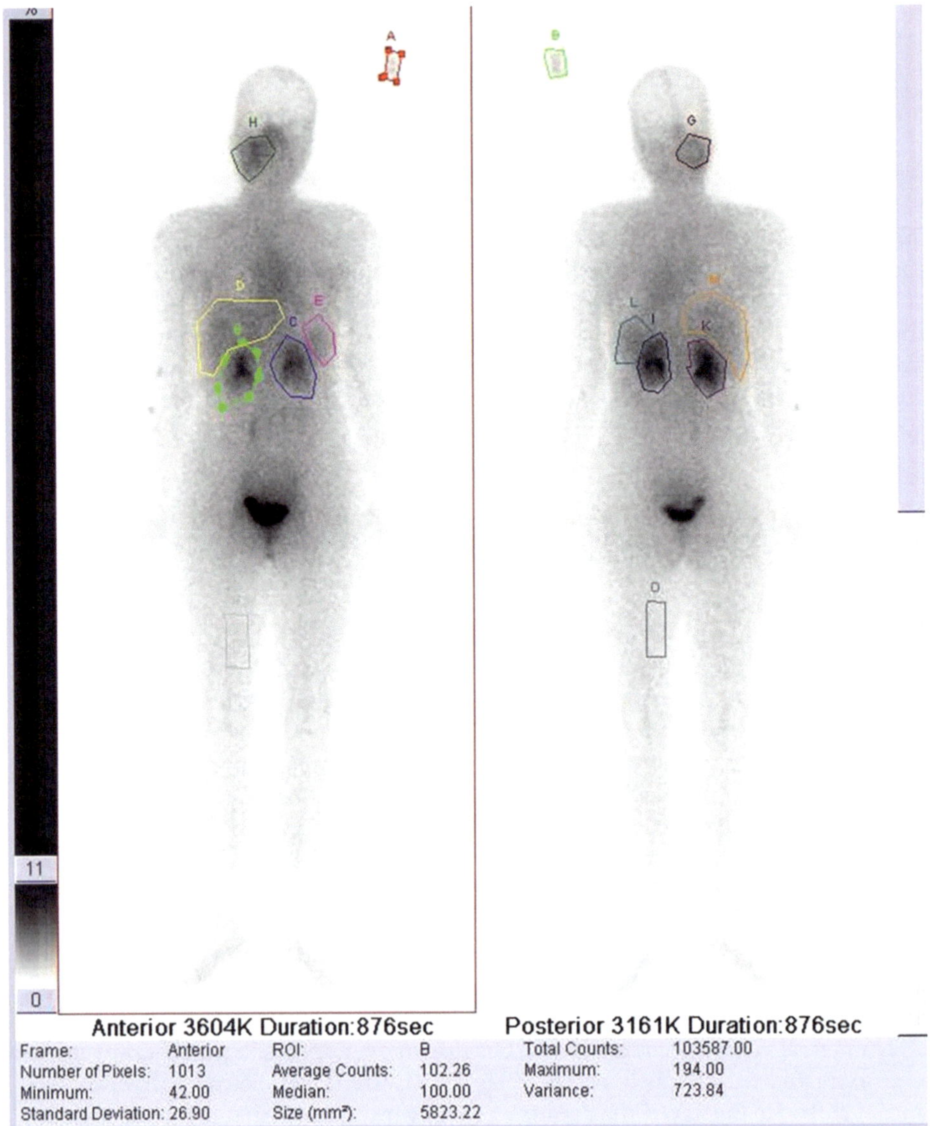

Figure 7.
The anterior and posterior images of post therapy scan with ^{177}Lu-DOTATATE.

10. Stepwise methodology for the calculation of radiation absorbed dose using OLINDA/EXM1 software

A. Step-1
Analyze the series of patient images, times at which the images are acquired at various time point are calculated. These time points can be calculated simply by spreadsheet program by just subtracting one time from another.
B. Step-2
I_A and I_P were calculated as explained above.
C. Step-3
The system calibration factor "C" can be calculated as explained in Calibration Factor paragraph.
D. Step-4

Activity in the source organs and fraction of administered activity in the source organs were calculated. The percentage of administered activity (% IA) at each time point of images of various organs and tumors were calculated and used in OLINDA/EXM software for absorbed dose calculation.
E. Step-5
Total number of disintegrations of source organs can be calculated with the help of percentage of injected activity at various time points. Depending on the data collected i.e. % IA of organs, mono-exponential or bi-exponential curve can be fitted in kinetic input form of OLINDA/EXM software and total number of disintegration can be calculated selecting the particular organs. For tumor and pituitary organs "remainder body" was selected and curve was fitted for the calculation of total number of disintegration (cumulated activity).

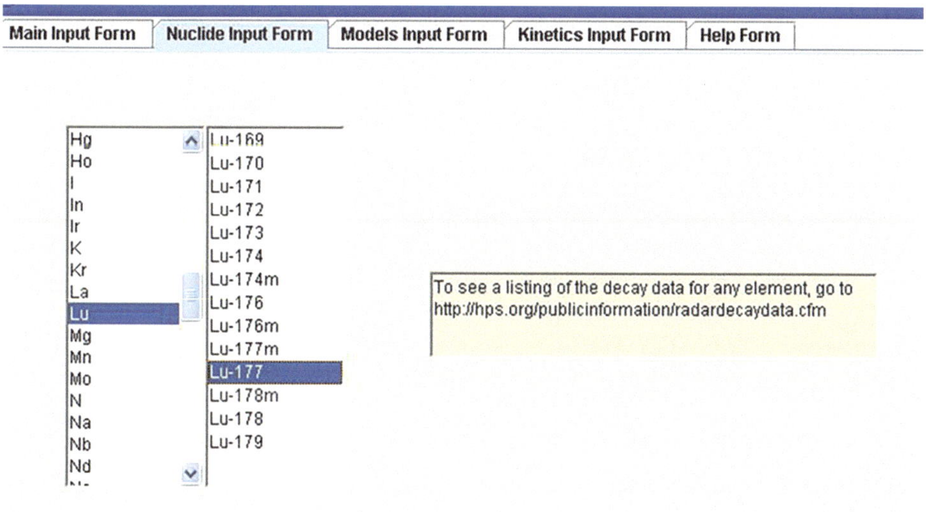

Figure 8.
The selection of radionuclide in OLINDA EXM 1 software.

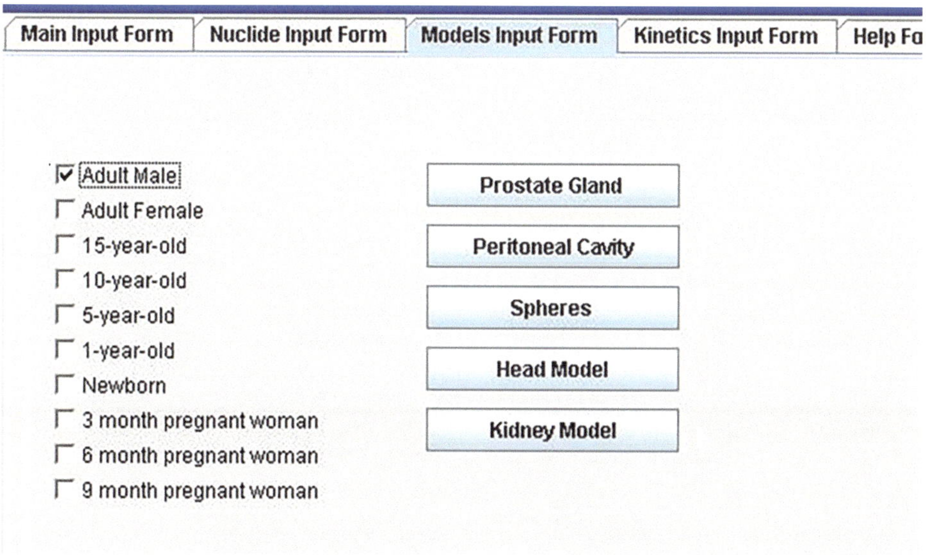

Figure 9.
The selection of models in OLINDA EXM 1 software.

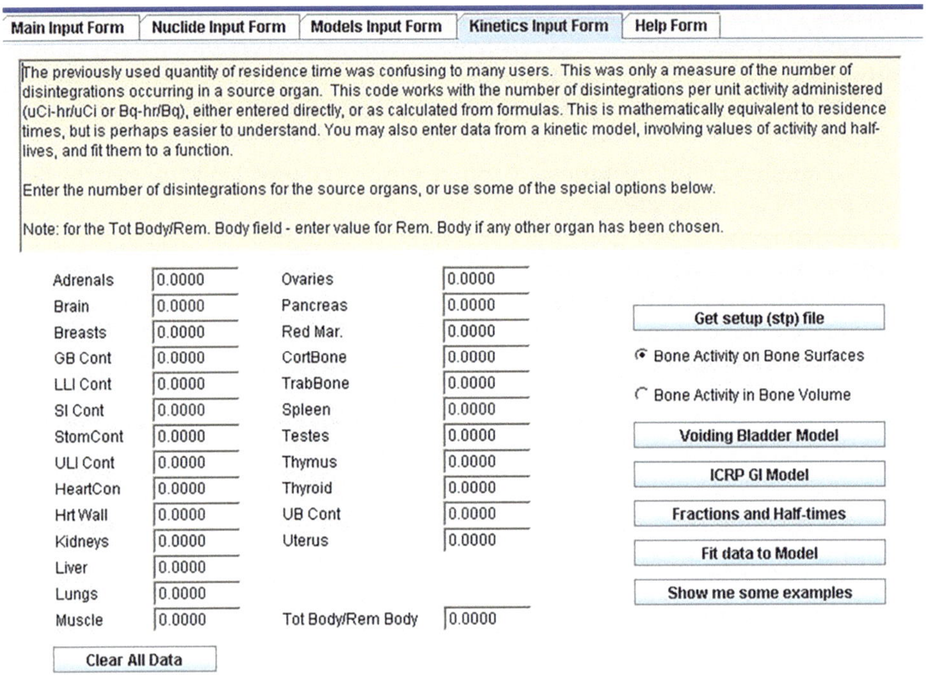

Figure 10.
Data fitting curve in OLINDA EXM 1 software.

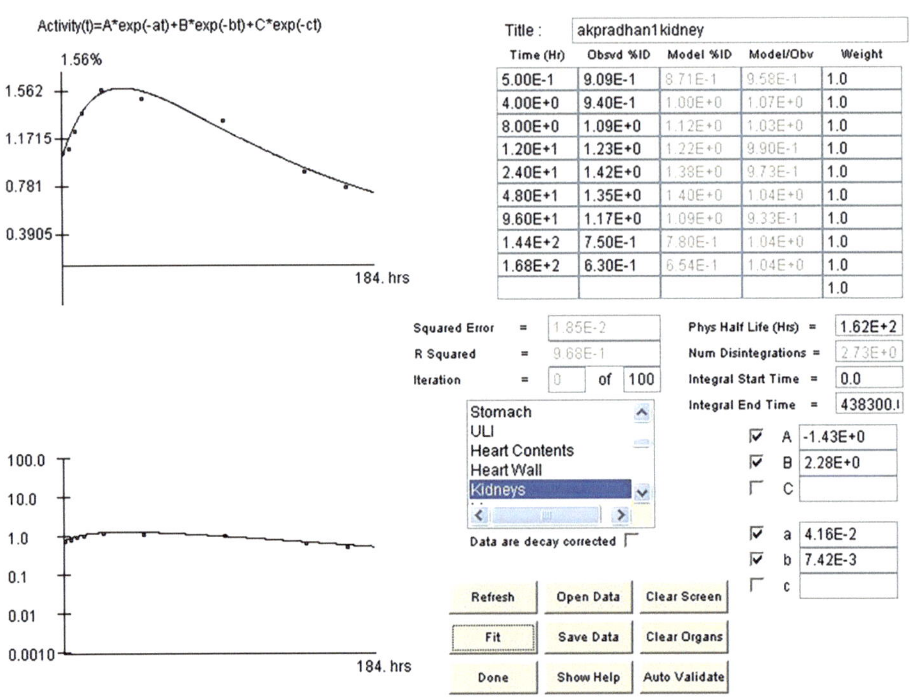

Figure 11.
Input of cumulated activity in OLINDA EXM 1 software.

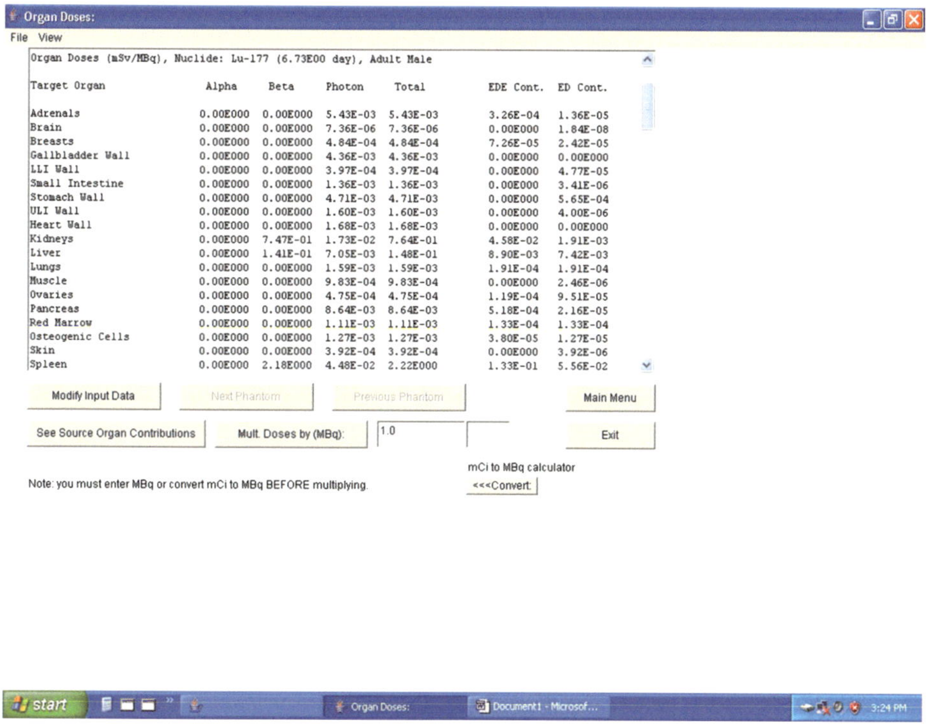

Target Organ	Alpha	Beta	Photon	Total	EDE Cont.	ED Cont.
Adrenals	0.00E000	0.00E000	5.43E-03	5.43E-03	3.26E-04	1.36E-05
Brain	0.00E000	0.00E000	7.36E-06	7.36E-06	0.00E000	1.84E-08
Breasts	0.00E000	0.00E000	4.84E-04	4.84E-04	7.26E-05	2.42E-05
Gallbladder Wall	0.00E000	0.00E000	4.36E-03	4.36E-03	0.00E000	0.00E000
LLI Wall	0.00E000	0.00E000	3.97E-04	3.97E-04	0.00E000	4.77E-05
Small Intestine	0.00E000	0.00E000	1.36E-03	1.36E-03	0.00E000	3.41E-06
Stomach Wall	0.00E000	0.00E000	4.71E-03	4.71E-03	0.00E000	5.65E-04
ULI Wall	0.00E000	0.00E000	1.60E-03	1.60E-03	0.00E000	4.00E-06
Heart Wall	0.00E000	0.00E000	1.68E-03	1.68E-03	0.00E000	0.00E000
Kidneys	0.00E000	7.47E-01	1.73E-02	7.64E-01	4.58E-02	1.91E-03
Liver	0.00E000	1.41E-01	7.05E-03	1.48E-01	8.90E-03	7.42E-03
Lungs	0.00E000	0.00E000	1.59E-03	1.59E-03	1.91E-04	1.91E-04
Muscle	0.00E000	0.00E000	9.83E-04	9.83E-04	0.00E000	2.46E-06
Ovaries	0.00E000	0.00E000	4.75E-04	4.75E-04	1.19E-04	9.51E-05
Pancreas	0.00E000	0.00E000	8.64E-03	8.64E-03	5.18E-04	2.16E-05
Red Marrow	0.00E000	0.00E000	1.11E-03	1.11E-03	1.33E-04	1.33E-04
Osteogenic Cells	0.00E000	0.00E000	1.27E-03	1.27E-03	3.80E-05	1.27E-05
Skin	0.00E000	0.00E000	3.92E-04	3.92E-04	0.00E000	3.92E-06
Spleen	0.00E000	2.18E000	4.48E-02	2.22E000	1.33E-01	5.56E-02

Figure 12.
Display of calculated absorbed dose in OLINDA EXM 1 software.

F. Step-6
Radiation absorbed dose of source organs can be calculated using the total number of disintegration of source organs from Step-5 and S-value of selected radionuclide in OLINDA/EXM software.
First radionuclide will be selected in OLINDA/EXM for data processing as shown in **Figure 8**. Then, adult male or adult female will be selected according to patient's data for Kidney, Liver and Spleen but Sphere model can be used for the tumors as shown in **Figure 9**.
Figures 10–12 of OLINDA/EXM software is shown the fitting the curve for calculation of cumulated dose or total number of disintegrations to dose calculation using the s-value from the software.

Author details

Santosh Kumar Gupta[1*] and Venkatesh Rangarajan[2]

1 Mahamana Pandit Madanmohan Malviya Cancer Center and Homi Bhabha Cancer Center (a TMC Unit), Varanasi, Uttar Pradesh, India

2 Tata Memorial Hospital (a TMC Unit), Mumbai, India

*Address all correspondence to: santoshaiims@gmail.com

References

[1] Stabin M. Nuclear medicine dosimetry. Physics in Medicine and Biology. 2006;**51**:R187-R202

[2] Frame PW. Radioactive curative devices and spas. Oak Ridger Newspaper, ID-3D. 1989

[3] Gupta SK, Singla S, Thakral P, Bal CS. Dosimetric analyses of kidneys, liver, spleen, pituitary gland and neuroendocrine tumors of patients treated with 177Lu-DOTATATE. Clinical Nuclear Medicine. 2013;**38**(3): 188-194

[4] Bolch WE et al. MIRD pamphlet No. 21: A generalized schema for radiopharmaceutical dosimetry—Standardization of nomenclature. Journal of Nuclear Medicine. 2009; **50**(21):477-484

[5] Siegel JA et al. MIRD pamphlet no. 16: Techniques for quantitative radiopharmaceutical biodistribution data acquisition and analysis for use in human radiation dose estimates. Journal of Nuclear Medicine. 1999;**40**(2):37S-61S

[6] Bolch WE et al. MIRD pamphlet No. 17: The dosimetry of nonuniform activity distributions—Radionuclide S values at the voxel level. Journal of Nuclear Medicine. 1999;**40**(1):11S-36S

[7] Dewaraja YK et al. MIRD pamphlet No. 23: Quantitative SPECT for patient specific 3-dimensional dosimetry in internal radionuclide therapy. Journal of Nuclear Medicine. 2012;**53**(8):1310-1325

[8] Ljungberg M et al. MIRD Pamphlet No. 26: Joint EANM/MIRD guidelines for quantitative 177Lu SPECT applied for dosimetry of radiopharmaceutical therapy. Journal of Nuclear Medicine. 2016;**57**:151-162

[9] Stabin MG. A model of the prostate gland for use in internal dosimetry. Journal of Nuclear Medicine. 1994;**35**: 516-520

[10] Bouchet LG, Bolch WE, Weber DA, Atkins HL, Poston JW Sr. MIRD pamphlet no.15: Radionuclide S values in a revised dosimetric model of the adult head and brain. Journal of Nuclear Medicine. 1999;**40**:62S-101S

[11] Mardirossian G, Tagesson M, Blanco P, Bouchet LG, Stabin M, Yoriyaz H, et al. A new rectal model for dosimetry applications. Journal of Nuclear Medicine. 1999;**40**:1524-1531

[12] Bouchet LG, Bolch WE, Howell RW, Rao DV. S values for radionuclides localized within the skeleton. Journal of Nuclear Medicine. 2000;**41**:189-212

[13] Bouchet LG, Bolch WE, Blanco HP, Wessels BW, Siegel JA, Rajon DA, et al. MIRD pamphlet no. 19: Absorbed actions and radionuclide S values for 6 agedependent multiregion models of the kidney. Journal of Nuclear Medicine. 2003;**44**:1113-1147

[14] Goddu SM, Howell RW, Rao DV. Cellular dosimetry: Absorbed fractions for monoenergetic electron and alpha particle sources and S-values for radionuclides uniformly distributed in different cell compartments. Journal of Nuclear Medicine. 1994;**35**:303-316

[15] Goddu SM, Howell RL, Bouchet LG, Bolch WE, Rao DV. MIRD Cellular S Values. Reston, VA: Society of Nuclear Medicine; 1997. p. 19

[16] Williams LE, Liu A, Raubitschek AA, Wong JY. A method for patient-specific absorbed dose estimation for internal beta emitters. Clinical Cancer Research. 1999;**5**:3015s-3019s

[17] McKay E. A software tool for specifying voxel models for dosimetry

estimation. Cancer Biotherapy & Radiopharmaceuticals. 2003;**18**:379-392

[18] Guy MJ, Flux GD, Papavasileiou P, Flower MA, Ott RJ. RMDP: A dedicated package for I-131 SPECT quantification, registration and patient-specific dosimetry. Cancer Biotherapy & Radiopharmaceuticals. 2003;**18**:61-69

[19] Stabin MG. Uncertainties in internal dose calculations for radiopharmaceuticals. Journal of Nuclear Medicine. 2008;**49**:853-860

[20] Stabin MG. MIRDOSE: Personal computer software for internal dose assessment in nuclear medicine. Journal of Nuclear Medicine. 1996;**37**:538-546

[21] ICRP. ICRP-103. The 2007 recommendations of the International Commission on Radiological Protection. Annals of the ICRP. 2007;**2–4**:1-334

[22] IAEA. Nuclear Medicine Physics: A Handbook for Students and Teachers. Vienna: IAEA; 2014

[23] Cherry S, Sorenson J, Phelps M. Physics in Medical Biology. Philadelphia: Elsevier; 2012

[24] Zaidi H. Quantitative Analysis in Nuclear Medicine Imaging. New York: Springer; 2006

[25] Chang LT. A method for attenuation correction in radionuclide computed tomography. IEEE Transactions on Nuclear Science. 1978;**25**(1):638-643

[26] Zhao W et al. Determination of gamma camera calibration factors for quantitation of therapeutic radioisotopes. EJNMMI Physics. 2018;**5**:8

Chapter 4

Focal Increased Radiopharmaceutical Uptake Differentiation Using Quantitative Indices

V. Sivasubramaniyan and K. Venkataramaniah

Abstract

Focal increased radiopharmaceutical uptake in a lesion results in focal Hot Spots in the scans. This can occur in benign infective or inflammatory disorders and cancerous diseases as well. Comparison between malignant and benign lesions is important. The Hot spots can be classified into benign and malignant lesions by Spatial Scintimetry or Temporal Scintimetry. Spatial Scintimetry compares the uptake in the region of interest with the adjacent tissue or the unaffected contra-lateral site. The quantitative indices are lesion/non lesion ratio, lesion/background activity and lesion to Bone ratio etc. The Temporal Scintimetry relies on the changes in the counts or uptake in the Hotspot lesion with reference to the dual point time of acquisition. The Hotspot in the bone scan can be classified using the quantitative index of retention ratio by Dr. V. Siva and Israel. In PET studies the focal hot spots can be differentiated into benign and malignant lesion using the dual phase PETCT evaluation using the Rong's Retention ratio and Dr. V. Siva's modified RRI values.

Keywords: radiopharmaceutical uptake, scintimetric characterization, spatial scintimetry, temporal scintimetry, quantitative indices

1. Introduction

The uptake of the Radiopharmaceuticals in the organ of interest makes the functional evaluation of that organ feasible. Not only that the radiopharmaceutical uptake in the pathological conditions depends on the blood supply to the organ, bolus injection of the radiopharmaceutical and the functional integrity of the organ. When there is increase in blood supply and integral functionality in a lesion will lead to focal increase in radiopharmaceutical uptake resulting in the Hot spots. In those situations where there is reduction in the blood supply to the organ and decreased functional integrity will result in photopenic or photon void lesions. Conventionally scintigraphic imagery is being inferred by graphical inspection of the photographic imprints and comparing with the known normal distribution pattern in the organ of interest.

The advancement of digital scanning technologies have made it easier to measure the scintillations by quantifying the per pixel counts of the intended regions. In addition, the post-processing and PACS transmission characteristics have been the major reason behind the Dicom compatible graphics. The phrase "SCINTIMETRY" means the number of scintillations taking place in intended regions in scintigraphic imagery that has been covered in the study. Basically, "Scintimetry" is the combined term of "Scintillation + Metric".

2. Scintimetric characterization

The scintillations in a focal hot spot can be counted using Scintimetry. Depending upon the method of comparison there are TWO types of Scintimetry:

1. Regional: The process of drawing the region of interest (ROI), picking the ROI, and comparing the same with either equivalent or neighboring site on the contra lateral part by marking the same region of interest is known as Spatial Scintimetry.

2. Temporal: The ROI is drawn above the lesion of interest or the site at a time and evaluating the same with a region of interest on the acquired imagery after some time from the first study is known as "Time Bound Scintimetry" or the scintimetry of same ROI regarding time.

2.1 Regional scintimetry methods

Scintimetric evaluations can be performed with several quantitative approaches. Some of the most popular methods are: a. Local Uptake; b. bone soft tissue ratio; c. Lesion bone ratio; d. Standardized Uptake Ratio (SUV); and e. Percentage uptake.

a. Local uptake ratio: It is the easiest way to quantify the tracer's uptake in an ROI to determine the count rate calculated in the form of ratio of count rate in a region in a closest area in identical image (Rosenthall and Kaye, 1975) [1]. On the other hand, it is also possible to use a line profile curve at lesion area (Lentle et al., 1977) [2], **Figure 1**.

b. Lesion Bone (L/B) Ratio: Here, "lesion" means focal region of abnormality and "bone" refers to the suitable region of a bone. Its utility has been best described by (Condon et al., 1981) [3] and (Vellenga et al., 1984) [4] when it comes to detect rib lesions and almost indiscernible lesions.

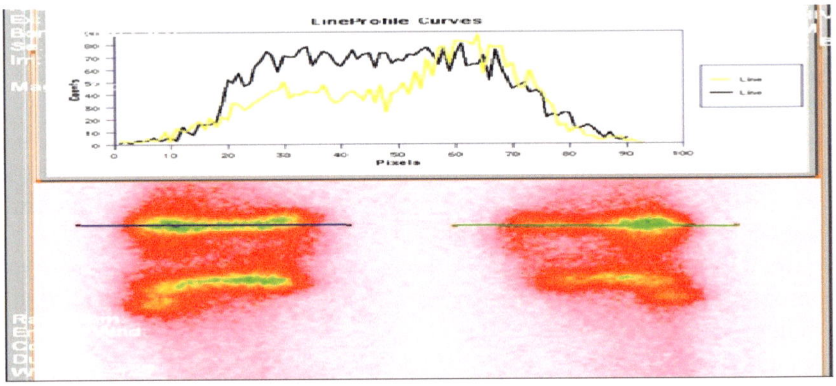

Figure 1.
Line profile curve.

c. Bone/Soft Tissue: There are some measurements that can help detect hematological malignancies in patients (Pfeifer et al., 1983) [5]. This ratio has been used by (Constable and Cranage, 1980) [6] to verify the prostatic super scans.

d. Percentage uptake: The uptake is referred in the area of interest to the given dose to calculate the percentage uptake (Hardly et al., 1980) [7] or to the given external activity by Meindok et al., 1985 [8].

2.2 Methods of temporal scintimetry

There are two methods to do it:

a. Retention Ratio and

b. Change in the regional uptake ratios with reference to time.

- Retention Ratio: Israel et al., 1985 [9] measured Lesion Bone uptake with this clue at 4 and 24 hours and suggested that the ratio of 24/4-h was lower among patients who have been through metastasis treatment and who have degenerative disease. Dr. V. Siva et al., 1995 [10] devised a retention ratio of 4/24 hr. to distinguish the focal hotspots into Metabolic, Benign, and Malignant characteristics. In that study it has been demonstrated that the Retention ratio 0–5 indicates benign nature of the lesion, 5–10 denotes indeterminate or metabolic or degenerative nature and 10 and above confirms the malignant nature of the lesions. The concept is being depicted in **Figure 2**.

- Change in Regional uptake ratio: The change in the Regional uptake ratio with reference to time is currently used in the evaluation of healing potential of Fracture neck of Femur [10].

3. Scintimetric classification of skeletal hot spot in bone scan

X-ray is not sufficient to diagnose bone metastases. Nuclear scintigraphy imaging has always been helpful for early diagnosis of bone disease. The diphosphonates

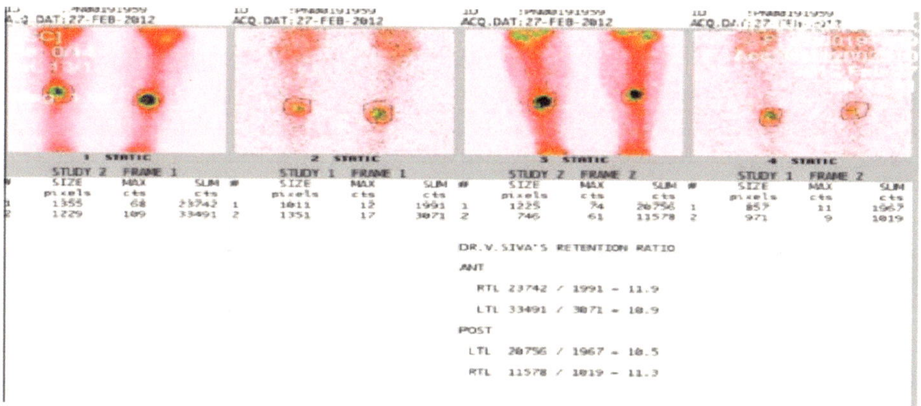

Figure 2.
Dr. V. Siva's retention ratio.

labeled as "99mTechnetium" in Bone scan detects the osteoblastic response that takes place in malignant cells. This method is best suited for the entire body scan at affordable cost and with high sensitivity and availability. But there is a problem with specificity [11]. The crystal immature bone surfaces absorb the "99mTc-polyphosphate" along with its variants through ionic deposition.

The rise in bone vascularity raises this process along with matrix localization. Hence, the focal hotspots or abrupt scintiscan area is the region of elevated osteoblastic activity. The Scintiscan bone has been shown to be more sensitive than x-rays to detect bone's focal illness. The major flaw in this process is the non-specificity of the study [12].

There are reasons Prostatic Carcinoma metastasis, which is usually found in bone, has gained a lot of attention for investigation. The anatomical aspects of the prostate gland are the first reason. Baston's plexus is the venous drainage of the prostate gland with a unique range of venous plexus. The Lumbosacral plexus of veins is directly connected with it. In the advanced stage of prostate cancer, this metastatic lesion occurs especially in the axial skeleton [13].

It is not possible to cover the metastatic association in ribs, skull and the bones with this anatomical elaboration. According to Paget, there have been mutations in carcinoma prostate cells in osteotropic cells either with activation of particular proteases and cytokine or with genetic form. They can be latent till an expected change takes place around them like a seed. Hence, there is some clue in the 'seed and soil' theory from the next standpoint [14]. The elevated levels of TGF-β and "bone morphogenetic proteins (BMPs)" had been established in metastasis of bones in prostate cancer cells [15–18]. These cells of "osteotropic metastatic seeds" are combined to the endothelium of bones better than other tissues' endothelium [19].

The skeletal tissue contains Tc-99 mm MDP as the ionic radiopharmaceutical radius is much like the same of "Calcium Hydroxy-appetite crystal". Hence, it is added to the skeletal tissue. Hence, even Osteomyelitis, Paget's disease and Post Traumatic skeletal disorders occur with focal skeletal hotspots. For skeletal hotspots, the major cause must be determined with invasive procedure and further scanning as well. Several quantitative measures are there to improve the specificity of bone scan. Along with fusion imaging procedures like PET-CT and SPECT–CT, BONE SPECT and other cross-sectional techniques have been introduced. We have proposed a novel Scintimetric technique in this work for bone scanning to verify and rule out metastatic or malignant nature of skeletal areas in the non-invasive bone imaging.

The bone scans have focal hotspot margins of 4 and 24 h followed by injecting radiopharmaceutical drawings with a tool and experts tabulate the maximum per-pixel counts in such scans. The ratio of two values is taken to determine the focal hotspot changes in the scan with time interval. It is defined as Scintimetry of one region regarding time and is termed "Time Bound Scintimetry". In addition, it is possible to infer the metabolic turnover in hotspots.

4. Temporal scintimetry method and Dr. Siva's retention ratio

A method named "Temporal Scintimetry" has been proposed by Israel et al. [9]. The Non lesion (NL) and Lesion (L) count ratio has been measured over the bone at 4 h in bone imaging. It is also performed again in bone scan at 24 h as well.

$$\text{"Israel's ratio} = \text{L / N 24 h / L / N 4 h"} \tag{1}$$

There has been too negligible variation in measurements among patients who have been treated with metastasis and with degenerative disease and it was steep in metastatic lesions. The decimal values came up in the result only as the indicator is high according to the "Radioactive decay law". We also presented Dr. V. Siva's 4/24 h retention ratio in this work to classify the 'focal hot spots' and to find the difference between benign lesions and metastatic lesions with this procedure [10]:

1. Only the maximum counts at the Lesion or Focal hot spot were taken rather than L/N ratio.

2. Thc 4/24 h ratio of Dr. V. Siva is taken rather than Israel's 24/4 h ratio.

5. Dr. V. Siva's retention ratio = 4/24 h focal hot spot count

5.1 Clinical applications of scintimetric characterization of the skeletal hotspots in the differentiation of benign and metastatic lesion

The bone scan was performed 4 h following the 15–25 mCi of IV injection containing "Tc-99 m Methylene Di-Phosphonate "with proper hydration with the entire body acquisition of dual head gamma camcorder of Siemen's eCAM. Next day, the full-body bone imaging is done again with the same protocol and injection. The General Display protocol is used to select both images of 4 h and 24 h. The 4 h anterior and 24 h posterior scans are selected with Region Ratio protocol and the experts tabulate the maximum counts at a focal area. The region ratio protocol is used to calculate Dr. V. Siva 4/24 h retention ratios and it is also tabulated.

In a study, a group of 32 patients with proven and known Paget's disease, Avascular Necrosis, Osteomyelitis, and degenerative problems and 75 patients with proven Carcino Prostate biopsy reports were included. There was metastatic involvement in 53 people in a Carcinoma Prostate group, out of which 22 were reported negative for metastases. The "11.5 ± 2.8" is the mean value of the 4/24 retention ratio of Dr. V. Siva in malignant bone lesions and "0.08 ± 0.02" is the mean value of Israel's 24/4 ratio in the group with Carcinoma Prostate. The mean value of "4.8 ± 2.5" was found in benign bone lesions in Dr. V Siva's 4/24 retention ratio and "-0.06 ± 0.02" was the mean value of Israel's 24/4 ratio. The statistical values are estimated using the online "Social Sciences Statistics" calculator. The T value comes out to be 17.1 from the two independent values of the student T test. There was a significant result at $p < 0.05$ value and < 0.00001 is the p value. There was a significant outcome at $p < 0.05$ value. **Figure 3** illustrates the graphical calculation of dispersion and major difference between metastatic and benign lesions:

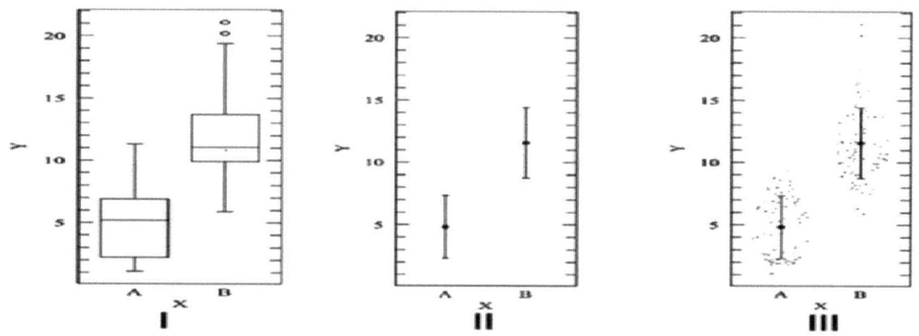

Figure 3.
The graphical representation of difference between A – Benign and B – Malignant lesions.

The Quantitative and non-invasive classification of "Skeletal Metastasis" with Tc99m MDP scans in Carcinoma prostate was presenting good values with Retention Ratio of Dr. V. Siva as per Serum PSA levels [20].

6. Evaluating pathological/non-healing fractures using scintimetry

The authors in [21] have documented the "Scintimetric" assessment of "delayed union of skeletal fractures". The retention values of 4/24 for all cases were characterized into benign fracture and metastatic fracture as per the scientometric classification of skeletal hot spots. Around 37% (11) were pathological fractures and 63% (19) were benign ones due to benign bone tumors and stress fracture out of 30 non-union/delayed skeletal fractures reported. Dr. V. Siva's 4/24 h retention ratio had 12.5 ± 3.1 of mean value for pathological group with typical estimation of ± 0.61 for errors and the error estimation (±0.38) was measured with mean value "6.68 ± 2.8" of benign group. The statistical calculation found a major difference between two values with <0.0001 of p value.

The authors in [22] also reported the comparative study of Scintimetric classification by the "Triple Phase Bone Scan" and Retention Ratio by Dr. V Siva in skeletal fracture as compared to the entire body counts. The authors in [23] also described the use cases of "scientometric classification of skeletal hotspots" also in a diagnostic facility.

7. Scintimetry in rheumatoid arthritis

The bone imaging of two-sided hands is helpful to determine the severity of afflictions in interphalangeal joints. The accumulation of delayed 24 h imaging of hands and quantitative retention ratio measurements was helpful. The authors in [24] also published a groundwork report on Scintimetric assessment of the involvement of rheumatoid arthritis by retention ratio of Dr. V Siva. The mean of "5.91 ± 0.35" was found in the maximum counts of skeletal zones of patients in 3 h and 24 h scans as well as the 4/24 h ratio with means of 0.3496 in standard error. The 8.8408 was the estimated variance and 2.9734 was the standard and estimated deviation. The 6.6306 was the estimated variance for the sample size and 2.575 was the standard estimated deviation by modification from HOJO. The sample population was very small and it was totally unavoidable. It opens further research paths on a global scale.

8. Diastolic dysfunction assessment, characterization and identification

The left ventricle has the diastolic function that plays an important role in efficacy and preservation of left systolic ventricular function. Hence, there have been a lot of concerns on determining the "Left Ventricular Diastolic function" as well as the management and detection of left heart failure. The "M-mode echocardiography" is usually taken to evaluate the same at the mitral valve orifice with "E/A ratio" tracing. The "Left Ventricular Diastolic function" Stage I is represented by <0.8 of E/A ratio, Stage II by >1.4, and Stage III by >1.8 [25, 26]. The tissue characterization and "Color Doppler echocardiography" are the methods to refine these parameters [27].

The advancement of studies related to "ECG-Gated SPECT" has given great insights for its evaluation. The visual insights to "Regional Wall Motion Abnormalities" and "Ejection Fraction" with "Gated SPECT Myocardial Perfusion Studies" are widely used and popular. However, it is still important to explore

DOI: http://dx.doi.org/10.5772/intechopen.99065

the portal to extract and analyze vital info from the analysis of "Phase image" of systolic and diastolic phases in cardiac cycle. After the use of "Gated SPECT Myocardial Perfusion Imaging" described by Morgan and Mannting [28] in the year 1993, Raymond Taillefer et al. [29] explained the "Diastolic image analysis" and its utility in early diagnosis of C.A.D. among women over "Summed Image Analysis" in the year 1999.

A "Gated SPECT Perfusion Processing" protocol has been developed by Siemens on the basis of Depuey et al. [30] who have covered individual image analysis in "Ejection fraction calculation", "Diastole and Systole", and "Regional Wall Thickness". With "phase image analysis" in processing of "Gated SPECT Perfusion", the "Irregular, In-homogenous, and Insufficient Tracer distribution" incidence is inferred having regular, homogenous and even tracer distribution in summed scans to show diastolic dysfunction. The "SNMICON" presentation [31] also highlights the association with the markers of "echocardiographic diastolic dysfunction", especially "Diabetes Mellitus and Hypertension" and E/A ratio.

The ideal correlation between S/D ratio and rate of Peak flow is estimated by considering the "Time Volume" curves that are obtained from E/A ratio and ECG-gated SPECT [32]. The "Time To Peak Flow" and "Peak Flow Rate" are the parameters of diastolic dysfunction. Their normal values have been documented to determine diastolic function with total agreement between "Echocardiographic assessment and QGSPECT" using 16-frame "99mTc-Sestamibi Gated Myocardial Perfusion SPECT" [33]. According to RD Lele et al., diastolic dysfunction was 92/121 (76) and "echocardiographic E/A ratio" detected only 53/121 (43%) [29]. The common individual risk factor was "Left Ventricular Hypertrophy (LVH)" with heavy risk related to unfavorable results [34, 35]. Some of the major causes are hypertension and hypertrophic cardiomyopathy (HCM) [36] and aortic stenosis, obesity, and chronic kidney problems are responsible for the thickness of the left LV wall [37–40].

There were 75 males aged 31 to 67 years participated in a study to evaluate the left "ventricular diastolic dysfunction" with average age of 51.9 ± 7.4 years and there were 25 females from 31 to 55 years with mean 45.9 ± 6.6 years of mean age. The patients using "Thallum-201 Bruce protocol 2-mCi" on a treadmill were injected after exercise with "Gated SPECT MPI" through IV. They were equipped with E-Cam Dual Head Gamma cam by Siemens. The "Gated SPECT PERFUSION ANALYSIS" protocol was used by the ICON software to analyze the images. The irregular, in-homogenous and insufficient tracer distribution was found in diastolic phase scans instead of usual Systolic phase scans. These images show changes in diastolic dysfunction in "left ventricular muscle tissue" (**Figure 4**).

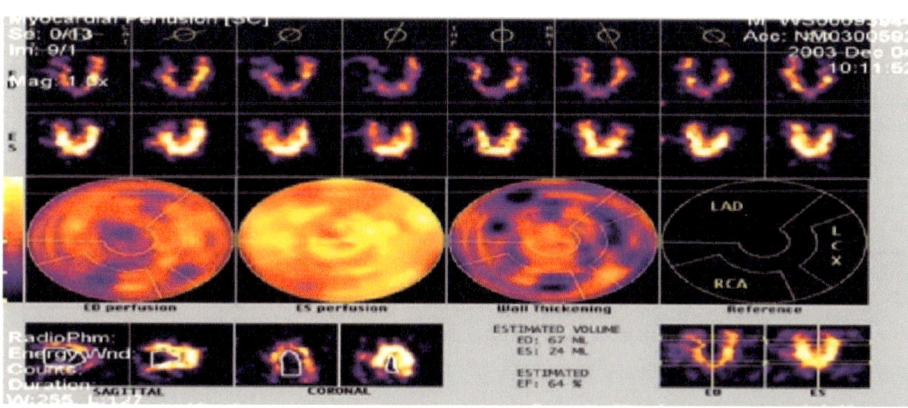

Figure 4.
Diastolic images – Upper row, systolic images middle row, Bull's eye maps third row.

The images on the upper row show diastolic phase in various angles. These scans show in-homogenous, constantly decreased, irregular, and insufficient distribution of tracer, which indicate perfusion absence. The images on the lower row of the systolic phase illustrate stable and normal tracer distribution. In this study, the discordance between systolic and diastolic phases has been displayed and it is related to straight changes because of diastolic dysfunction in the "left ventricular muscle mass". These images display Bull's eye map assessment and 'left ventricular ejection fraction' of the end systolic perfusion, end diastolic perfusion, and wall thickening. The systolic and diastolic phases are described in the images on the lower and upper row, respectively. The bull's eye map of "diastolic phase ED perfusion" describes affliction from moderate to severe levels as per the ES perfusion on systolic phase and color scale that displays color and normal scale. The left ventricular ejection which is calculated from the "end systolic ES volumes" and derived end diastolic ED" is normal.

The research findings have been noted as below. The researchers have tabulated the echocardiographic grading of "left ventricular diastolic dysfunction" apart from the findings given above. They saved the scan data of systolic and diastolic pictures in H.L.A., S.A., and V.L.A. views. The inner and outer margins are drawn by the "ventricular wall outline" in the systolic and diastolic phase and counts were calculated in the area of interest with the ICON software's region ratio count protocol (**Figure 5**).

The S/D ratio was used to tabulate the diastolic and systolic counts in female and male patients in this study. We also analyzed the S/D ratios of diastolic dysfunction stage II and Stage III individually. We found the discordance between systolic and diastolic pictures in 98/100 (98%). The Grade II and Grade III classify the echocardiographic images of this disorder with E/A ratio in 87/100 (87%). Similarly, hypertension was reported in 63% and diabetes in only 16%. There was no major statistical change in S/D ratio between both groups (**Figure 6**).

The Grade II LVDD has 1.47 ± 0.32 of S/D ratio and Grade III LVDD has 1.81 ± 0.03 of S/D ratio. With "Paired Student t-test", the statistical data found a major difference between Stage II and Stage III in S/D ratio (**Figure 7**).

The visual analysis of the images of systolic and diastolic phases led to interpretation and identification of heart's "Left ventricular diastolic dysfunction". This method identified 98% (98/100) people with this condition. On the other hand, the E/A echocardiographic test detected only 87% of patients. The direct changes

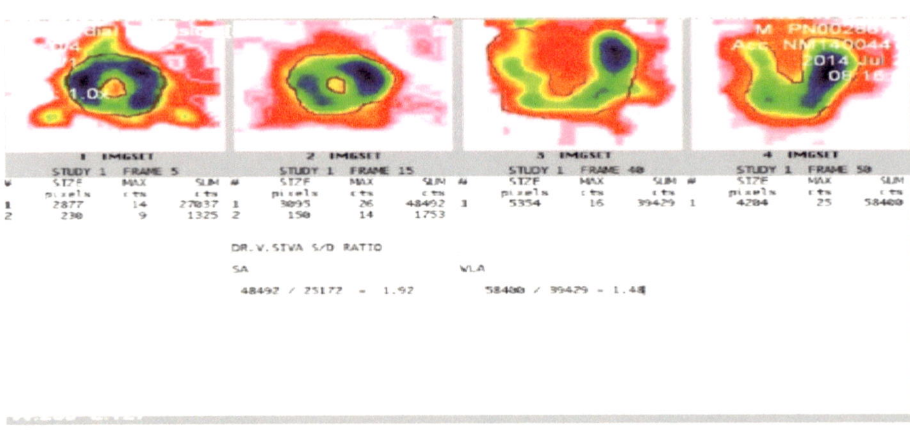

Figure 5.
Scintimetric method of calculating Distolic and systolic for deriving S/D ratio.

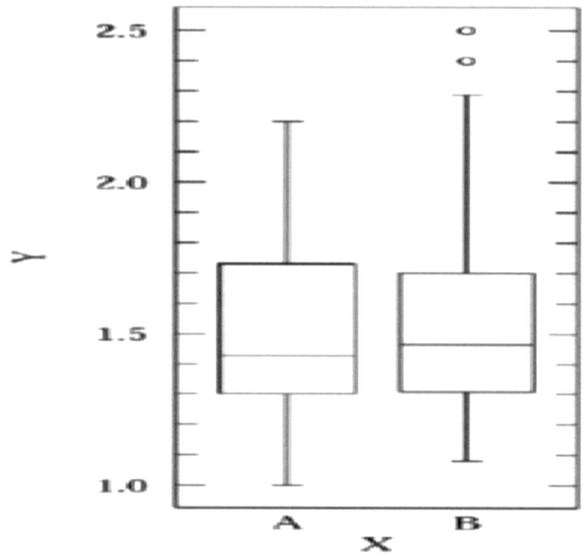

Figure 6.
No difference between A-male and B-female scintimetric S/D values.

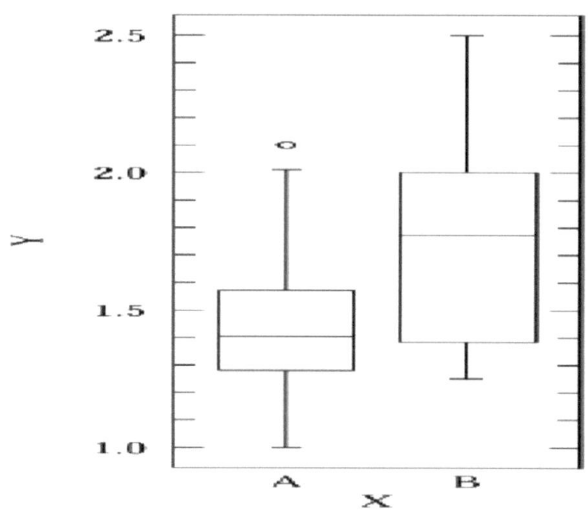

Figure 7.
Significant difference between A-stage II and B-stage III scintimetric S/D values.

in "Left ventricular cardiac myocytes" base the visual analysis to diagnose diastolic dysfunction. Hence, they could detect 98% of cases with diastolic dysfunction. RD Lele et al. [34] detected only 76% (92/121) cases with diastolic heart function by using "16-Gated Myocardial Perfusion SPECT" and "time volume curve" analysis.

On the other side, diastolic dysfunction is detected in 98% patients with "direct visual image interpretative assessment" of systolic and diastolic phases. However, there is a need to extend this study further to all the rest of "Gated SPECT" research for a large number of patients. It is also important to contemplate the separated comparison of ES and ED perfusions in both rest and stress gated myocardial imaging results. Along with it, the normal population should also be included as this study group covered only patients.

9. Scintimetric characterization of primary tumors by dual phase PETCT study

The utility and advantage of the dual phase PETCT evaluation in the tumor detection was reported by Kuboto K et al. [41]. The optimal time interval between the early and delayed phase PETCT scans had been proved to be 3 hr. post injection by Chen YM et al. [42]. In our study protocol the delayed PETCT was conducted at 4 hours post injection due to logistic reasons. Rong et al. reported a quantitative estimation to differentiate between the benign and malignant bone lesions using the dual phase PETCT evaluation termed as Rong's Retention Index [43]. The Rong's retention index (RRI), computed as follows:

$$\text{RRI} = (\text{SUVmaxD-SUVmaxE})\text{X } 100 \qquad (2)$$

Even though there is a noticeable difference between the malignant and benign bone lesions, they also have a major overlap in between.

$$\text{Dr.V.Siva's modified Retention ratio} = \text{SUV max Delayed} / \text{SUV max Early X } 100 \qquad (3)$$

We have focused on the clinical and technical aspects of a novel method in this oncologic utility of "Positron Emission Tomography (PET)". In this method, the PET scanner is combined with a CT scanner in a single device [44–47].

In May 2019, this study was conducted among 19 patients aged 9 to 76 years (12 females, 7 males) with a median of 46 ± 18 years with active primary and metabolically lesions of several types of cancers. Permission was taken from each volunteer before they joined the study for delayed 4 h PET/CT scan without injecting F18-FDG any further. The protocol of "F-18 FDG PET image reconstruction and acquisition" was approved by the ethics group and all cases have obtained official consent.

Patients did not drink or eat anything for 4 to 6 hours before IV injection of "F-18 FDG (185 to 375 MBq, i.e. 4 MBq/kg of weight of the body)". Before getting injected, patients received the concentration of serum glucose and all patients had glucose levels below 200 mg/dl. After the injection at 1 hour early and PET/CT scans at 4 hour (delayed) after injection with PET/CT scanner (from PETCT and Wipro GE), the patients settled down in a silent room. The Spiral CT was used for acquiring CT image at 0.75 s per rotation with 4 mm of section thickness, 4 mm of interval, and 40mAs and 120 kVp.

No IV contrast injection was used. We obtained the early images of PET emission from thigh to cranium, usually with 6–7 positions with acquisition of 2 minutes in each bed position. We acquired the images of delayed PET emission of abnormal spots at 4 h after F-18 FDG injection, with 2 minutes of interval between 2 to 3 bed positions. We used the LOR algorithm to reconstruct all PET scans while applying CT-based correction of attenuation. We used the "Advantage 4.7 Volume Viewer"program to obtain the images. The F-18 FDG uptake was evaluated with delayed and early PET images, evaluation of parameters and interpretation of PET image, semi quantitatively. A circular ROI was positioned above the detected bone lesion for semi-quantitative analysis with transverse PET picture.

The ROI was positioned above the whole "F18 FDG lesion" for visualized lesions on PET, including utmost radioactivity. The following formula was used to estimate the "Standardized Uptake Value":

$$\text{"SUV} = \text{tissue concentration}\left(MBq/\text{g}\right)/\left[\text{injected dose}\left(MBq\right)/\text{body weight}\left(\text{g}\right)\text{"}$$

For each region of interest, the SUVmax or maximal SUV was calculated in lesion ROI. The variations in the lesions' uptake were measured as retention index:

$$\text{“RI} = (\text{SUVmaxD} - \text{SUVmaxE}) \times 100 / \text{SUVmaxE”} \quad (4)$$

Here is the formula to calculate RRI modification by Dr. V. Siva:

$$\text{“RRI} = \text{SUVmaxD} / \text{SUVmaxE} \times 100\text{”} \quad (5)$$

The dual time point based quantifications of metabolic uptake rate in 18F-FDG PET had been reported by den Hoff et al. [48]. The potential diagnostic role of dual phase 18F-FDG PETCT scanning was reported by Jones c et al. [49]. This is the first study reporting the findings of the dual phase PETCT in the evaluation and characterization in various primary lesions. The Rong's Retention values showed a wide ranging value and no definite cut off value could be arrived at. But Dr. V. Siva's modification of Rong's Retention Ratio revealed that the cut off value to be 100 and above for confirming the malignant nature of the lesions. The statistical evaluation of the values by Student t Test showed good p value confirming the significance that the two values were significantly different. There is a strong positive correlation in the "Pearson evaluation". It means a high y variable with high x scores and vice versa (**Figure 8**). The inclusion of the various primary malignancies in both the sexes adds advantage to the study. However the non-inclusion of primary benign lesions in the study is the greatest disadvantage. The other limitations being the single institutional study and the small number of patient population.

Scintimetric Characterization of metastatic lymph nodes in various primary malignancies by Dual Phase PETCT study.

In the proven cases of various primary malignancies like Ca. Breast, Ca. Prostate, Lymphomas and alveolar tumors the SUV max values of the metastatic lymph nodes were calculated in both the Early and Delayed phase scans. The PETCT study was performed using the GE Discovery IQ PETCT in those patients with positive lymph node uptake. The early scan was done One hour post injection of 5 to 10 mCi of F18-FDG tracer in the fasting state with their informed consent with optimal serum blood

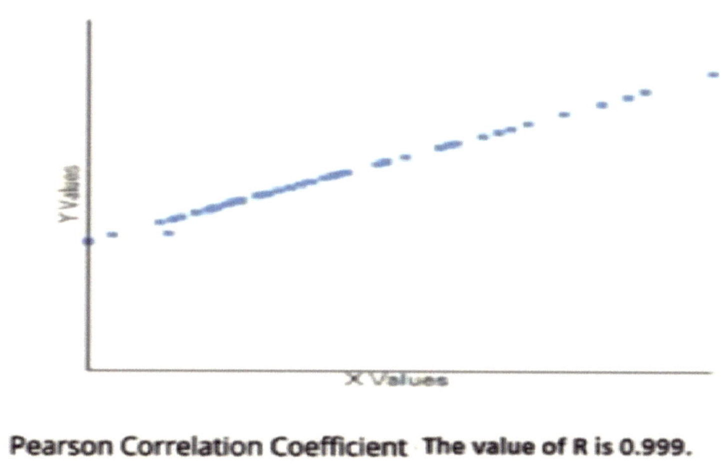

Figure 8.
Pearson correlation coefficient test.

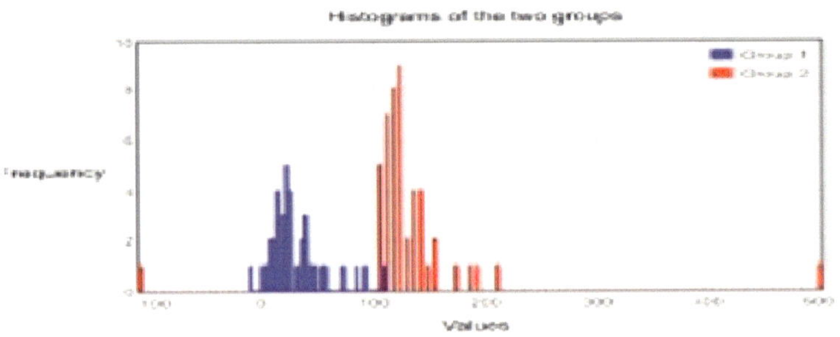

Figure 9.
The difference between group 1 Rong's ratio group 2 Dr. V. Siva's modification.

sugar level of 150 mg/dl. The delayed PETCT was done Four hours after the post injection time with voluntary consent of the patients without any additional injection of the tracer or contrast medium. The SUV max values were obtained utilizing the Advantage 4.4 software provided by the GE. Total of Forty eight lymph nodes at various locations were included in the study. The calculated SUV max values were used to arrive at the Rong's Retention Ratio and the Dr. V. Siva's modification of RRI.

The Rong's retention ratio in the Metastatic lymph nodes group showed the mean value of 37.2 ± 17.0. Dr. V. Siva's modification of the Rong's Ratio showed the mean value of 132.7 ± 19.8. The Dr. V. Siva'a modification of Rong's Retention ratio resulted in the increase in value by 100 with no significant overlap.

In the previous study of dual PETCT scintimentric characterization of the various primary malignancies the Rong's Retention ratio showed the mean value of 35.8 ± 8 and the Dr. V. Siva's modification of RRI showed the mean value of 135 ± 8.1 as reported confirming that the definitive cut of value of 100 and above could be assigned to indicate the malignant and metastatic lesions in the Dual Phase PETCT scans in the Dr. V. Siva's modification method. By eliminating the subtraction of early SUV max value from the delayed SUV max value the negative values were avoided. The statistical analysis of the data using student t test evaluation showed that there is clear cut demarcation between the original Rong's Retention Ratio values and the Dr. V. Siva's modification of Rong's Ratio as shown in the **Figure 9**.

The p value is < 0.0001 indicating the validity of Dr. V. Siva's modification of Rong's Ratio in the Scintimetric characterization of the metastatic lymph nodes of various primary cancers. However the homogeneous population of cancer patients and non-inclusion of the benign lymph nodal enlargement is a definitive limitation of this study. Further evaluation of this concept is warranted as this is a single institutional study of short duration and small number of cases.

10. Conclusions

The Scintimetric Characterization of the skeletal hot spots helps in the differentiation of benign and malignant lesions that might coexist in a carcinoma prostate patient and treat them accordingly. This has been proved to be useful in the assessment of non healing fractures and pathological fractures as well. The usefulness of this in the evaluation of Rheumatoid Arthritis opens up a new era of research on clinical utilization in both the diagnostic and prognostic aspects of the disease process. The identification and characterization of the diastolic dysfunction directly by applying the Systolic/Diastolic count ration in the gated SPECT myocardial viability studies remains to be explored further.

The advent and quantification of FDG uptake in a hot spot in the Dual Phase PETCT scan helps in the identification and differentiation of various primary malignant processes and the Metastatic involvement of the lymph nodes. The clinical application of the quantitative indices like the Israel's ratio, Dr. V. Siva's retention ratio in the conventional nuclear medicine studies must see the light of clinical utilization of day to day practice. Similarly in the case of PETCT evaluation of Oncology the utilization of the Rong's retention ratio and the Dr. V. Siva's modification of Rong's Ratio should reach the daily practice mode from the bench [50–52].

11. Future perspectives

In the current era of large volume Data handling and DATAMATIC scenario this quantitative approach will be more suitable for the QBOT establishment for qualitative standardization of the Nuclear Medicine studies [53]. These quantitative indices can be incorporated into the automatic report generation aspect of the Artificial Intelligence in Nuclear medicine as reported by Cumali Aktolun and Felix Nensa [54, 55]. The recent explosion in DATA sciences and ARTIFICIAL INTELLIGENCE provide a new arena worth exploring in the future.

Conflict of interest

The authors declare no conflict of interest.

Notes/thanks

The authors express their gratitude and fervent references at the divine lotus feet of Bhagawan Sri Sathya Sai Baba varu with whose sole blessings alone this work had become a reality.

Author details

V. Sivasubramaniyan[1,2]* and K. Venkataramaniah[1]

1 Department of Physics, Sri Sathya Sai Institute of Higher Learning, Puttaparthi, Andhra Pradesh, India

2 Department of Nuclear Medicine, Sri Aurobindo Institute of Medical Sciences, Indore, Madhya Pradesh, India

*Address all correspondence to: drvssm@gmail.com

References

[1] Rosenthall L, Kaye M (1975) Technetium 99m pyrophosphate kinetics and imaging inmetabolic bone disease. J Nucl Med 16:33-39.

[2] Lentle BC, Russell AS, Percy JS, Jackson FI (1977) The scintigraphic investigation of sacroiliac disease J Nucl Med 18:529-533.

[3] Condon BR, Buchanan R, Garvie NW et al (1981) Assessment of secondary bone lesionsfollowing cancer of the breast or prostate using serial radionucleide imaging. Br. J Radiol 54:18-23.

[4] Vellenga CJLR, Pauwels EKJ, Bijvoet OLM (1984) Comparison between visual assessment and quantitative measurement of radioactivity on the bone scintigram in Paget's disease of bone. Eur J Nucl Med 9:533-537.

[5] Pfeifer JP, Hill W, Bull U, Burkhardt R, Kirsch CM (1983) Improvement of bone scintigraphy by quantitative evaluation compared with X-ray studies and iliaccrest biopsy in malignant disease. Eur J Nucl Med 8: 342-345.

[6] Constable AR, Cranage RW (1980) Recognition of superscan in prostatic bone scintigraphy. Br J Radiol 54: 122-125.

[7] Hardy JG, Kulatilake AE, Wastie ML (1980) An index for monitoring bone metastases from carcinoma of the prostate. Br J Radiol 53: 869-873.

[8] Mendiok H, Rapoport A, Oreopoulos DG, Rabinovich S, Meema HF, Meema S (1985) Quantitative radionucleide scanning in metabolic bone disease. Nucl Med Comm 6: 141-148.

[9] Israel O, Front D, Frenkel A, Kleinhaus U (1985) 24 hour/4 hour ratio of technetium 99mmethylene diphosphonate uptake in patients with bone metastases and degenerative bonechanges. J Nucl Med 26: 237-240.

[10] V. Sivasubramaniyan and K. Venkataramaniah, Temporal Scintimetric Characterizationof Skeletal Hotspots in Bone Scan by Dr. V. Siva's Retention Ratio S.C. Satapathy et al. (eds.), Information Systems Design and Intelligent Applications, Advances in Intelligent Systems and Computing 433, DOI 10.1007/978-81-322-2755-7_31

[11] Langsteger W, Haim S, Knauer M, Waldenberger P, Emmanuel K, Loidl W, Wolf I, Beheshti M. Imaging of bone metastases in prostate cancer: An update. Q J Nucl Med Mol Imaging. 2012 Oct; 56(5):447-458.

[12] Brian C. Lentle, M.D., F.R.C.P. (C); Anthony S. Russell, M.B., F.R.C.P (C); John S. Percy, M.D., F.R.C.P. (Edin) (C); John R. Scott, M.Sc.; and Frank I. Jackson, M.B., C.R.C.P. (C) Bone Scintiscanning Updated. (Ann Intern Med. 1976; 84(3):297-303. doi:10.7326/0003-4819-84-3-297.

[13] Batson OV: The function of the vertebral veins and their role in the spread of metastases. Clin Orthop Relat Res 312: 4-9, 1995.

[14] Paget S: The distribution of secondary growths in cancer of the breast. Cancer Metastasis Rev 8: 98-101, 1989.

[15] Masuda H, Fukabori Y, Nakano K, Takezawa Y, T CS and Yamanaka H: Increased expressionof bone morphogenetic protein-7 in bone metastatic prostate cancer. Prostate 54: 268-274, 2003.

[16] De Pinieux G, Flam T, Zerbib M, Taupin P, Bellahcene A, Waltregny D, Vieillefond A and Poupon MF: Bone

sialoprotein, bone morphogenetic protein 6 and thymidine phosphorylaseexpression in localized human prostatic adenocarcinoma as predictors of clinical outcome: Aclinicopathological and immunohistochemical study of 43 cases. J Urol 166: 1924-1930, 2001.

[17] Shariat SF, Shalev M, Menesses-Diaz A, Kim IY, Kattan MW, Wheeler TM and Slawin KM: Preoperative plasma levels of transforming growth factor beta(1) (TGF-beta(1)) stronglypredict progression in patients undergoing radical prostatectomy. J Clin Oncol 19: 2856-2864, 2001.

[18] Klaus Strobel, Cyrill Burger, Burkhardt Seifert, Daniela B. Husarik, Jan D. Soyka1, Thomas F. Hany Characterization of Focal Bone Lesions in the Axial Skeleton: Performanceof Planar Bone Scintigraphy Compared with SPECT and SPECT Fused with CT AJR: 188, 467-474, May 2007.

[19] Lehr JE and Pienta KJ: Preferential adhesion of prostate cancer cells to a human bone marrowendothelial cell line. J Natl Cancer Inst 90: 118-123, 1998.

[20] Sivasubramaniyan V* and Venkataramaniah K, Non-invasive Quantitative Characterization of Skeletal Metastasis in Carcinoma Prostate by Tc99m MDP Bone Scans Using Dr. V. Siva's Retention Ratio in Correlation with Serum PSA Levels, Med Surg Urol Volume 5 Issue 2 1000164

[21] Rahul Namdeo, Dr. V. Sivasubramaniyan, Dr. K. Vijaya Sai, Dr. K. Venkataramaniah Scintimetric Evaluation in the Assessment of Delayed Union of Skeletal Fractures, International Journal of Innovative Research and Development, www.ijird.com July, 2015 Vol 4 Issue 8.

[22] Sivasubramaniyan n, Venkataramaniah K, Comparative Evaluation of the role of Scintimetric Characterization by Dr. V. Siva'sRetention Ratio and the Triple Phase Bone Scan in the Skeletal Fracture Assessment. J Trauma Treat 7: 421. doi:10.4172/2167-1222.1000421,2018.

[23] Sivasubramaniyan V. K Venkataramaniah. Scintimetric Characterization of Skeletal Hotspots by Dr. V. Siva's Retention Ratio in A Diagnostic Referral Center. Biomed J Sci and Tech Res 6(5)2018. BJSTR. MS.ID.001420. DOI: 10.26717/BJSTR.2018.06.001420.

[24] Sivasubramaniyan V and Venkataramaniah K, Scintimetric Evaluation of the Rheumatoid Arthritis Involvement by Dr. V. Siva's Retention Ratio-(Preliminary Report). J Arthritis 6: 231. doi:10.4172/2167-7921.1000231 2017.

[25] Sherif F. Nagueh, Christopher P. Appleton, Thierry C. Gillebert, Paolo N. Marino, Jae K. Oh, Otto A. Smiseth, Alan D. Waggoner, Frank A. Flachskampf, Patricia A. Pellikka, Arturo Evangelisa. Recommendations for the evaluation of left ventricular diastolic function by echocardiography – Houston, Texas; Phoenix, Arizona; Ghent, Belgium; Novara, Italy; Rochester, Minnesota; Oslo, Norway; St. Louis, Missouri; European Journal of Echocardiography. 2009;10:165-193.

[26] Thomas Mathew, Rick Steeds, Richard Jones, Prathap Kanagala, Guy Lloyd, Daniel Knight, KevinO' Gallagher, David Oxborough, Bushra Rana, Liam Ring, Julie Sandoval, Gill Whart, Richard Wheeler. A guideline protocol for the echocardiographic assessment of diastolic dysfunction. Published November; 2013.

[27] Juan Lacalzada, et al. Evaluation of left ventricular diastolic function by echocardiography. Hospital Universitario de Canarias, La Laguna, Santa Cruz de Tenerife Chapter 6,

Establishing Better Standards of Care in Doppler Echocardiography, Computed Tomography and Nuclear Cardiology Edited by Dr. Richard M. Fleming; 2011.

[28] Morgan MG, Mannting F, et al. Gated SPECT with Tc99m SESTAMIBI for assessment of myocardial perfusion abnormalities. JNM. 1993;21:13.

[29] Raymond Taillefer, Gordon Dupey E, et al. Comparison between end diastolic and the summed images of gated Tc99m MIBI SPECT in the detection of C.a.D in women. JNC; 1999.

[30] Depuey EG, Nicholas K, et al. Left ventricular ejection fraction assessed from gated Tc99m sestamibi SPECT. JNM. 1993;34.

[31] Sivasubramaniyan V, Dash PK, Iyer VR, Prasad RD, Purantharan N. Role of gated SPECT myocardial perfusion imaging in the evaluation of diastolic dysfunction of the heart oral. Paper Presentation Session 1 (Parallel) (Cardio Vascular System) Abstracts of SNMICON; 2003.

[32] Ichiro Nakae, Shinro Matsuo, Terue Koh, Kenichi Mitsunami, Minoru Horie. Left ventricular systolic/diastolic function evaluated by quantitative ECG-gated SPECT: Comparison with echocardiography and plasma BNP analysis. Annals of Nuclear Medicine. 2005;19(6):447-454.

[33] Cigdem Akincioglu, Daniel S. Berman, Hidetaka Nishina, Paul B. Kavanagh, Piotr J. Slomka, Aiden Abidov, Sean Hayes, John D. Friedman, Guido Germano. Assessment of diastolic function using 16Frame 99mTc-Sestamibi gated myocardial perfusion SPECT: Normal values. J Nucl Med. 2005;46:1102-1108.

[34] Lele KarunaLuthra, Yogini Sawant. Assessment of diastolic heart function – Experience with 16-gated myocardial perfusion SPECT RD. JAPI. 2008;56:763-767.

[35] Vakili BA, Okin PM, Devereux RB. Prognostic implications of left ventricular hypertrophy. American Heart Journal. 2001;141(3):334-341.

[36] Agabiti-Rosei E, Muiesan ML. Left ventricular hypertrophy and heart failure in women. Journal of Hypertension. Supplement: Official Journal of the International Society of Hypertension. 2002;20(2):S34.

[37] Torpy JM, Lynm C, Glass RM. JAMA patient page. JAMA. 2010;303(15).

[38] Woodiwiss AJ, Norton GR. Obesity and left ventricular hypertrophy: The hypertension connection. Current Hypertension Reports. 2015;17(4):28.

[39] Di Lullo L, Gorini A, Russo D, Santoboni A, Ronco C. Left ventricular hypertrophy in chronic kidney disease patients: From pathophysiology to treatment. Cardiorenal Medicine. 2015;5(4):254-266.

[40] Shah AS, Chin CW, Vassiliou V, Cowell SJ, Doris M, Kwok TN, Semple S, Zamvar V, White AC, McKillop G, Boon NA. Left ventricular hypertrophy with strain and aortic stenosis. Circulation. 2014;130(18):1607-1616.

[41] Tsai SY, Wang SY, Shiau YC, Wu YW. Mechanical dyssynchrony and diastolic dysfunction are common in LVH: A pilot correlation study using Doppler echocardiography and CZT gated-SPECT MPI. Scientific Reports. 2018;8(1):1-2.

[42] Kubota K, Itoh M, Ozaki K, et al. Advantage of delayed whole-body FDG-PET imaging for tumour detection. Eur J. Nucl Med. 2001;28:696-703.

[43] Chen YM, Huang G, Sun XG, et al. Optimizing delayed scan time for FDG

PET: Comparison of the early and late delayed scan. Nucl Med Commun. 2008;29:425-430.

[44] Rong Tian, Minggang Su, Ye Tian, Fanglan Li, Lin Li, Anren Kuang, Jiancheng Zeng. Dual-time point PET/CT with F-18 FDG for the differentiation of malignant and benign bone lesions. Skeletal Radiol. 2009;38:451-458.

[45] Griffeth LK. Use of PET/CT scanning in cancer patients: Technical and practical considerations. In Baylor University Medical Center proceedings. Taylor and Francis. 2005;18(4):321-330.

[46] Sachpekidis C, Thieke C, Askoxylakis V, Nicolay NH, Huber PE, Thomas M, Dimitrakopoulou G, Debus J, Haberkorn U, Dimitrakopoulou-Strauss A. Combined use of 18F-FDG and 18F-FMISO in unresectable non-small cell lung cancer patients planned for radiotherapy: A dynamic PET/CT study. American Journal of Nuclear Medicine and Molecular Imaging. 2015;5(2):127.

[47] Li K, Sun H, Guo Q. Combinative evaluation of primary tumor and lymph nodes in predicting pelvic lymphatic metastasis in early-stage cervical cancer: A multiparametric PET-CT study. European Journal of Radiology. 2019;113:153-157.

[48] Du S, Sun H, Gao S, Xin J, Lu Z. Metabolic parameters with different thresholds for evaluating tumor recurrence and their correlations with hematological parameters in locally advanced squamous cell cervical carcinoma: An observational 18F-FDG PET/CT study. Quantitative Imaging in Medicine and Surgery. 2019;9(3):440.

[49] den Hoff J, Hofheinz F, Oehme L, et al. Dual time point based quantification of metabolic uptake rates in 18F-FDG PET. EJNMMI Res. 2013;3:1-6.

[50] Jones C, Badger S, Lynch T. A potential diagnostic role of dual phase 18F-FDG PET/CT scanning. Ulster Med J. 2014;83:52-54.

[51] Dr. V. Sivasubramaniyan, Sai Shivnarayan, Dr. K. Venkataramaniah, Scintimetric Characterization of Primary Tumors by Dual Phase PETCT study, INDIAN JOURNAL OF APPLIED RESEARCH, Feb. 2020. Volume 10/ Issue 2/61-62

[52] Dr. V. Sivasubramaniyan, Dr. Vinod Bhandari, Dr. K. Venkataramaniah, Scintimetric Characterization of metastatic lymph nodes in various primary malignancies by Dual Phase PETCT study, MODERN APPLIED MEDICAL RESEARCH 1(1): 01-03

[53] Nagy et al. EJNMMI Physics (2021)8:2. doi:10.1186/ s40658-021-00371-w

[54] Cumali Aktolun, Artificial intelligence and radiomics in nuclear medicine: Potentials and challenges, European Journal of Nuclear Medicine and Molecular Imaging (2019) 46:2731-2273. doi:10.1007/s00259-019-04593-0

[55] Felix Nensa1, Aydin Demircioglu1, and Christoph Rischpler2, Artificial Intelligence in Nuclear Medicine, THE JOURNAL OF NUCLEAR MEDICINE Vol. 60 No. 9 (Suppl. 2) September 2019.

Chapter 5

Strategies for Site-Specific Radiolabeling of Peptides and Proteins

Ingrid Dijkgraaf, Stijn M. Agten, Matthias Bauwens and Tilman M. Hackeng

Abstract

Although anatomical imaging modalities (X-ray, computed tomography (CT), magnetic resonance imaging (MRI)) still have a higher spatial resolution (0.1–1 mm) than molecular imaging modalities (single-photon emission computed tomography (SPECT), positron emission tomography (PET), optical imaging (OI)), the advantage of molecular imaging is that it can detect molecular and cellular changes at the onset of a disease before it leads to morphological tissue changes, which can be detected by anatomical imaging. During the last decades, noninvasive diagnostic imaging has encountered a rapid growth due to the development of dedicated imaging equipment for preclinical animal studies. In addition, the introduction of multimodality imaging (PET/CT, SPECT/CT, PET/MRI) which combines high-resolution conventional anatomical imaging with high sensitivity of tracer-based molecular imaging techniques has led to successful accomplishments in this exciting field. In this book chapter, we will focus on chemical synthesis techniques for site-specific incorporation of radionuclide chelators. Subsequently, radiolabeling based on complexation of a radionuclide with a chelator will be discussed, with focus on: diethylenetriaminepentaacetic acid (DTPA), 1,4,7,10-tetraazacyclododecane-tetraacetic acid (DOTA), 1,4,7-triazacyclononane-triacetic acid (NOTA), hexa-histidine (His-tag), and 6-hydrazinonicotinic acid (HYNIC) that allow the production of peptides labeled with ^{18}F, ^{68}Ga, ^{99m}Tc, and ^{111}In – the currently most widely used isotopes.

Keywords: radiolabeled peptides, chelator, PET, SPECT, radionuclide, peptide synthesis, protein synthesis

1. Introduction

1.1 Application of peptides and proteins as molecular imaging agents

The concept of using radiolabeled receptor-binding peptides and proteins to target receptor-(over)expressing tissues *in vivo* has stimulated a large body of research in nuclear medicine. Peptides and small proteins for receptor imaging and targeted radiotherapy have particular advantages over antibodies and antibody fragments. Peptides are small molecules and show rapid diffusion in target tissue. They rapidly clear from the blood and non-target tissues, resulting in high target-to-background ratios. Furthermore, peptides have a low toxicity and are generally not immunogenic. However, ubiquitously occurring amino- and carboxypeptidases in the circulation will rapidly degrade most peptides preventing intact imaging agents to reach the target tissue in sufficient quantities. Thus, to prevent rapid enzymatic degradation of peptide-based imaging agents, most peptides have to be modified [1, 2]. Several methods to prevent enzymatic peptide proteolysis have been developed, including substitution of L- by D-amino acids, replacement of amino moieties by imino groups, substitution of peptide bonds, insertion of unusual amino acids or side chains, amidation, cyclization, *C*-terminal amidation or reduction, *N*-terminal acylation or methylation, and use of peptidomimetics. Cyclization of peptides results not only in resistance to enzymatic degradation, it can also lead to conformationally more constrained compounds with enhanced receptor affinity and biological activity [1, 3].

Besides stability toward enzymes, lipophilicity is very important. The preferred route of clearance of a peptide-based radiopharmaceutical is via the kidneys. For targeting of tumors, cardiovascular diseases, and infections or inflammation, the lipophilicity of the compound should not be too high ($\log P < 1$) as lipophilic compounds result in non-specific binding and slower blood clearance via mainly the hepatobiliary route. In contrast, molecular imaging tracers that target brain diseases such as Alzheimer require a higher lipophilicity ($\log P > 1$) in order to cross the blood–brain barrier (BBB). Lipophilicity of molecular imaging tracers can be reduced by linking them to polyethylene glycol (PEG) chains, a technique called PEGylation. An alternative method to reduce lipophilicity of a tracer is attachment of carbohydrates, as this enhances the hydrophilicity, resulting in reduced hepatobiliary uptake, enhanced urinary excretion, and reduced nonspecific binding [4].

Furthermore, conjugation of chelators like DOTA (1,4,7,10-tetraazacyclododecane-tetraacetic acid), NOTA (1,4,7-triazacyclononane-triacetic acid), or DTPA (diethylenetriaminepentaacetic acid) also reduce the lipophilicity of an imaging agent. However, modification of a tracer by for example PEGylation, glycosylation or conjugation to a chelator, can also affect the affinity of a peptide for the receptor and thus the effectiveness of the radiotracer.

1.2 Introduction of bifunctional chelating agents (BFCAs) into the peptide or protein

A chelating agent will not only influence the hydrophilicity of a peptide or protein, but it will also increase the overall size of the radiotracer and thus the pharmacokinetics. To preserve biological activity and receptor-binding affinity, conjugation of a chelator must be performed at a site remote from the active and receptor-binding region of the tracer [5]. Total chemical protein synthesis enables single site-specific protein modification, which cannot be achieved through regular labeling methods of biologically obtained proteins. To prevent interference of the chelator with the active and receptor-binding region of the peptide, introduction of a linker may be necessary. These linkers (PEG chains, amino acids, aliphatic hydrocarbon chains, etc.) can be used as pharmacokinetic modifiers (PKMs) to adjust the pharmacokinetics of the probe.

Several acyclic and cyclic bifunctional chelators have been developed for both diagnostic and therapeutic applications (**Figure 1**). A bifunctional chelator is a molecule which can be covalently coupled to the targeting compound and has the ability to chelate a (radio)metal. The most widely used chelators are DTPA, DOTA, and NOTA or derivatives thereof. A chelator should effectively sequester the radionuclide in high-yields (quantitative) and with high stability. Unstable complexation of the radionuclide by the chelator can lead to trans-chelation of the radionuclide

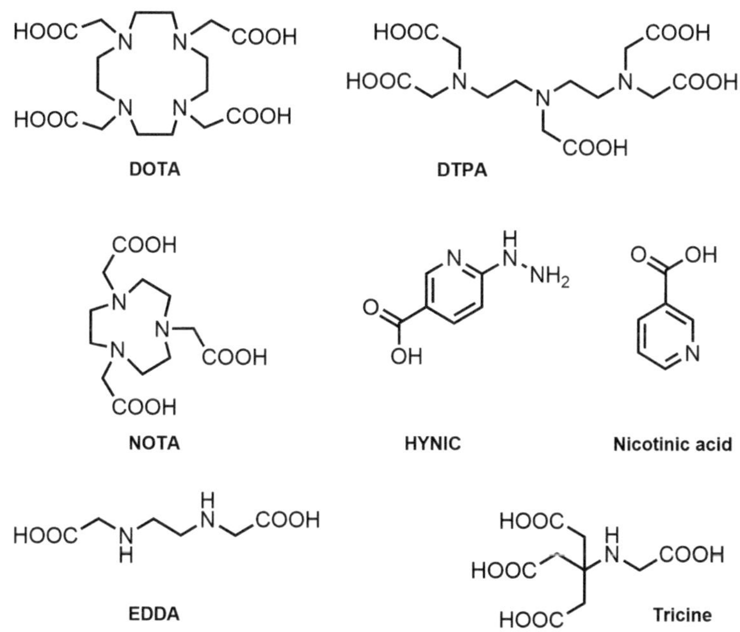

Figure 1.
Structural formula of different chelators and co-ligands for radiolabeling peptides and proteins.

to blood proteins and enzymes (e.g. transferrin, ceruloplasmin, superoxide dismutase). For a detailed review of chelating agents and the optimal match between chelator and radionuclide see Price *et al*. 2014 [6] and references therein.

The introduction of BFCA in proteins or peptides can be achieved using bioconjugation methods based on reactive functional groups, such as amide coupling (carboxylic acids and their activated *N*-hydroxysuccinimide (NHS) esters), thiol couplings (maleimides), oxime bond formation (ketones or aldehydes with aminooxy), and Cu(I) catalyzed azide-alkyne Huisgen 1,3-dipolar cycloaddition "click reactions". We will discuss some of the methods in detail in Section 2.3.

1.3 Radionuclide imaging

Apart from planar imaging, SPECT and PET are the two main imaging modalities in nuclear medicine. SPECT imaging is much more widely available than PET imaging and the radionuclides used for SPECT are easier to prepare, financially generally more accessible, and usually have a longer half-life than those used for PET (**Table 1**). Commonly used gamma emitters are: ^{123}I (E_{max} 529 keV, $t_{1/2}$ 13.0 h), ^{111}In (E_{max} 245 keV, $t_{1/2}$ 67.2 h), and ^{99m}Tc (E_{max} 141 keV, $t_{1/2}$ 6.02 h). Compared to SPECT, PET has the possibility to more accurately quantitate the *in vivo* concentration of a tracer labeled with a positron emitting radionuclide, such as for (pre)clinical applications ^{18}F (E_{max} 635 keV, $t_{1/2}$ 1.83 h), ^{68}Ga (E_{max} 1.90 MeV, $t_{1/2}$ 68.1 min), ^{64}Cu (657 keV, $t_{1/2}$ 12.7 h), and ^{124}I (E_{max} 2.13 MeV; 1.53 MeV; 808 keV, $t_{1/2}$ 4.18 days).

PET is independent of the location depth of the reporter probe of interest and is able to detect picomolar concentrations of tracer [7]. This high sensitivity of PET can only be matched to some degree by optical imaging (OI) techniques, but not by MRI, CT or ultrasound (US). In addition, compared to MRI and conventional optical imaging techniques, PET has the advantage of being quantitative. Though, with the introduction of fluorescence mediated tomography (FMT), quantitative measurements are also possible with OI techniques [8].

	Isotope	Half-life (h)	Decay type
γ-emitter (SPECT)	^{99m}Tc	6.02	IT
	^{111}In	67.2	EC, γ
	^{123}I	13.0	EC, γ, e^-
β^+-emitter (PET)	^{18}F	1.83	β^+, EC
	^{64}Cu	12.9	β^-, EC
	^{68}Ga	1.14	β^+, EC
	^{124}I	76.8	EC, β^+, γ
β^--emitter (therapy)	^{90}Y	64.1	β^-
	^{177}Lu	161	β^-
	^{186}Re	91	β^-, EC, γ
	^{188}Re	17.0	β^-
	^{131}I	192	β^-, γ, e^-

Half-life is given in hours, unless stated otherwise. β^- = negative beta decay, β^+ = positive beta decay, γ = gamma transition, IT = isometric transition, EC = electron capture.

Table 1.
Half-life and decay type of several radionuclides.

Recent developments also allow semi-quantitative measurements with SPECT, but these developments are not yet widespread and still show higher uncertainties compared to PET.

The spatial resolution of PET and SPECT scanners depends on several factors: the type of isotope (PET or SPECT), the energy of the isotope emissions, and the object being scanned. The type of isotope (positron-emitting or single-photon emitting) has a strong impact, as the image reconstruction techniques for PET are superior to those of SPECT due to physical characteristics in large objects, but this is reversed for small objects. The energy of the isotope emissions is negatively correlated to the spatial resolution: the stronger the energy, the poorer the spatial resolution. The object being scanned has a substantial impact: spatial resolution in mice is vastly superior to that in humans, and even within humans spatial resolution in obese people is worse compared to healthy subjects. Some typical spatial resolutions are: ^{99m}Tc, mouse: 0.5 mm; ^{99m}Tc, human: 10 mm; ^{18}F, mouse: 0.8 mm; ^{18}F, human: 2 mm; ^{68}Ga, human and mouse: both 4 mm. The spatial resolution should be taken into account when designing studies.

2. Peptide and protein synthesis

2.1 Protein production by expression systems

Nowadays, recombinant protein expression is a routine laboratory technology that enables fast and high-yield protein production. The choice of bacterial, yeast, insect or mammalian cellular-based expression system depends on several factors such as, cell growth characteristics, intracellular and extracellular expression, posttranslational modifications, and regulatory issues of proteins used as diagnostics and therapeutics. Recently, even cell-free expression systems using purified RNA polymerase, ribosomes, tRNA and ribonucleotides have been developed [9]. Each expression system has its particular advantages and disadvantages that are relevant for the purpose of use. Several review papers give a good description of the variety of expression systems and their pros and cons. However, for development of target-specific radiotracers, fluorescent probes, or multimodality molecular imaging agents, chemical protein synthesis is the method of choice because of reasons described below. Therefore, this book chapter does not cover recombinant expression systems further.

2.2 Solid-phase peptide synthesis

Total chemical protein synthesis is an attractive alternative to biological protein production. Chemical peptide synthesis can be divided in: (I) liquid-phase peptide synthesis and (II) solid-phase peptide synthesis. Liquid-phase peptide synthesis is a classical approach to peptide synthesis and since the beginning of the 20th century this technique has developed considerably. Although liquid-phase peptide synthesis has some limitations due to its time consuming nature, solubility issues and the need for lengthy purification procedures, it is still useful for large-scale peptide production and for specialized laboratory applications [10].

Solid-phase peptide synthesis (SPPS) is currently the preferential technique to establish access to synthetic peptides. The general process for SPPS is based on sequential addition of α-amino and reactive side chain protected amino acids to a solid support (resin). The *C*-terminal residue is coupled to the resin and after removal of the N^{α}-protecting group, the next *C*-terminally activated N^{α}-protected amino acid is coupled and so on, until full chain assembly is reached. The most commonly used N^{α}-protecting groups are the acid-labile Boc (*tert*-butyloxycarbonyl) group and the base-labile Fmoc (9-fluorenylmethoxycarbonyl) group. Side chain protecting groups are ideally orthogonal to the N^{α}-protecting group, which means that they are removable under completely different reaction conditions.

The use of synthetic chemistry allows infinite variation of the polypeptide chain by for example incorporation of unnatural amino acids such as β-amino acids, *N*-methyl amino acids, peptoids, stable isotope-labeled amino acids, and D-amino acids. Furthermore, the use of orthogonal amino acid side chain protecting groups during the sequential elongation of the peptide chain in SPPS, allows conjugation of fluorescent tags, chelators, biotin, etc., at single specific sites. Current optimized SPPS chemistry protocols enable effective peptide synthesis of 30–50 amino acids. For the synthesis of peptides and proteins bigger than 30–50 amino acids, various chemical ligation techniques were developed that enable the formation of a peptide bond between two unprotected peptides resulting in larger synthetic proteins with a fully native peptide backbone [11, 12].

2.3 Site-specific incorporation of chelators and/or fluorescent tags

Functionalization of peptides and proteins still heavily relies on amine or thiol functionalities, present in proteins as lysine and cysteine side chains, respectively. New ligation techniques are emerging that are moving away from amines or use of protected thiols. The functionalization of lysine side chains can be achieved by reacting them with activated esters such as NHS-DTPA or –DOTA that are commercially available (**Figure 2**). The most appropriate derivatives of these chelators for conjugation to a peptide or protein are those which are *t*Bu (*tert*-butyl)-protected at all functional acid groups, except one. This acid group can either be activated *in situ* using a proper coupling agent or be obtained as a preactivated NHS ester in DOTA-tris(*t*Bu)ester NHS ester, NOTA-bis(*t*Bu) ester NHS ester, or DTPA-tetrakis(*t*Bu) ester NHS ester.

The main advantage of these activated ester chelators is their ease of use, while the main disadvantage of this technique is their unspecific labeling. A protein generally contains more than one lysine residue and thus more than one position for chelator conjugation. It is difficult to predict the site of coupling, which will

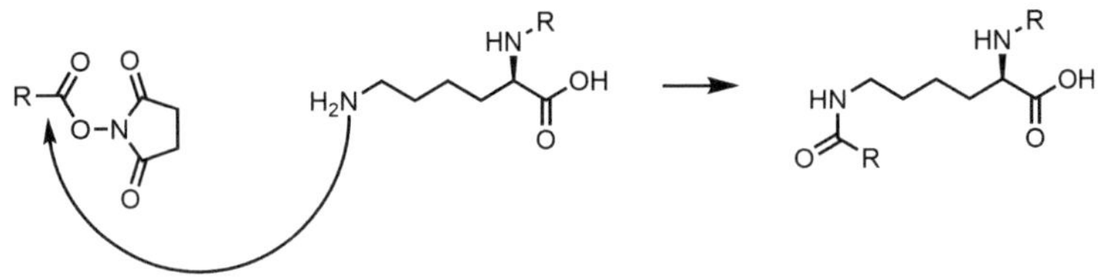

Figure 2.
Conjugation at N^{ε}-amine group of a lysine residue with an amine reactive NHS ester (N-hydroxysuccinimide ester) resulting in an amide bond.

often lead to heterogenous labeling of the compound of interest. With the use of Boc SPPS this problem can be circumvented by using orthogonally ε-amino Fmoc-protected lysine residues. Deprotection of the Fmoc group can be performed on resin and directly be followed by functionalization of the desired lysine with an NHS-activated label of choice. In case of Fmoc SPPS, orthogonally ε-amino allyloxycarbonyl (Alloc) protected lysine residues can be used.

Conjugation at cysteine residues can be realized by reactions with maleimide containing compounds or 2-azidoacrylate-derivatives [13]. Similar to the amine reactive NHS esters, commercial compounds with maleimides are widespread. Maleimide-DOTA or –DTPA are coupled to free cysteine-containing proteins (**Figure 3**). Although the reaction is specific and easy to use, maleimides have their disadvantages. The first being the availability of a free cysteine in a protein of interest; the major part of cysteines present in proteins are paired with a second cysteine to form a disulfide bridge. Moreover, these cysteines are often buried within the core of the protein making them inaccessible for maleimides. To overcome this problem an additional cysteine can be incorporated into the protein specifically for labeling. This will, however, lead to problems with oxidative folding of the protein and can lead to improperly folded proteins with loss of activity.

However, this does not mean that thiol reactive compounds cannot be useful in protein labeling. The introduction of an encrypted cysteine that can be deprotected after correct folding of the protein can offer a solution. Recently N^{ε}-(thiazolidine carboxyl)-lysine was applied for this purpose [14], the thiazolidine carboxylic acid (Thz) that was originally designed to facilitate sequential one-pot native chemical ligation (NCL) [15–17], was used as a handle for late stage site-specific modification of proteins under mild conditions [14]. The encrypted cysteine was introduced on a lysine side chain which after opening under mild conditions with $MeONH_2$ or NH_2OH resulted in a free cysteine enabling reactions with maleimide groups (**Figure 4**).

Furthermore, it was shown that this technique is fully compatible with established techniques of peptide synthesis and NCL. The chemokine CCL5 was synthesized from an *N*- and *C*-terminal part that were joined by native chemical ligation. The *C*-terminus contained a lysine with an orthogonal Fmoc protective group. After completion of the synthesis of the *C*-terminus, the Fmoc group was removed and the thiazolidine residue was site-specifically introduced. After cleavage from resin and

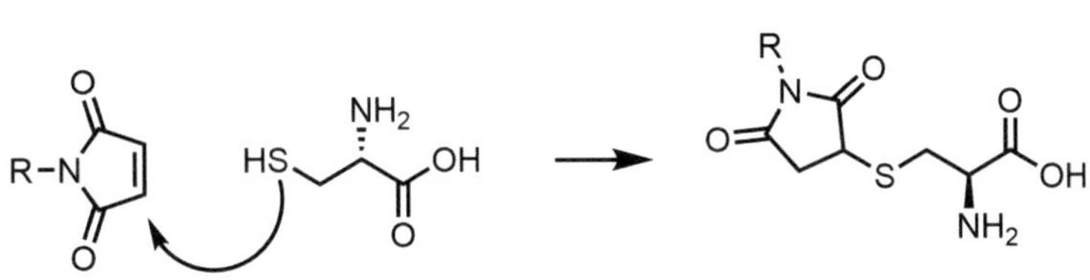

Figure 3.
Conjugation at a free thiol moiety present in cysteine using a maleimide resulting in a thioether bond.

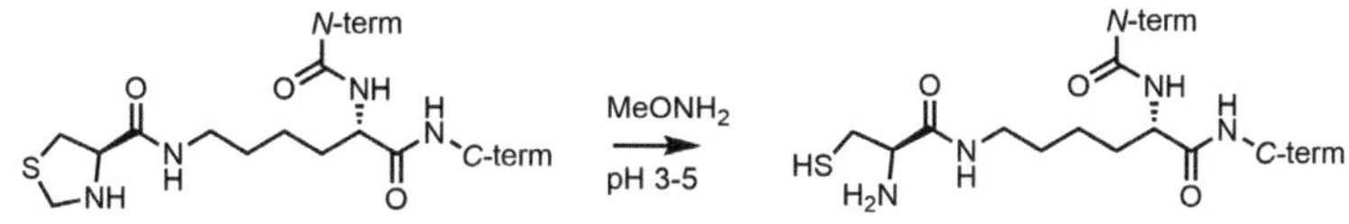

Figure 4.
Deprotection of thiazolidinecarboxyl coupled to N^{ε}-amine group of a lysine residue using methoxylamine.

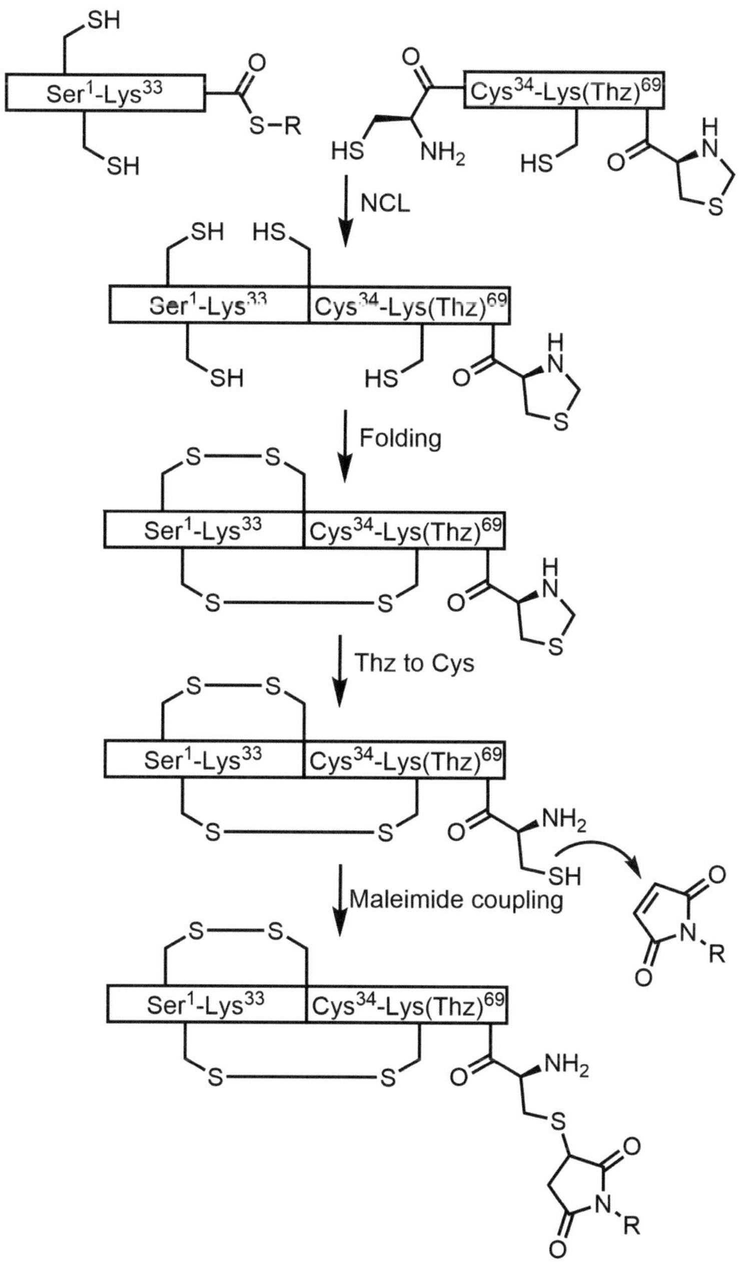

Figure 5.
Schematic representation of the synthesis of chemokine CCL5. In the first step two unprotected peptide fragments are ligated using native chemical ligation. Subsequently, the peptide is folded into an active protein. In the last step the thiazolidine ring is opened while simultaneously the newly formed thiol moiety is modified with a maleimide.

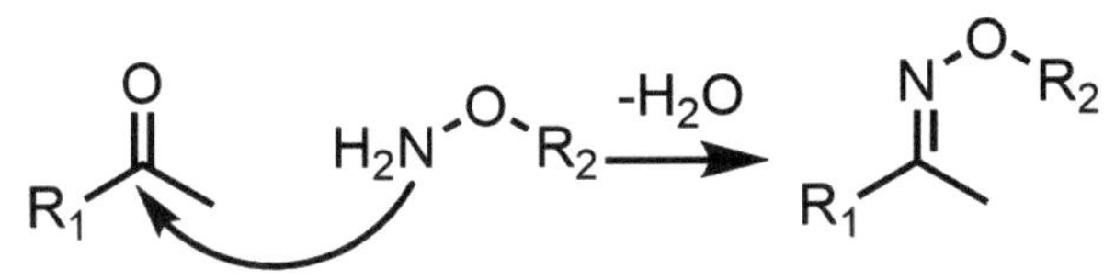

Figure 6.
Reaction of an aminooxy with a ketone which results in an oxime bond.

subsequent purification, the two parts were ligated to obtain the full length protein and subsequently the protein was folded under oxidative conditions. After obtaining the folded protein, the thiazolidine ring was opened by treatment with $MeONH_2$.

Upon treatment with $MeONH_2$ to convert the thiazolidine functionality into a free cysteine and subsequent modification with a maleimide label, unwanted disulfide shuffling can occur in proteins containing disulfide bonds [18]. To circumvent this problem a synchronized protocol for thiazolidine deprotection and maleimide coupling can be best used (**Figure 5**).

A chemoselective conjugation approach that does not use any of the naturally occurring functional groups in proteins is oxime ligation. The reaction is comprised of a ketone or aldehyde reacting with an aminooxy group to yield an oxime bond (**Figure 6**). The reaction can be performed in aqueous media at neutral pH but is faster at slightly acidic pH [19]. The reaction can be catalyzed with aniline or derivatives thereof, to facilitate fast reactions [20, 21].

Although the oxime reaction itself can be performed relatively easy, the more challenging part is the incorporation of a ketone or aminooxy in the peptide/protein of interest. Since a ketone is virtually inert to most chemical reactions, the ketone is mostly chosen over the aminooxy component to be incorporated in the protein of choice, while the aminooxy component is used to modify the label. The increased attention for the oxime bond in the last decade has led to the development of several methods to incorporate ketones or aldehydes in proteins. An overview of the available techniques was previously reviewed, here we will briefly highlight methods useful in chemical synthesis [22]. Historically, oxidation of peptides/proteins containing an *N*-terminal 2-amino alcohol residue (serine/threonine) is among the most used to obtain an aldehyde in the form of a glyoxyloyl moiety [23]. Site-specific incorporation using chemical synthesis, however, can be achieved using suitably protected unnatural amino acids such as p-acetylphenylalanine or keto-proline [24, 25]. A large amount of flexibility in both site of introduction and distance from active regions can be achieved with modification of amine moieties with keto-acids [26, 27]. Care has to be taken, however, in the choice of keto-acid as some are less efficient in subsequent oxime formation [28].

In summary, several techniques are available for the modification of proteins to include chelators used for PET and SPECT. Amine and thiol reactive compounds are easy to use through orthogonally protected lysine side chains or through thiazolidine deprotection in pre-folded proteins. Oxime conjugation can be used for chelator incorporation but is also used for covalent radiolabeling approaches, such as introducing ^{18}F-containing prosthetic groups (see for an overview [29]).

3. Radiolabeling of peptides

A variety of labeling techniques can be applied to peptides and proteins, but according to George De Hevesy's definition of a tracer the radiolabeling procedure should not affect the biological properties, the affinity to the target, or the physicochemical properties (e.g. charge, hydrophilicity, size). In the following part a list of radiosynthesis techniques for commonly used isotopes is described, omitting isotopes that are used less frequently. For example, ^{11}C is a widespread isotope for labeling small organic compounds, but it is used less frequently in peptides or larger structures and so will therefore not be further discussed here.

3.1 Radioiodination

Radioiodination of peptides with ^{125}I, ^{123}I, ^{124}I, or ^{131}I can be performed by either direct labeling or indirect labeling via an auxiliary group. During direct radioiodination, radioactive iodine is incorporated covalently into the side chains of tyrosyl or histidyl residues in the presence of an oxidizing agent such as chloramine-T or iodogen. If no tyrosyl or histidyl residue is available, free amino groups in the peptide may be radioiodinated by auxiliary groups, including *N*-succinimidyl-3-(4-hydroxyphenyl)propionate, known as Bolton-Hunter reagent [30]. Other auxiliary groups for radioiodination of peptides are *N*-succinimidyl-3-iodobenzoate (SIB), *N*-succinimidyl-5-iodo-3-pyridinecarboxylate (SIPC), and *N*-succinimidyl 4-guanidinomethyl-3-iodobenzoate (SGMIB) (**Figure** 7) [31–34].

As none of the radioiodination methods is based on complexation with a chelator, we will not focus on this labeling method in this book chapter further.

3.2 Radiofluorination

For routine PET imaging, fluorine-18 represents the near ideal radionuclide with its half-life of 109.8 min and low β^+-energy (0.64 MeV). Due to this low positron energy, it has a short positron linear range in tissue, leading to particularly high spatial resolution in PET imaging. Furthermore, compared to other short lived radionuclides, such as ^{11}C, its half-life is long enough to allow syntheses and imaging procedures to be extended over hours, enabling kinetic studies and high-quality metabolite and plasma analysis.

Efficient ^{18}F-labeling of peptides and proteins often comprises a multistep process involving labeling and purification of a prosthetic group (synthon) and subsequent conjugation of the ^{18}F-labeled synthon to the peptide/protein with or without activation. If necessary, the ^{18}F-conjugate is purified by a final purification step. Over the years, a variety of prosthetic groups have been developed ranging from amine-reactive groups such as *N*-succinimidyl-4-[^{18}F]fluorobenzoate ([^{18}F]SFB) [35] to chemoselective groups like 4-[^{18}F]fluorobenzaldehyde and [^{18}F]FDG ([^{18}F]

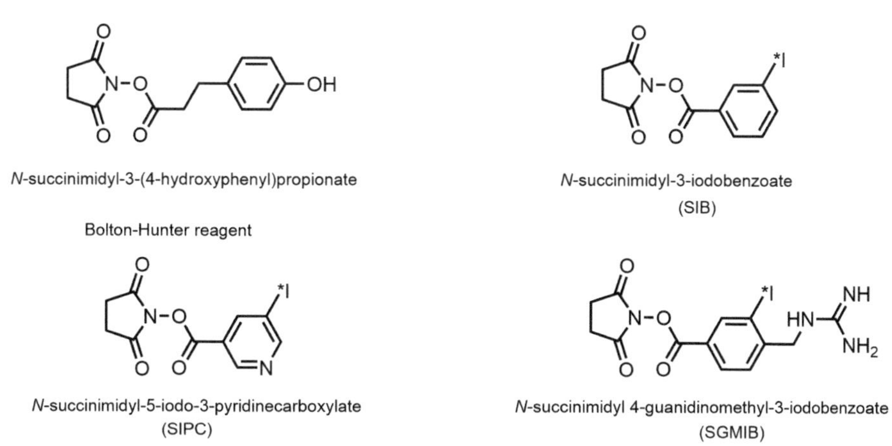

Figure 7.
The auxiliary groups Bolton-hunter reagent, SIB, SIPC, and SGMIB for the radioiodination of peptides.

fluorodeoxyglucose) [36, 37] that react with an aminooxy- or hydrazine-modified peptides. A special prosthetic group approach that has been explored in ^{18}F-labeling chemistry is the click chemistry methodology. Click chemistry appeared to be an effective method to radiolabel peptides and proteins, because the click reaction is fast, bioorthogonal, chemo- and regioselective, results in relatively high yields and can be performed in aqueous media. This copper(I)-catalyzed azide-alkyne cycloaddition reaction has been exploited in radiopharmaceutical chemistry by several research groups [38–44]. A variant of the copper(I)-catalyzed click reaction is the copper-free click reaction that does not require the use of the cytotoxic metal. Reactions of electron-deficient tetrazines with ring-strained trans-cyclooctenes or norbenes have been investigated [45–49]. Click reactions, Cu(I)-catalyzed and copper-free, appeared to be powerful and versatile reactions for the synthesis of ^{18}F-labeled peptides and proteins.

In spite of the variety of possibilities for introducing ^{18}F, a major drawback of the ^{18}F-labeling methods described above is that they are laborious, (require azeotropic drying of the fluoride and multiple purification steps) and are thus time consuming. In search of a kit-based ^{18}F-labeling method, new ^{18}F-labeling strategies based on fluorine-silicon [50–56], fluorine-boron [57–59], and fluorine-phosphorus [60] have been developed.

A facile chelator-based approach was developed wherein ^{18}F is first attached to aluminum as $Al^{18}F$, which is then complexed in a chelating agent attached to the peptide, forming a stable $Al^{18}F$–chelate peptide complex in an efficient 1-pot process [61].

3.3 Radiolabeling with ^{68}Ga

Gallium-68 is an interesting positron-emitter, because of its well established radiochemistry and its easy access and availability from commercial available $^{68}Ge/^{68}Ga$-generators ($t_{1/2}$ ^{68}Ge = 268 days) which renders it independent of an on-site cyclotron. The application of ^{68}Ga-labeled peptides and proteins has attracted considerable interest for molecular imaging, because of its physical characteristics. The high positron emission fraction, 89% through positron emission of 1.9 MeV (max. energy), and half-life of 68 min allows short scanning times with sufficient amounts of radioactivity for high quality images. Generally, DOTA and NOTA are very suitable chelators and are commonly used for $^{68}Ga^{3+}$-complexation. Though, recently TRAP (Tri-azacyclononane-phosphinic acid) and its derivatives revealed to be powerful ^{68}Ga chelators which possess valuable utility in nuclear medicine and molecular imaging [62].

DOTA has a larger cavity than NOTA and, thus, needs higher ring distortion for complexation of $^{68}Ga^{3+}$. Therefore, higher temperatures are required for ^{68}Ga-DOTA complex formation compared to ^{68}Ga complex formation with NOTA. Typically, DOTA-conjugated peptides are radiolabeled with ^{68}Ga at 90–100°C, whereas NOTA-conjugated peptides can be labeled at room temperature [62].

Generally, ^{68}Ga is obtained by eluting a $^{68}Ge/^{68}Ga$ generator with a 0.01–1 M HCl solution. The eluate can be added directly to the NOTA- or DOTA-conjugated compound dissolved in a suitable buffer system such as HEPES (4-(2-hydroxyethyl)piperazine-1-ethanesulfonic acid), phosphate, or ammonium acetate. It is important that the resulting pH of the reaction mixture is a pH value <4 to prevent formation of colloidal hydroxide $[^{68}Ga(OH)_3]_n$ which begins at a pH value above 4.

3.4 Radiolabeling with ^{111}In

The SPECT isotope indium-111 is a frequently used radionuclides in diagnostic nuclear medicine. It has a physical half-life of 67 hours and is produced by a cyclotron. The principle photons are 173 keV (89%) and 247 keV (94%). The most commonly used chelators for ^{111}In-labeling of peptides and proteins are DTPA and DOTA. DTPA chelates ^{111}In at room temperature with sufficient efficiency and stability. This DTPA chelator is used in the commercially available somatostatin analog OctreoScan®. DOTA forms a more stable complex with ^{111}In, but requires heating of the reaction mixture which can lead to protein denaturation, especially for larger proteins. Labeling of DTPA- and DOTA-conjugated peptides and proteins is a one pot, one step procedure in which the compound is incubated with ^{111}InCl3 at a pH between 4 and 6. Ammonium and sodium acetate buffers are commonly used as buffer for labeling of DTPA- and DOTA-conjugated compounds with ^{111}In. However, it was shown that ^{111}In-labeling efficiency and specific activity of DTPA- and DOTA-conjugated peptides was significantly improved in MES (2-(*N*-morpholino)ethanesulfonic acid) and HEPES buffer compared to acetate buffers [63]. The enhanced labeling efficiency appeared to be due to the reduced competitive chelation of cadmium, the decay product of ^{111}In. These observations made MES and HEPES the buffers of choice for ^{111}In-labeling.

3.5 Radiolabeling with ^{99m}Tc

Technetium-99 m is the most widely used isotope due to its ideal half-life of 6 hours, its low cost, and excellent imaging characteristics. Similar to ^{68}Ga, ^{99m}Tc can be obtained from a generator (^{99}Mo/^{99m}Tc, with a half-life of 66 hours for ^{99}Mo) which is easily shipped, allowing worldwide use. Since the 1960s, ^{99m}Tc has been used in a variety of applications, including cancer research and cardiac assessment. ^{99m}Tc is a nearly pure gamma-emitter (88%), with the remaining 12% yielding internal conversion electrons. The application is therefore restricted to SPECT imaging (although research into therapeutic applications is also performed).

Possibilities for coupling of ^{99m}Tc to small organic compounds, peptides or proteins are nearly unlimited, in part due to the many oxidation states that ^{99m}Tc can have, ranging from +I to +VII. The isotope is obtained from the generator in a pH-neutral and isotonic saline solution, ensuring computability with nearly any peptide or protein.

One solution to radiolabel proteins is, instead of chemically modifying the protein, synthesizing it with an additional hexa-histidine chain at the *N*-terminus (His-tag). This addition mostly does not interfere with recognition sites and allows for site-specific labeling of ^{99m}Tc (in the form of $^{99m}Tc(CO)_3$) [64]. This is a two-step reaction, where $^{99m}TcO_4$- (Technetium pertechnetate, as it is eluted from the generator) is first converted to $^{99m}Tc(CO)_3$ (thereby changing the oxidation state from +VII to +I, under relatively harsh conditions) and subsequently coupling $^{99m}Tc(CO)_3$ to the His-tag.

An alternative for ^{99m}Tc-labeling of peptides and proteins is conjugating them with the bifunctional chelator HYNIC (6-hydrazinonicotinic acid). HYNIC has been introduced to radiolabel an IgG antibody with ^{99m}Tc for infection imaging [65]. HYNIC is an established and appropriate BCA for ^{99m}Tc-labeling, because it allows rapid and efficient labeling of proteins. In addition, ^{99m}Tc-labeled HYNIC-conjugates can be produced with high specific activities. However, conjugation of HYNIC to a peptide of protein can be complex as the hydrazine group of HYNIC is highly nucleophilic and, when unprotected, undergoes unwanted side reactions with electrophiles. Protecting the hydrazine group of HYNIC-conjugated compounds with for example Fmoc, Cbz, and Boc, has been investigated by several research groups and is still subject of current research [66–71].

Since the HYNIC group can only coordinate to a metal through 2 donor groups at most, it is unable to saturate the technetium coordination sphere. To complete the coordination sphere, an additional coligand, such as EDDA (ethylenediamine diacetic acid), tricine (*N*-[Tris(hydroxymethyl)-methyl]glycine), or nicotinic acid is required. However, the choice of the coligand has significant influence on the pharmacokinetics, and thus, biologic properties of the radiotracer [72]. Because the chemistry of HYNIC conjugation to a peptide or protein remains a challenge and the coordination mode of the ^{99m}Tc-HYNIC complex is still undefined, it is not possible to give a standard HYNIC-conjugation and ^{99m}Tc-radiolabeling protocol. For a review about ^{99m}Tc-HYNIC coordination chemistry see Meszaros *et al*. and references herein [73].

4. Conclusions

Improvements in effective nuclear imaging are not only dependent on progression in imaging equipment and technology, but is also strongly dependent on the availability of powerful probes with optimal pharmacokinetic and imaging characteristics. The diversity of methods for syntheses of peptides and proteins and the variety of possibilities for modification, stabilization, labeling (radiolabeling and labeling for other modalities), and construction of more complex multivalent and multimodal constructs, make radiolabeled peptides and proteins a flexible class of tracers and meaningful molecules for nuclear imaging of several diseases such as cancer, thrombosis, infection, and inflammation in pre-clinical and clinical research.

Radiotracers enable early diagnosis and thus early treatment of disease and they enable better stratification of patients with disease-stage-adapted therapy instead of escalating to the most aggressive and costly therapy. Moreover, radiolabeled compounds are used to monitor the therapeutic effect of drugs and are used as therapeutic radiopharmaceuticals when labeled with either β^- - or α-emitting radionuclides such as ^{90}Y, ^{186}Re, ^{188}Re, ^{131}I, ^{177}Lu and ^{211}At and ^{213}Bi, respectively.

The growth of the world population and the overall rise in life expectancy in the last decades will increase the demand for radiopharmaceuticals, including basic research into and the development of new radiopharmaceuticals.

Conflict of interest

The authors declare no conflict of interest.

Author details

Ingrid Dijkgraaf[1,2]*, Stijn M. Agten[1], Matthias Bauwens[2]
and Tilman M. Hackeng[1]

1 Department of Biochemistry, Maastricht University, The Netherlands

2 Department of Radiology and Nuclear Medicine, Maastricht University Medical Centre, Maastricht, The Netherlands

*Address all correspondence to: I.Dijkgraaf@maastrichtuniversity.nl

References

[1] Weiner RE, Thakur ML. Radiolabeled peptides in diagnosis and therapy. Semin Nucl Med. 2001;31:296-311.

[2] Powell MF, Grey H, Gaeta F, Sette A, Colón S. Peptide stability in drug development: A comparison of peptide reactivity in different biological media. J Pharm Sci. 1992;81:731-735.

[3] Okarvi SM. Peptide-Based Radiopharmaceuticals: Future Tools for Diagnostic Imaging of Cancer and Other Diseases. Medicinal Research Reviews. 2004;24:357-397.

[4] Wester HJ, Schottelius M, Poethko T, Bruus-Jensen K, Schwaiger M. Radiolabeled Carbohydrated Somatostatin Analogs: A review of the Current Status. Cancer Biother Radiopharm. 2004;19:231-244.

[5] Okarvi SM. Recent developments in ^{99m}Tc-labelled peptide-based radiopharmaceuticals: An overview. Nucl Med Commun. 1999;20:1093-1112.

[6] Price EW, Orvig C. Matching chelators to radiometals for radiopharmaceuticals. Chem Soc Rev. 2014;43:260-290.

[7] Weber WA. Positron emission tomography as an imaging biomarker. J Clin Oncol. 2006;24:3282-3292.

[8] Jaffer FA, Weissleder R. Molecular Imaging in the Clinical Arena. JAMA. 2005;293:855-862.

[9] Rosenblum G, Cooperman BS. Engine out of the chassis: cell-free protein synthesis and its uses. FEBS Letters. 2014;588:261-268.

[10] Wentworth P Jr. Recent developments and applications of liquid-phase strategies in organic synthesis. Trends Biotechnnol. 1999;17:448-452.

[11] Dawson PE, Kent SBH. Synthesis of native proteins by chemical ligation. Ann Rev Biochem. 2000;69:923-960.

[12] Kulkarni S, Sayers J, Premdjee B, Payne RJ. Rapid and efficient protein synthesis through expansion of the native chemical ligation concept. Nat Rev Chem. 2018;2:0122.

[13] Ariyasu S, Hayashi H, Xing B, Chiba S. Site-Specific Dual Functionalization of Cysteine Residue in Peptides and Proteins with 2-Azidoacrylates. Bioconjug Chem. 2017;28:897-902.

[14] Van de Vijver P, Suylen D, Dirksen A, Dawson PE, Hackeng TM. Nepsilon-(thiaprolyl)-lysine as a handle for site-specific protein conjugation. Biopolymers. 2010;94:465-474.

[15] Dawson PE, Muir TW, Clark-Lewis I, Kent SB. Synthesis of proteins by native chemical ligation. Science. 1994;266:776-779.

[16] Hackeng TM, Griffin JH, Dawson PE. Protein synthesis by native chemical ligation: expanded scope by using straightforward methodology. Proc Natl Acad Sci U S A. 1999;96:10068-10073.

[17] Bang D, Kent SB. A one-pot total synthesis of crambin. Angew Chem Int Ed Engl. 2004;43:2534-2538.

[18] Van de Vijver P, Schmitt M, Suylen D, Scheer L, Thomassen MC, Schurgers LJ, Griffin JH, Koenen RR, Hackeng TM. Incorporation of disulfide containing protein modules into multivalent antigenic conjugates: generation of antibodies against the thrombin-sensitive region of murine protein S. J Am Chem Soc. 2012;134:19318-19321.

[19] Cordes EH, Jencks WP. General Acid Catalysis of Semicarbazone Formation. J Am Chem Soc.1962;84:4319-4328.

[20] Dirksen A, Hackeng TM, Dawson PE. Nucleophilic catalysis of oxime ligation. Angew Chem Int Ed Engl. 2006;45:7581-7584.

[21] Rashidian M, Mahmoodi MM, Shah R, Dozier JK, Wagner CR, Distefano MD. A highly efficient catalyst for oxime ligation and hydrazone-oxime exchange suitable for bioconjugation. Bioconjug Chem. 2013;24:333-342.

[22] Agten SM, Dawson PE, Hackeng TM. Oxime conjugation in protein chemistry: from carbonyl incorporation to nucleophilic catalysis. J Pept Sci. 2016;22:271-279.

[23] Gaertner HF, Rose K, Cotton R, Timms D, Camble R, Offord RE. Construction of protein analogues by site-specific condensation of unprotected fragments. Bioconjug Chem. 1992;3:262-268.

[24] Wang L, Zhang Z, Brock A, Schultz PG. Addition of the keto functional group to the genetic code of *Escherichia coli*. PNAS. 2003;100:56-61.

[25] Choudhary A, Kamer KJ, Shoulders MD, Raines RT. 4-ketoproline: An electrophilic proline analog for bioconjugation. Biopolymers. 2015;104:110-115.

[26] Sohma Y, Kent SB. Biomimetic synthesis of lispro insulin via a chemically synthesized "mini-proinsulin" prepared by oxime-forming ligation. J Am Chem Soc. 2009;131:16313-16318.

[27] Kochendoerfer GG, Chen SY, Mao F, Cressman S, Traviglia S, Shao H, Hunter CL, Low DW, Cagle EN, Carnevali M, Gueriguian V, Keogh PJ, Porter H, Stratton SM, Wiedeke MC, Wilken J, Tang J, Levy JJ, Miranda LP, Crnogorac MM, Kalbag S, Botti P, Schindler-Horvat J, Savatski L, Adamson JW, Kung A, Kent SB, Bradburne JA. Design and chemical synthesis of a homogeneous polymer-modified erythropoiesis protein. Science. 2003;299:884-887.

[28] Agten SM, Suylen D, Ippel H, Kokozidou M, Tans G, van de Vijver P, Koenen RR, Hackeng TM. Chemoselective oxime reactions in proteins and peptides by using an optimized oxime strategy: the demise of levulinic acid. Chembiochem. 2013;14:2431-2434.

[29] Li XG, Haaparanta M, Solin O. Oxime formation for fluorine-18 labeling of peptides and proteins for positron emission tomography (PET) imaging: A review. J Fluor Chem. 2012;143:49-56.

[30] Bolton AM, Hunter RM. The labeling of proteins to high specific radioactivities by conjugation to a ^{125}I-containing acylating agent. Biochem J. 1973;133:529-538.

[31] Khawli LA, Kassis AI. Synthesis of ^{125}I labeled N-succinimidyl p-iodobenzoate for use in radiolabelling antibodies. Nucl Med Biol. 1989;16:727-733.

[32] Zalutsky MR, Narula AS. A method for radiohalogenation of proteins resulting in decreased thyroid uptake of radioiodine. Appl Radiat Isot. 1987;38:1051-1055.

[33] Garg PK, Zalutsky MR. N-succinimidyl 5-(trialkylstannyl)-3-pyridinecarboxylates: A new class of reagents for protein radioiodination. Bioconjugate Chem. 1991;2:50-56.

[34] Vaidyanathan G, Affleck DJ, Li J, Welsh P, Zalutsky MR. A polar substituent-containing acylation agent for the radioiodination of internalizing monoclonal antibodies: N-succinimidyl 4-guanidinomethyl-3-[^{131}I]iodobenzoate ([^{131}I]SGMIB). Bioconjugate Chem. 2001;12:428-438.

[35] Vaidyanathan G, Zalutsky MR. Labeling proteins with fluorine-18 using N-succinimidyl 4-[^{18}F]fluorobenzoate. Int J Rad Appl Instrum B. 1992;19:275-281.

[36] Hultsch C, Schottelius M, Auernheimer J, Alke A, Wester HJ. (18)F Fluoroglucosylation of peptides, exemplified on cyclo(RGDfK). Eur J Nucl Med Mol Imaging. 2009;36:1469-1474.

[37] Namavari M, Cheng Z, Zhang R, De A, Levi J, Hoerner JK, Yaghoubi SS, Syud FA, Gambhir SS. A novel method for direct site-specific radiolabeling of peptides using [^{18}F]FDG. Bioconjug Chem. 2009;20:432-436.

[38] Marik J, Sutcliffe JL. Click for PET: Rapid preparation of [^{18}F] fluoropeptides using CuI catalyzed 1,3-dipolar cycloaddition. Tetrahedron Lett. 2006;47:6681-6684.

[39] Ramenda T, Kniess T, Bergmann R, Steinbach J, Wuest F. Radiolabelling of proteins with fluorine-18 via click chemistry. Chem Commun (Camb). 2009;48:7521-7523.

[40] Glaser M, Arstad E. "Click labeling" with 2-[^{18}F]fluoroethylazide for positron emission tomography. Bioconjugate Chem. 2007;18:989-993.

[41] Thonon D, Kech C, Paris J, Lemaire C, Luxen A. New strategy for the preparation of clickable peptides and labeling with 1-(azidomethyl)-4-[(18) F]-fluorobenzene for PET. Bioconjugate Chem. 2009;20:817-823.

[42] Li ZB, Wu Z, Chen K, Chin FT, Chen X. Click chemistry for (18) F-labeling of RGD peptides and microPET imaging of tumor integrin alphavbeta3 expression. Bioconjugate Chem. 2007;18:1987-1994.

[43] Maschauer S, Einsiedel J, Haubner R, Hocke C, Ocker M, Hübner H, Kuwert T, Gmeiner P, Prante O. Labeling and glycosylation of peptides using click chemistry: A general approach to (18)F-glycopeptides as effective imaging probes for positron emission tomography. Angew Chem Int Ed. 2010;49:976-979.

[44] Li Y, Liu Z, Harwig CW, Pourghiasian M, Lau J, Lin KS, Schaffer P, Benard F, Perrin DM. (18) F-click labeling of a bombesin antagonist with an alkyne-(18) F-ArBF(3) (−): In vivo PET imaging of tumors expressing the GRP-receptor. Am J Nucl Med Mol Imaging. 2013;3:57-70.

[45] Arumugam S, Chin J, Schirrmacher R, Popik VV, Kostikov AP. [^{18}F]azadibenzocyclooctyne ([^{18}F] ADIBO): A biocompatible radioactive labeling synthon for peptides using catalyst free [3+2] cycloaddition. Bioorg Med Chem Lett. 2011;21:6987-6991.

[46] Hausner SH, Carpenter RD, Bauer N, Sutcliffe JL. Evaluation of an integrin αvβ6-specific peptide labeled with [^{18}F]fluorine by copper-free, strain-promoted click chemistry. Nucl Med Biol. 2013;40:233-239.

[47] Campbell-Verduyn LS, Mirfeizi L, Schoonen AK, Dierckx RA, Elsinga PH, Feringa BL. Strain-promoted copper-free "click" chemistry for ^{18}F radiolabeling of bombesin. Angew Chem Int Ed. 2011;50: 11117-11120.

[48] Selvaraj R, Liu S, Hassink M, Huang CW, Yap LP, Fox JM, Li Z, Conti PS. Tetrazine-trans-cyclooctene ligation for the rapid construction of integrin αvβ3 targeted PET tracer based on a cyclic RGD peptide. Bioorg Med Chem Lett. 2011;21:5011-5014.

[49] Knight JC, Richter S, Wuest M, Way JD, Wuest F. Synthesis and evaluation of an ^{18}F-labelled norbornene derivative for copper-free click

chemistry reactions. Org Biomol Chem. 2013;11:3817-3825.

[50] Schirrmacher E, Wangler B, Cypryk M, Bradtmoller G, Schafer M, Eisenhut M, Jurkschat K, Schirrmacher R. Synthesis of p-(di-tert-butyl[(18)F]fluorosilyl)benzaldehyde ([(18)F]SiFA-A) with high specific activity by isotopic exchange: a convenient labeling synthon for the (18) F-labeling of N-amino-oxy derivatized peptides. Bioconjug Chem. 2007;18:2085-2089.

[51] Schirrmacher R, Wangler C, Schirrmacher E. Recent developments and trends in F-18-radiochemistry: syntheses and applications. Mini-Rev Org Chem. 2007;4:317-329

[52] Mu L, Hohne A, Schubiger PA, Ametamey SM, Graham K, Cyr JE, Dinkelborg L, Stellfeld T, Srinivasan A, Voigtmann U, Klar U. Silicon-based building blocks for one-step ^{18}F-radiolabeling of peptides for PET imaging. Angew Chem Int Edn Engl. 2008;47:4922-4925.

[53] Hohne A, Mu L, Honer M, Schubiger PA, Ametamey SM, Graham K, Stellfeld T, Borkowski S, Berndorff D, Klar U, Voigtmann U, Cyr JE, Friebe M, Dinkelborg L, Srinivasan A. Synthesis, ^{18}F-labeling, and in vitro and in vivo studies of bombesin peptides modified with silicon-based building blocks. Bioconjug Chem. 2008;19:1871-1879.

[54] Iovkova L, Wangler B, Schirrmacher E, Schirrmacher R, Quandt G, Boening G, Schurmann M, Jurkschat K. Para-functionalized aryl-di-tert-butylfluorosilanes as potential labeling synthons for (18)F radiopharmaceuticals. Chemistry. 2009;15:2140-2147.

[55] Rosa-Neto P, Wangler B, Iovkova L, Boening G, Reader A, Jurkschat K, Schirrmacher E. [^{18}F] SiFA-isothiocyanate: a new highly effective radioactive labeling agent for lysine-containing proteins. Chem Biochem. 2009;10:1321-1324.

[56] Wangler B, Quandt G, Iovkova L, Schirrmacher E, Wangler C, Boening G, Hacker M, Schmoeckel M, Jurkschat K, Bartenstein P, Schirrmacher R. Kit-like ^{18}F-labeling of proteins: synthesis of 4-(di-tert-butyl[^{18}F]fluorosilyl) benzenethiol (Si[^{18}F]FA-SH) labeled rat serum albumin for blood pool imaging with PET. Bioconjug Chem. 2009;20:317-321.

[57] Ting R, Harwig C, auf dem Keller U, McCormick S, Austin P, Overall CM, Adam MJ, Ruth TJ, Perrin DM. Toward [18F]-labeled aryltrifluoroborate radiotracers: in vivo positron emission tomography imaging of stable aryltrifluoroborate clearance in mice. J Am Chem Soc. 2008;130:12045-12055.

[58] Liu Z, Pourghiasian M, Radtke MA, Lau J, Pan J, Dias GM, Yapp D, Lin KS, Bénard F, Perrin DM. An organotrifluoroborate for broadly applicable one-step ^{18}F-labeling. Angew Chem Int Ed Engl. 2014;53:11876-11880.

[59] Liu Z, Radtke MA, Wong MQ, Lin KS, Yapp DT, Perrin DM. Dual mode fluorescent (18)F-PET tracers: efficient modular synthesis of rhodamine-[cRGD]$_2$-[(18)F]-organotrifluoroborate, rapid, and high yielding one-step (18) F-labeling at high specific activity, and correlated in vivo PET imaging and ex vivo fluorescence. Bioconjug Chem. 2014;25:1951-1962.

[60] Studenov AR, Adam MJ, Wilson JS, Ruth TJ. New radiolabelling chemistry: synthesis of phosphorus-[F-18]fluorine compounds. J Labelled Compd Rad. 2005;48: 497-500.

[61] McBride WJ, Sharkey RM, Karacay H, D'Souza CA, Rossi EA, Laverman P, Chang CH, Boerman OC, Goldenberg DM. A novel method of ^{18}F

radiolabeling for PET. J Nucl Med. 2009;50:991-998.

[62] Notni J, Šimeček J, Hermann P, Wester HJ. TRAP, a powerful and versatile framework for gallium-68 radiopharmaceuticals. Chemistry. 2011;17:14718-14722.

[63] Brom M, Joosten L, Oyen WJ, Gotthardt M, Boerman OC. Improved labelling of DTPA- and DOTA-conjugated peptides and antibodies with ^{111}In in HEPES and MES buffer. EJNMMI Res. 2012;2:4.

[64] Alberto R. New Organometallic Technetium Complexes for Radiopharmaceutical Imaging. Top Curr Chem. 2005;252:1-44.

[65] Abrams MJ, Juweid M, tenKate CI, Schwartz DA, Hauser MM, Gaul FE, Fuccello AJ, Rubin RH, Strauss HW, Fischman AJ. Technetium-99m-human polyclonal IgG radiolabeled via the hydrazino nicotinamide derivative for imaging focal sites of infection in rats. J Nucl Med. 1990;31:2022-2028.

[66] Greenland WE, Howland K, Hardy J, Fogelman I, Blower PJ. Solid-phase synthesis of peptide radiopharmaceuticals using Fmoc-N-epsilon-(hynic-Boc)-lysine, a technetium-binding amino acid: application to Tc-99m-labeled salmon calcitonin. J Med Chem. 2003;46:1751-1757.

[67] Schwartz DA, Abrams MJ, Hauser MM, Gaul FE, Larsen SK, Rauh D, Zubieta JA. Preparation of hydrazino-modified proteins and their use for the synthesis of ^{99m}Tc-protein conjugates. Bioconjugate Chem. 1991;2:333-336.

[68] Rajopadhye M, Harris TD, Yu K, Glowacka D, Damphousse PR, Barrett JA, Heminway SJ, Edwards DS, Carroll TR. Synthesis, evaluation and Tc-99m complexation of a hydrazinonicotinyl conjugate of a gp IIb/IIIa antagonist cyclic peptide for the detection of deep vein thrombosis. Bioorg Med Chem Lett. 1997;7:955-960.

[69] Edwards DS, Liu S, Harris AR, Poirier MJ, Ewels BA. ^{99m}Tc-labeling of hydrazones of a hydrazinonicotinamide conjugated cyclic peptide. Bioconjugate Chem. 1999;10:803-807.

[70] Harris TD, Sworin M, Williams N, Rajopadhye M, Damphousse PR, Glowacka D, Poirier MJ, Yu K. Synthesis of stable hydrazones of a hydrazinonicotinyl-modified peptide for the preparation of ^{99m}Tc-labeled radiopharmaceuticals. Bioconjugate Chem. 1999;10:808-814.

[71] Surfraz MB, Biagini SC, Blower PJ. A technetium intermediate specifically promotes deprotection of trifluoroacetyl HYNIC during radiolabelling under mild conditions. Dalton Trans. 2008;22:2920-2922.

[72] Babich JW, Fischman AJ. Effect of "co-ligand" on the biodistribution of ^{99m}Tc-labeled hydrazine nicotinic acid derivatized chemotactic peptides. Nucl Med Biol. 1995;22:25-30.

[73] Meszaros LK, Dose A, Biagini SCG, Blower PJ. Hydrazinonicotinic acid (HYNIC) -Coordination chemistry and applications in radiopharmaceutical chemistry. Inorg Chim Acta. 2010;363:1059-1069.

Chapter 6

Dose Rates Comparative Study for Workers Involved in the Hot-Cells Clean-Up Activities of the VVR-S Nuclear Research Reactor under Decommissioning

Carmen Tuca and Ana Stochioiu

Abstract

The present study consists in the assessment of the dose rates potentially received by the workers involved in Hot Cells decontamination from a VVR-S type Nuclear Research Reactor under decommissioning. Two exposure scenarios were considered: the dosimetrist performing contamination scanning measurements (H*(10) inside of the Hot Cell prior decontamination and the mechanical worker performing floor decontamination. The dose rates were calculated based on the floor hot spots activity concentration using a standard and a numerical method (RESRAD Build code) assuming that the highest radiological risks are from these surfaces. It was noticed that the external dose rate is relatively high both for the floor scanning and decontamination and the internal committed effective dose is relatively low for floor decontamination due to fact that the worker is equipped with a high filter efficiency mask. By comparing the two methods results it is noticed that the dose rate obtained using the numerical method is 32% lower than the dose rate evaluated with the standard method, due to model complexity.

Keywords: Reactor, Hot Cell, decommissioning, decontamination, dose rate

1. Introduction

The VVR-S (water cooled and moderated) type, nuclear research reactor) from "Horia Hulubei" National Institute for R&D in Physics and Nuclear Engineering (IFIN-HH), Romania was operated between 1957 and 1997 without any radiological major incident. The reactor main purposes were the radioisotopes production for medical and industrial applications and the research in physics, biophysics, and biochemistry.

Due to the reactor' components and systems aging the specialists and the Romanian Government decided to decommission the facility. Thus, the reactor decommissioning was performed between 2010 and 2020.

During the operation period, the radioisotopes production was performed using four Hot Cells located in the Reactor Building basement (see **Figure 1**). A detailed description of the Hot Cells design, purpose and usage is presented in paper [2].

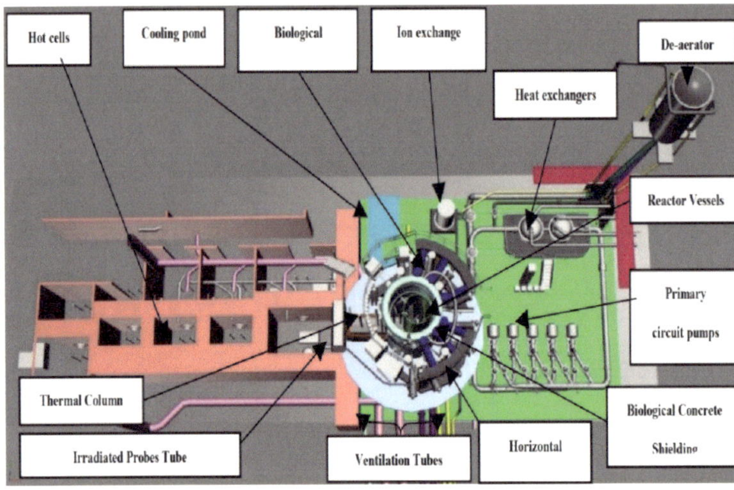

Figure 1.
Reactor overview [1].

The reactor decommissioning process was split in 3 main phases. The Hot Cells were decommissioned in the 3-rd one. The main tasks performed during Hot Cells decommissioning consisted of waste evacuation, internal surfaces decontamination and internal components dismantling (equipment's and stainless-steel lining). The wastes from the Hot Cells no. 3, 2 and 1 were remotely controlled evacuated using the mechanical arms and a trolley [2].

The wastes from the Hot Cell no. 4 were manually evacuated due to the mechanical arms malfunction. Also, the internal surfaces decontamination was performed manually. After the waste's evacuation the Hot Cell internal surfaces were scanned to identify the contamination level [2].

The measurements revealed that the main contamination is located on the Hot Cell floor because of the irradiated substances spilling from vials or capsules during the operation period [2].

Prior the Hot Cells decontamination the dose rate equivalent was assessed by two different methods to prevent over exposure for the workers involved in this process.

2. Methods for dose assessment

Dose rate equivalent was calculated using a standard and a numerical calculation method, RESRAD-BUILD code modeling, based on in-situ activity concentration measurements. For this purpose, we considered the worst potentially over exposure scenario, the Hot Cell no. 4 decontaminations, because the process should be performed manually.

2.1 Standard method

To determine the potential exposure of the dosimetrist and mechanical worker during the Hot Cell decontamination a standard calculation method was used.

For dose rate calculation we assumed that the dosimetrist performs 5 minutes of the Ambiental Dose Equivalent H*(10) direct measurements inside of the Hot Cell, being positioned outside at about 70 cm from the hot area along the horizontal axis (see **Figure 2**) [2].

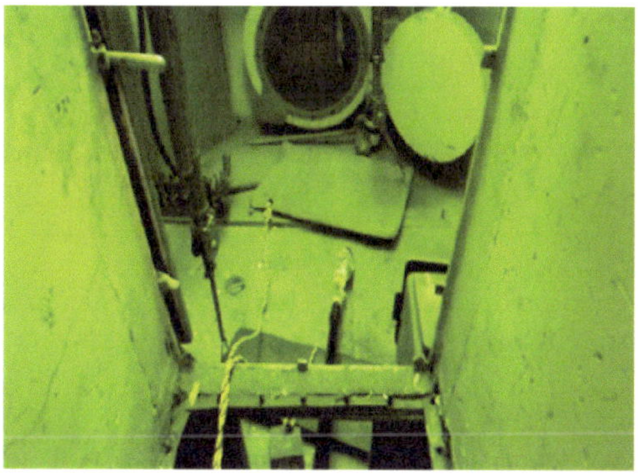

Figure 2.
Floor scanning [2].

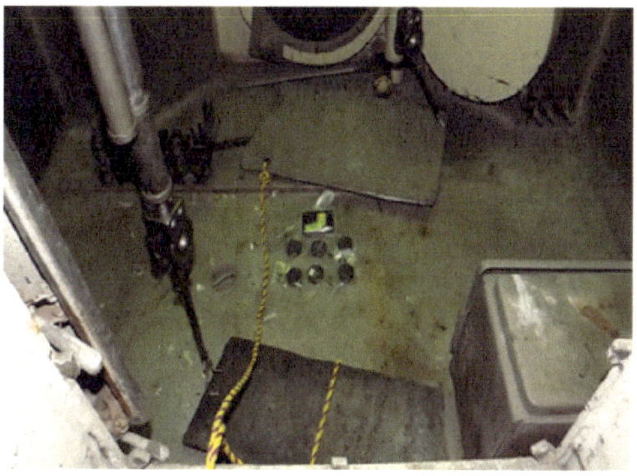

Figure 3.
TLD-s position [2].

For this purpose, a Thermo Scientific™ FH 40 G type, portable digital survey meter, with FHZ 612–10 gamma dose rate probe was used according with the specific procedure [3]. In order to determine the hot spots, the detector was placed less than 1 cm above the surface. Seven hot spots were identified on the Hot Cell no. 4 floor [2].

Parallel measurements were performed using dosimeters with thermo-luminescent detectors (TLDS), GR-200A type high sensitivity tissue equivalent [4].

The TLDS were placed on each hot spot for an hour (see **Figure 3**). A detailed description of the equipment used, and laboratories is presented in paper [2].

The hot spots activities used for dose rate calculation were estimated by indirect measurement of the samples sampled on 100 cm^2 surface around each hot spot, using a gamma-ray spectrometry system with a GEM60P4–95 high-purity germanium coaxial detector (HPGe) [2].

The measurements were performed in compliance with EN/ISO IEC 17025:2005, according to the specific procedure [5–8].

The penetrant dose rate for the workers was calculated using the activity concentration of the radionuclides of each hot spot, according to the methodology presented in paper [2]. For this purpose, we assumed that the sampling yield for activity measurement is 10% and the activity is concentrated in the hottest point (with a total activity equal with the sum of all hot spots) [2].

The internal committed effective dose, E (50), was calculated considering that it was concentrated in the air only 10^{-4} floor total activity and that the worker wore a mask with 99% filter retention efficiency [2].

For the mechanical worker dose calculation, we considered that the decontamination process was performed in three steps (4 minutes each).

First, the worker sprayed decontaminant (DeconGel type 1108), from 90 cm (on vertical axis) respective 45 cm (on horizontal axis) relative to the contaminated area, on the floor (see **Figure 4a**) [2].

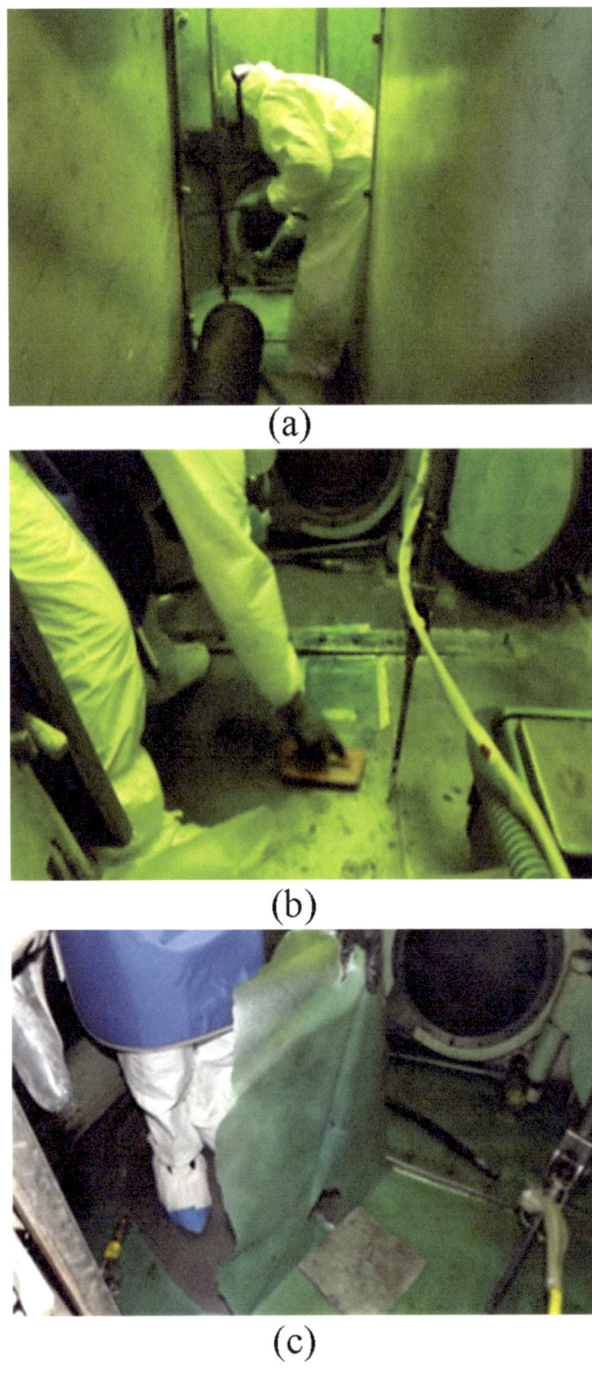

Figure 4.
(a) Decomtaminat spraying [2]. (b) Decontaminant spreading [2]. (c) Gel film removal [2].

Then, the hydro gel coating was spread with a V-tooth trowel, from 40 cm (on vertical axis) and 45 cm (on the horizontal axis) relative to the contaminated area (see **Figure 4b**) [2]. Finally, the worker removed the gel film after drying it, from a similar position to the first step (see **Figure 4c**) [2].

2.2 Numerical method: RESRAD-BUILD code modeling

Considering that the mechanical worker exposure could be much higher than the dosimetrist, a supplementary assessment was performed using RESRAD Build computer code (3.5 version).

The code is specifically designed for radiation doses and risks estimation of RESidual RADioactive materials on radioactively contaminated sites [9].

The external radiation penetrating the walls, ceilings or floors is calculated based on the input parameters for shielding material type, thickness and density. Shielding material can be specified between each source-receptor pair. The internal exposure is calculated based on the air quality model that considers the air exchange between compartments (rooms) and with outdoor air [9]. The code takes into consideration following exposure pathways: the external exposure due to the source, materials deposited on the floor as well as air submersion, the internal exposure due to the airborne radioactive particulates' inhalation, inhalation of the aerosol's indoor radon progeny, the inadvertent ingestion of the radioactive material directly from the source or materials deposited on the surfaces (see **Figure 5**) [9].

The total external dose at time t, over the exposure duration, ED, to a volume source containing radionuclide n in compartment i, $D_{iV}^{n}(t)$, was calculated using (Eq. (1)) [9]:

$$D_{iV}^{n}(t)=\left(\frac{ED}{365}\right)F_{in}\cdot F_{i}\cdot\overline{C_{sV}^{n}}\cdot DCF_{V}^{n}\cdot F_{G}^{n} \tag{1}$$

where:

ED is the exposure duration (days), total length of time considered by the dose assessment, including intervals during which receptors may be absent from the building or a contaminated indoor location; 365 is time conversion factor (days/year);

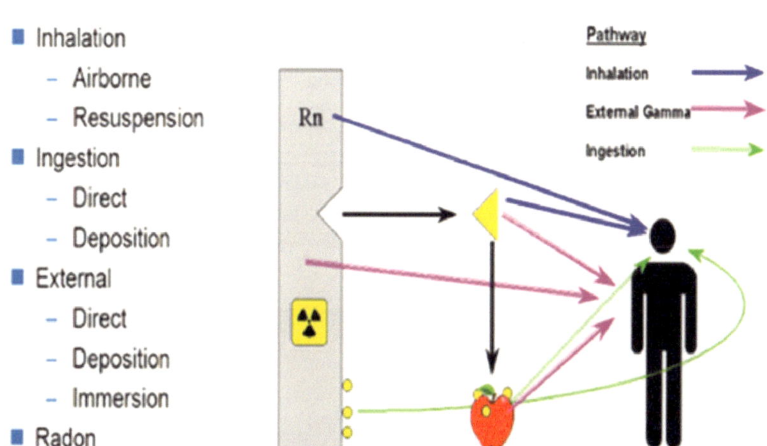

Figure 5.
RESRAD Build code exposure pathway [9].

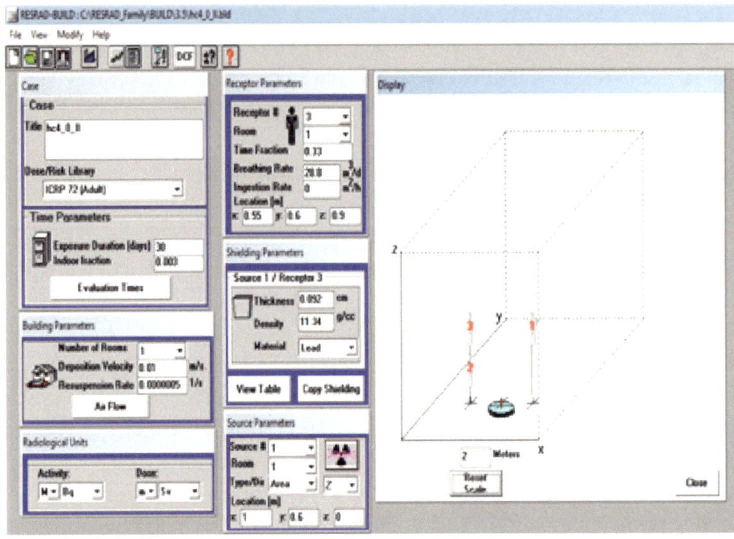

Figure 6.
RESRAD Build code input parameters on floor decontamination.

Fin is the fraction of time spent indoors; Fi is the fraction of time spent in compartment i; DCF_V^n is the FGR-12 dose conversion factor for infinite volume source [(mrem/yr)/(pCi/g)]; F_G^n is the geometrical factor for finite area, source thickness, shielding, source material, and position of receptor relative to the source for radionuclide n; C_{sV}^n is the average volume source concentration (pCi/g) of radionuclide n over the exposure duration, ED, starting at time t [9].

For the studied case (Hot Cell no. 4), the following input data and parameters was taken into consideration (see **Figure 6** and **Table 1**): 1 compartment, the hot cell itself, the source, a 2 m radius circle located in the Hot Cell center. The RESRAD Build considers the area source as being a small thickness volume source (0.01 cm) with up to five layers any one contaminated [9]. Three distinct receptor (the mechanical workers) (x, y, z) positions relative to the source were also considered: R1 (1.45 m, 0.60 m, 0.90 m) – receptor 1 performing decontaminant spraying, R2 (0.55 cm, 0.60 cm, 0.45 cm) - receptor 2 spreading the decontaminant, R3 (0.55 m, 0.40 m, 0.90 m) – receptor 3 removing the gel film.

Parameter	Unit	Building renovation scenario	Remarks
Exposure duration	days (d)	30.00	Total length of time considered for dose assessment, including intervals during which receptors may be absent from the contaminated indoor location
Indoor fraction	dimensionless	0.003	Fraction of the exposure duration spent by one or more receptors inside a building [9] (working time/exposure duration)
Receptor location	m	R1 (1.45, 0.60, 0.90) R2 (0.55, 0.60, 0.45) R3 (0.55, 0.40, 0.90)	Position relative to source center

Parameter	Unit	Building renovation scenario	Remarks
Receptor inhalation rate	m^3/d	28.8 [2]	For building renovation scenario, the breathing rate of moderate activity is 1.6 m^3/h in 24 hours, (breathing rate x 24 h) [10]
Receptor indirect ingestion rate	m^2/h	0.00001	Due to the mask wearing [2]
Source type -	—	Area	Source geometry
Direct ingestion rate	1/h (area) g/h (volume)	0.052	Calculated from the default ingestion rate of 1.1 x 10^{-4} m^2/h in NUREG/ CR-5512 building occupancy scenario [11]
Air release fraction	—	0.0001	Fraction of mechanically removed or eroded material that becomes airborne. For building renovation scenario, a smaller fraction is breathable [9]
Removable fraction	—	Not Required for our analysis	According with NUREG/CR-5512, 10% of the contamination is removable. For the volume source is null [12]
Time for source removal or source lifetime	d	Not Required for our analysis	Value for the building occupancy scenario is the most likely value from the parameter distribution [9]. The parameter is not required for the volume source.
Source erosion rate	cm/d	0	Due to very short time of decontamination process

Table 1.
Input parameters for case study.

The receptor inhalation rate is 28 m^3/day (1.2 m^3/h x 24 h) [2]; the receptor ingestion rate is 0 (the workers wearing respiratory mask) [2] and the air release fraction (fraction of mechanically removed material that becomes airborne) is 0.0001. The removable fraction and time for source removal (source lifetime) are not required for this kind of scenario - building renovation; the source erosion rate (cm/day) is 0 due to very short time of the decontamination [9].

We assume that is necessary to perform 3 decontamination cycle, 12 min. Each. The dose rate was calculated based on hottest spot activity (A_7) considering a 30-day exposure duration [13] and the indoor fraction (report between the working time and the exposure duration) of 0.003.

The assessment was performed: initially, after 7 days, 14 days, 21 days and 28 days respectively considering that the initial activity (Ai) decreased in time from 100–15%.

3. Results

The mean values of the Ambiental Dose Equivalent H*(10) are presented in **Table 2** [2]. For the six hot spots the mean value, determined by floor contamination scanning is 15.6 mSv/h and respectively 28.6 mSv/h for TLDs measurements [2].

Hot spots	$H^*(10)_{scan}$ [mSv/h]	$H^*(10)_{TLD}$ [mSv/h]	Probe position above the hot spot [cm]	TLD position toward the hot spot [cm]
A_1	23.00 ± 2.76	31.70 ± 4.08	1.22	1.04
A_2	9.40 ± 1.13	31.80 ± 4.54	0.90	0.49
A_3	17.00 ± 2.04	31.87 ± 4.71	0.83	0.61
A_4	15.00 ± 1.08	41.40 ± 7.63	0.89	0.53
A_5	18.00 ± 2.16	23.97 ± 2.37	0.57	0.50
A_6	11.00 ± 1.32	10.70 ± 0.94	0.90	0.91
A_7	400.00 ± 20.00	782.00 ± 6.07	6.49	4.64

Table 2.
Ambiental dose equivalent H(10) [2].*

The main risk for dosimetrist during contamination scanning is due to A_7 hot spot. For this hot spot, the Ambiental Dose Equivalent is about 26 (27 for TLDs) times higher than the mean value of the other six hot spots [2].

In the hottest point, A_7, the ^{60}Co activity (4.57E+08 Bq) is 3 orders of magnitude higher than the mean value of the other six hot spots (3.60 E+05 Bq) thus, the results for the Ambiental Dose Rate measurements are confirmed [2]. The activities of the ^{134}Cs, ^{137}Cs and ^{108m}Ag are 3 and 2 times lower than ^{60}Co activity [2].

The penetrant dose rate for the workers was calculated by standard method assuming that the sampling yield for the activity measurement is 10% and that the entire activity is concentrated in the hottest point. The values are presented in **Table 3**. According to Romanian legislation the professional exposed dose limit is 20 mSv/year, and for 2000 working hours/year the dose rate is 10 μSv/hour [2].

For the dosimetrist, the penetrant dose rate is 3.39 mSv/h, respectively 0.28 mSv for five minutes exposure and the risk are quite high. Consequently, the working time for future activities must not be longer than 5.9 hours/year [2]. For the mechanical worker, the penetrant dose rate is 7.97 mSv/h, 1.59 mSv for 12 minutes. The risk is also very high, consequently the working time must be less than 2.5 hours/year for future activities [2].

The internal committed effective dose E (50) was calculated for mechanical worker performing floor decontamination. For this purpose, we assume that inside of the hot cell is spread only the 10^{-4} of the total activity and the worker wearing a mask with filter (99% retention efficiency) [2]. The values are presented in **Table 3**. The internal irradiation could be due to the A_7 the hottest point presence (1.62 μSv).

Hot spot	$\dot{H}_p(10)_{scan}$ [mSv/h]	$\dot{H}_p(10)_{decon.}$ [mSv/h]	$E(50)_{decon.}$ [mSv]
A_1	5.36E-03	1.12E-02	3.33E-06
A_2	1.18E-03	2.45E-03	7.48E-07
A	2.09E-03	4.71E-03	1.14E-06
A_4	2.41E-03	5.85E-03	1.16E-06
A_5	1.19E-03	2.87E-03	5.74E-07
A_6	2.45E-03	5.52E-03	8.55E-07
A_7	3.37E+00	7.93E+00	1.62E-03
Total	3.39E+00	7.97E+00	1.63E-03

Table 3.
Dose rate assessed by standard method [2].

Time [days]	Ai [%]	Ai	R1 [mSv/h]	R2 [mSv/h]	R3 [mSv/h]	Total [mSv/h]
0	100	4.57E+09	1.34E+00	2.86E+00	1.22E+00	5.42E+00
7	60	2.74E+09	8.04E-01	1.71E+00	7.30E-01	3.24E+00
14	40	1.10E+09	3.20E-01	6.80E-01	2.91E-01	1.29E+00
21	25	2.74E+08	7.97E-02	1.70E-01	7.25E-02	3.22E-01
28	15	4.11E+07	1.20E-02	2.54E-02	1.09E-02	4.82E-02

Table 4.
Dose rate assessed by numerical method.

The dose is low enough and the internal irradiation does not affect the worker due to the high filter efficiency [2].

The dose rates for mechanical workers (receptors) who performed the floor decontamination, assessed using RESRAD Build code modeling, are presented in **Table 4** as well as in the **Figure** 7.

At the inception of the decontamination process, the highest potential dose rate was received by the receptor 2 (R2) who spread the decontaminant on the floor. A similar behavior could be noticed for receptor 1 (R1) performing decontaminant spraying and receptor 3 (R3) performing decontaminant coating gel removal.

The potential dose received by R2 receptor is 2.1 times higher than the dose received by R1 and respectively 2.3 times higher for R3.

Although, dose rate decreased after 28 days (the end of floor surface decontamination) the value it is at about 5 times greater than the limit of 10 μSv/hour.

By comparing the total initial dose rates for the mechanical worker performing all decontamination steps, at the inception of the decontamination process, it can be noticed that the RESRAD dose (5.42 mSv/h) is 1.5 lower than the dose evaluated by standard method (7.97 mSv/h). The difference can be explained by RESRAD model complexity. Consequently, the working time of the mechanical worker must be less than 3.7 hours/year.

In the proposed scenario, according to the hot spot's activities, the greatest risk is presented by the ^{60}Co and ^{137}Cs [2]. The risk is very high because the decontamination scenario considers that the task is performed manually.

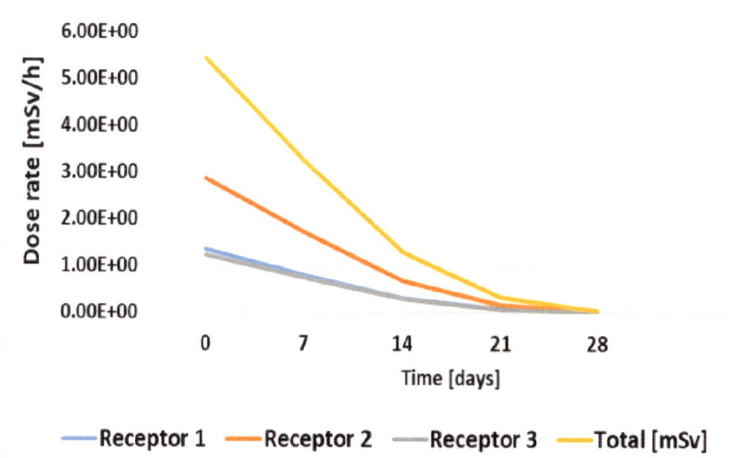

Figure 7.
RESRAD Build dose rate.

The radiation level remains significant after three decontamination cycles since the stainless-steel lining is activated.

4. Recommendation and future perspective

Due to high dose, the risks for the workers are considerable. In such circumstances we also consider that the clean-up process should be performed using robots [13] instead of the workers, according with the ALARA principle.

In order to avoid the dosimetrist and mechanical worker over exposure, prior decontamination, the sources located inside on the Hot Cell are extracted using a

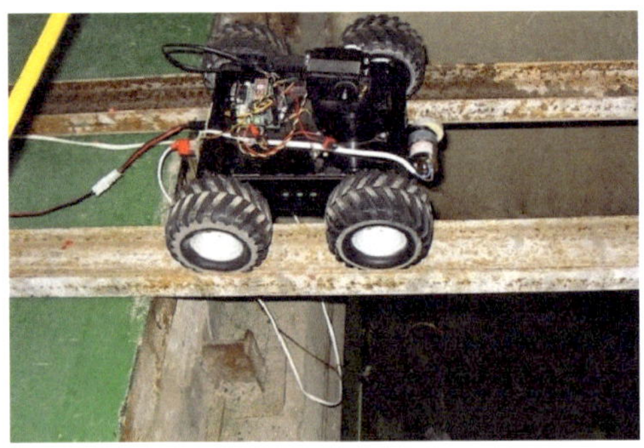

Figure 8.
Robot for sorce removal.

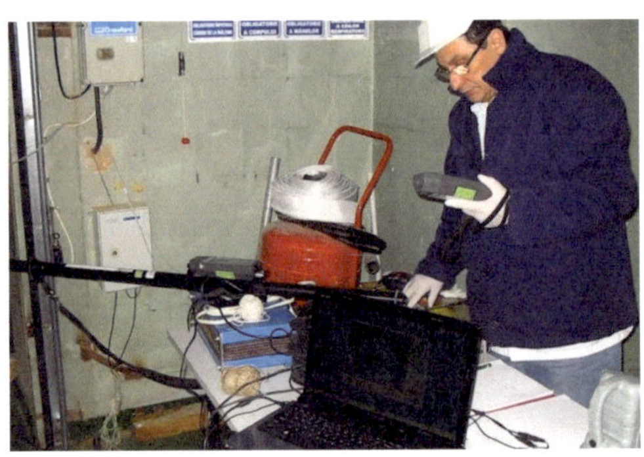

Figure 9.
Sources removal monitoring.

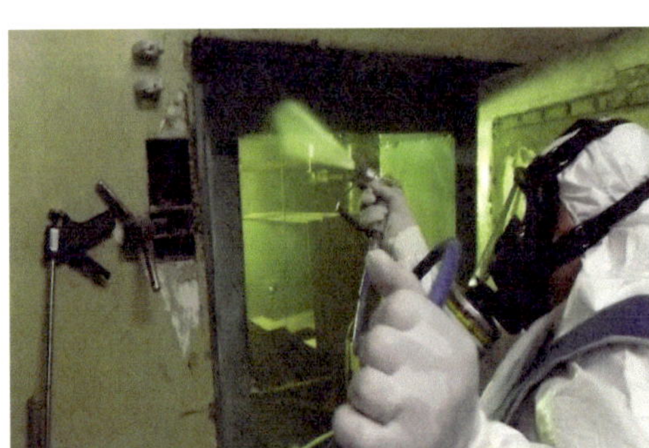

Figure 10.
Outside decontaminat spraying.

remote-controlled car (see **Figure 8**). The process is monitored by the dosimetrist from distance using a portable digital survey meter [2], (see **Figure 9**).

The decontaminant gel should be also sprayed from distance by the worker located outside of the Hot Cell (see the **Figure 10**). Then the decontamination should be performed using a Schunk robotic arm mounted on a Neobotix Platform [13, 14].

5. Conclusions

Dose rates received during a nuclear research reactor Hot Cells decontamination were assessed by a standard as well as a numerical method.

For both assessments resulted that the dose for professional exposed is higher than the limit. The risk is very high due to the fact that decontamination process was performed manually.

After three decontamination cycles, the radiation level remains significant because the stainless-steel lining is activated. The clean-up and decontamination should be performed by the robots in order to prevent workers over exposure.

The dose rates calculated with RESRAD Build code are lower and more accurately than the those obtained by standard method due to model complexity.

Despite small differences, it can conclude that both methodologies for dose assessment are in agreement and useful for similar exposure situations.

Acknowledgements

The authors offer many thanks to Dr. A.O. Pavelescu for his suggestions and feedback when clarifications of issues were required and also to Mr. Adrian Zorliu for his support for samples sampling.

Author details

Carmen Tuca* and Ana Stochioiu
"Horia Hulubei" National Institute for R&D in Physics and Nuclear Engineering, IFIN-HH, Magurele, Romania

*Address all correspondence to: tuca@nipne.ro

References

[1] Tuca C, Deju R. The assessment of the radioactive inventory for the solid wastes from VVR-S Nuclear Research Reactor Decommissioning. Acta Physica Polonica A. 2019; 135:1050-1054. DOI: 10.12693/APhysPolA.135.1050

[2] Tuca C, Deju R, Zorliu A. Radiological Risk Assessment for Hot Cell Decontamination, Romanian Journal of Physics. 2017;62:812. DOI10.4172/2155-9619.C1.008

[3] Ionescu E. Direct measurement of the surface contamination, control procedure PC-DEZ-401, 2012.

[4] Stochioiu A. The monitoring of the environmental radioactivity using thermo-luminescent dosimetry system, operational procedure, PL-UMRM-01, 2015.

[5] Gurau D. Gamma-ray spectrometry analysis with HPGe detector, model GEM60P4-95, control procedure, PC-DEZ-408, 2011.

[6] Radu D, Stanga D, Sima O. A method of efficiency calibration for disk sources in gamma-ray spectrometry, Rom. Rep. Phys. 2009; 61,2:203-213

[7] Sahagia M, Razdolescu A. C., Luca A., Macrin R. Volume standard sources in soil matrix, Rom. J. Phys. 1997; 42, 9-10: 659-663

[8] Luca A, Neacsu B, Antohe A, Sahagia M. Calibration of the high and low resolution Gamma- ray spectrometers, Rom. Rep. Phys. 2012;64,4:968-972

[9] C. Yu, A.J. Zielen, J.-J. Cheng, D.J. LePoire, E. Gnanapragasam, S. Kamboj, J. Arnish, A. Wallo III,* W.A. Williams,* and H. Peterson*. July 2001. User's Manual for RESRAD Version 6, by Environmental Assessment Division Argonne National Laboratory, 9700 South Cass Avenue, Argonne, Illinois 60439

[10] U.S. Environmental Protection Agency, Exposure Factor Handbook, EPA/600/P-95/002Fa, Office of Research and Development, National Center for Environmental Assessment, 1997

[11] Beyeler W.E. et al., Residual Radioactive Contamination from Decommissioning; Parameter Analysis, NUREG/CR-5512, Vol. 3, Nuclear Regulatory Commission, Office of Nuclear Regulatory Research, Oct. 1999.

[12] Wernig M.A., et al., Residual Radioactive Contamination from Decommissioning: User's Manual, NUREG/CR-5512, Vol. 2, Nuclear Regulatory Commission, Office of Nuclear Regulatory Research, May 1999

[13] Pavelescu A.O, Popa V, Drăguşin M. Modelling of the dose rates and risks arising from hot-cells clean-up activities in the decommissioning of the VVR-S research reactor; Rom. Rep. Phys. 2012; 64, 1:33-49

[14] Schunk GmbH & Co., LWA3 Lightweight Arm Modular Robotic Specification Sheet, Catalog Automation Highlights, 2009.

Chapter 7

Quality in Non-Licensed Radiopharmaceutical Products: Are We Achieving the Goal?

Estrella Moya Sánchez

Abstract

Radiopharmaceutical compounds, considered a special group of medicines, can be prepared outside the marketing authorisation track. Small-scale preparations at non-commercial sites thereby represent an important segment, however a lack of harmonisation in the regulation leads to extreme differences in the application and availability of radiopharmaceuticals across Europe. A number of guidelines and guidance documents have been issued by European Association of Nuclear Medicine (EAMN), Pharmaceutical inspection convention (PICs), European Directorate for the Quality of Medicines & HealthCare (EDQM) to achieve a good radiopharmacy practice for small-scale preparation. Nevertheless, in the case of non-licensed radiopharmaceuticals their consideration as magistral formulas, in some countries, makes it possible to waive regulatory inspections aimed to ensure those good practices enforcement. Moreover, special attention should be put on the quality assurance process for non-licensed starting materials, given that the final radiopharmaceuticals quality chiefly depends on it. This paper (chapter) will provide an insight into the quality standards applicable to starting materials, such as supplier qualification control, starting material re-test period, etc. in order to raise for discussion about how best to achieve a proven quality, efficacy, and safety for our radiopharmaceuticals (licensed or non-licensed).

Keywords: non-licensed, good radiopharmacy practice, magistral formulas, quality assurance process

1. Introduction

During the '80s radiopharmaceuticals were considered as tracers used in hospital centres under the responsibility of a person with a sound knowledge in the safe use of radiation. It was in 1989 when radiopharmaceuticals were considered for the first time in the European Union as medicinal products after entry into force the Council Directive 89/343/EEC [1]. In this Directive was stated the first official radiopharmaceutical definition as:

"any medicinal product which, when ready for use, contains one or more radionuclides (radioactive isotopes) included for a medicinal purpose."

Radiopharmaceuticals are used in major clinical areas for diagnosis and therapy. They usually have no pharmacologic effects, as they are used in tracer quantities. Consequently, there is no dose–response relationship, which thus differs significantly from conventional medicinal products. Radiation is an inherent characteristic of all radiopharmaceuticals, and patients always receive an unavoidable radiation dose. In the case of therapeutic radiopharmaceuticals, radiation is what produces the therapeutic effect.

The manufacturing and handling of radiopharmaceuticals is potentially hazardous. The level of risk depends in particular upon the types of radiation, the energy of radiation and the half-lives of the radioactive isotopes. The facilities and procedures for the production, use, and storage are subject to licencing by national and/or regional authorities. This licencing includes compliance both with regulations governing pharmaceutical preparations and with those governing radioactive materials.

Considering the special nature of radiopharmaceuticals, strict adherence to conventional good manufacturing practices is not possible in many scenarios where radiopharmaceuticals are handled. It is necessary to balance aseptic handling practices (patient safety) with radiation protection practices (worker safety) complying with the current *As Low As Reasonably Achievable* (ALARA) requirements. Moreover, a demanding technical difference and challenge is that in most cases, diagnostic radiopharmaceuticals need to be prepared, controlled and used within a short time of a few hours or even minutes due to the physical half life of the radionuclides.

Specific guidance is available on adaptations to the conventional regulatory framework to address challenges of the preparation of radiopharmaceuticals.

2. Medical uses of radiopharmaceuticals

A radionuclide may decay by emitting different types of ionising radiation: alpha (α), beta (β-), positron (β+) and gamma (γ) radiation.

Depending on the radiation characteristics of the radionuclide, the radiopharmaceutical is used either for diagnosis or for therapy. Diagnostic radiopharmaceuticals should decay by gamma emission like Technetium-99 m (99mTc), Iodine-123 (123I) and Galium-67 (67Ga) or positron emission like Fluorine-18 (18F), Oxygen-15 (15O), Carbon-11 (11C), Zirconium 89 (89Zr) and Gallium 68 (68Ga) and never emit alpha particles or even beta particles.

On the other hand, therapeutic radiopharmaceuticals should decay by particulate decay (alpha or beta) since the intended effect is in fact radiation damage to specific cell, examples of β -emitters are Rhenium-186/Rhenium-188 (186Re/188Re), Strontium-89 (89Sr), Lutetium-177 (177-Lu),Iodine-131 (131-I) and Yttrium-90 (90Y) and of therapeutic α-emitters are Actinium-225 (225Ac), Bismuth-213 (213Bi) and Astatine-211 (211At).

Moreover, there is an emerging field of nuclear medicine named theranostics (Therapeutics and diagnostics), that involves diagnostic and therapeutic agents to target diseased cells and tissues. The use of targeting molecules labelled either with diagnostic radioisotopes and with therapeutic isotopes enables a more complete approach to patient management, because the diagnosis can then serve several simultaneous functions: assessing disease, monitoring and selection for therapy. The prospects of identifying the disease and orienting treatment, provide an advance level in precision medicine.

One of the most common examples of theragnosis in nuclear medicine is the use of Gallium 68(68Ga) as a diagnostic radiopharmaceutical, followed by therapy with radionuclides such as Lutetium 177 (177-Lu) to label the same molecule in the context of personalised therapy.

3. Radiopharmaceutical's dosage forms. Alternative methods to control sterility in radiopharmaceuticals

Radiopharmaceuticals are medicinal products on prescription that can be delivered orally (in pill form), intravenously (injected into a patient's vein) or interstitially (inserted into a cavity in the body). The intravenous route of administration is the most used in Radiopharmaceuticals application. According to the European Pharmacopoeia monograph regarding Radiopharmaceutical preparations (01625) [2], these products must be sterile as stated in the following extract.

"Radiopharmaceutical preparations for parenteral administration comply with the test for sterility. They must be prepared using precautions designed to exclude microbial contamination and to ensure sterility. The test for sterility is carried out as described in the general method (2.6.1)." [3].

Moreover, the pharmacopoeia also considers the specific nature of radiopharmaceuticals, as specified in this other extract.

"Special difficulties arise with radiopharmaceutical preparations because of the short half-life of some radionuclides, the small size of batches and the radiation hazards. In the case that the monograph states that the preparation can be released for use before completion of the test for sterility, the sterility test must be started as soon as practically possible in relation to the radiation."

With the conventional sterility method (2.6.1) [3] the portions of the media should be incubated for 14 days. Though the test must be started as soon as practically possible in relation to the radiation, it will take several days to achieve a safe level of exposure. This means that sterility testing results would be available around three weeks after the radiopharmaceutical preparation. Consequently, the outcomes of the tests when following this method seldom enable proactive corrective actions to be taken in case a lack of sterility is detected.

Alternative methods for control of microbiological quality have been described in European Pharmacopoeia (5.1.6) [4]. They have shown potential for real-time o near real-time results with the possibility of earlier corrective action. Although this pharmacopoeia chapter is published for information, these new methods, if validated and adapted for routine use can also offer significant improvements in the quality of testing.

Similarly, USP has another monograph (1071) [5] where the following extract can be found.

"Rapid microbial tests for release of sterile short-life products: a risk-based approach".

In this chapter, positron emission tomographic (PET) products are mentioned as an example where these rapid methods could be applied.

"It is widely recognized that the current growth-based sterility tests with an incubation period of at least 14 days are not suitable for products with a short shelf-life or for products prepared for immediate use, which are usually infused into patients before the completion of the test (1). These short-life products include compounded sterile preparations (CSPs), **positron emission tomographic (PET) products,** *and cell and gene therapies, which require a new generation of risk-based approaches that include rapid microbial tests".*

The information provided in these pharmacopoeia chapters may be used as a supplement or as an alternative microbiological method and to give guidance on validation of the chosen method. It is neither the intention to recommend one method over another, nor to provide an exclusive list of alternative methods that can be used.

Rapid microbial tests described in USP (1071) • Adenosine triphosphate bioluminescence • Flow cytometry • Isothermal microcalorimetry • Nucleic acid amplification • Respiration • Solid phase cytometry
Alternative methods for control of microbiological quality described in Ph. Eur 5.16 There are 3 major types of determination specific to microbiological tests: 1. **Qualitative tests for the presence or absence of micro-organisms:** • Tests based on bioluminescence • Solid phase cytometry • Gas detection or autofluorescence • Nucleic acid amplification techniques (NAT) (2.6.21) may also be used for the detection of mycoplasmas (2.6.7) 2. **Quantitative tests for enumeration of micro-organisms:** • Autofluorescence • Flow cytometry • Direct epifluorescent filter technique (DEFT) • Solid phase cytometry 3. **Identification tests** • Biochemical and morphological characterisation

Table 1.
List with alternative methods of microbiological quality described in pharmacopoeia European and USP.

In both chapters, European Pharmacopoeia (5.1.6) [4] and USP monograph (1071) [5], it is stated that risk analysis tools may be used to determine which alternative method is to be implemented as well as to balance user requirement specification including time to result, specificity, limit of detection (LOD), sample size, and product attributes. The microbiological alternative methods proposed in European Pharmacopoeia and USP are described in **Table 1**.

4. Types of radiopharmaceutical marketing authorisations

Licensed radiopharmaceuticals manufactured under GMP requirements.

In the European Union, radiopharmaceutical compounds are considered a special group of medicines. Their manufacturing/preparing and uses are regulated by directives and regulations that must be adopted by Member States. (Directive 2001/83/EC [6] and Regulation (EC) No 726/2004 [7]).

For a radiopharmaceutical to be available on the market, sold and marketed, it needs to have a marketing authorisation. The marketing authorisation application must provide evidence of the efficacy, safety, and quality of the radiopharmaceutical. When applying for a marketing authorisation for a radiopharmaceutical, the marketing authorisation application is submitted to a regulatory authority, which will assess the medicinal product's pharmaceutical and chemical quality, efficacy, and safety, as well as its risk–benefit ratio.

In the EU, there are four types of marketing authorisation application procedures. These procedures can be found in European Medicines Agency (EMA) website [8] in its section devoted to medicine for human use marketing authorisations:

- National procedure: Used when applying for a marketing authorisation in one individual EU Member State, Norway, Iceland, and Liechtenstein.

- Centralised procedure: The centralised procedure allows manufacturers to submit a single Market Authorization Application (MAA) to the European Medicines Agency (EMA) who is responsible for the scientific evaluation. Once granted by the European Commission, the centralised marketing authorisation is valid in all European Union (EU) Member States, Iceland, Norway and Liechtenstein.

The centralised procedure is **compulsory for:**

- *Human medicines containing a new active substance to treat:*

    - *human* immunodeficiency *virus (HIV) or acquired immune deficiency syndrome (AIDS);*

    - *cancer;*

    - *diabetes;*

    - neurodegenerative diseases;

    - auto immune and other immune dysfunctions;

    - viral dise*ases.*

- *Medicines derived from biotechnology processes, such as genetic engineering.*

- *Advanced-therapy medicines, such as gene-therapy, somatic cell-therapy or tissue-engineered medicines.*

- *Orphan medicines (medicines for rare diseases).*

- *Veterinary medicines for use as growth or yield enhancers.*

It is optional for other medicines:

- *Containing new active substances for indications other than those stated above.*

- *That are a significant therapeutic, scientific, or technical innovation.*

- *Whose authorisation would be in the interest of public or animal health at EU level.*

Today, the great majority of new, innovative medicines pass through the centralised authorisation procedure in order to be marketed in the EU.

If a company wishes to request marketing authorisation in several EU Member States for a medicine that is outside the scope of the centralised procedure, it may use one of the following routes, as also clarified in the EMA website:

- Decentralised Procedure: The procedure for authorising medicines whereby a medicine that has not yet been authorised in the EU can be simultaneously authorised in several EU Member States.

- Mutual Recognition Procedure: The procedure for authorising medicines whereby a marketing authorisation granted in one Member State can be recognised in other EU countries.

In case of Radiopharmaceuticals, that are used extensively to treat people with cancer, centralised procedure will be the proceeding to be followed.

4.1 Radiopharmaceuticals within a clinical trial

On the other hand, the Radiopharmaceuticals can be used for research and development. All requirements to apply in Europe for a clinical trial are stated in *EudraLex - Volume 10 -* **Clinical trials guidelines** *Volume 10 of the publication "The rules governing medicinal products in the European Union"* [9].

The following four circumstances are possible for the use of Radiopharmaceutical within a clinical trial:

- Licensed radiopharmaceutical products used within their authorised indications,

- Licensed radiopharmaceutical products used outside their authorised indications,

- Radiopharmaceuticals having established clinical use that are prepared in accordance with approved regulations and meet approved quality requirements (e.g. as described in a monograph of a pharmacopoeia),

- New radiopharmaceuticals or tracer agents outside the previous categories.

4.2 Small scale preparations of radiopharmaceuticals

Radiopharmaceuticals may be prepared at small scale in healthcare establishments, and they may also be prepared outside the marketing authorisation track.

There are various types of radiopharmaceuticals prepared in healthcare establishments as it is described in PIC/S (Pharmaceutical inspection convention, pharmaceutical inspection co-operation scheme) [10] among which can remark:

- Sterile products with a marketing authorisation which are aseptically prepared in the healthcare establishment. These are typically used for routine diagnostic purposes in nuclear medicine and include:

- Technetium- 99 m radiolabelled ligands obtained by the combination of the kit component with [99mTc] pertechnetate from a radionuclide generator.

- Radionuclide precursors with a marketing authorisation, for example Yttrium-90 which are used as starting materials for synthesis.

- Sterile products without a marketing authorisation which are synthesised, radiolabelled, purified and formulated for diagnostic or therapeutic use.

- Oral products with marketing authorisation which are prepared as capsules or solutions which the patient takes for diagnosis or therapeutic. Use (e. g. Iodine-131 for thyroid treatment).

5. Preparation or manufacturing of radiopharmaceuticals?

The difference between radiopharmaceutical preparation and manufacture is a sensitive issue which calls for a consensus that, it seems not exist at present.

The following definitions for preparation and manufacturing can be found in the GMP Annex 3 [11]:

"Preparation: handling and radiolabelling of kits with radionuclide eluted from generators or radioactive precursors within a hospital. Kits, generators and precursors should have a marketing authorisation or a national licence".

"Manufacturing: production, quality control and release and delivery of radiopharmaceuticals from the active substance and starting materials".

As per the extract above, it becomes apparent that in a preparation, products with marketing authorisation should be used. Provided that the summary of product characteristics (SPC) instructions is followed, the ultimate responsibility for the radiopharmaceutical preparation with respect to its safety, quality, and efficacy, over its shelf live lies with the marketing authorisation holder (MAH). However, this requirement is not remarked in the case of manufacturing.

By contrast, if we regard the Pharmacopoeia European monograph (5.19) Extemporaneous preparation of radiopharmaceuticals [12], the following definition is stated:

"The preparation of radiopharmaceuticals is considered as a process involving some or all of the following steps: purchase of materials and products, production of radionuclides for radiolabelling, radiolabelling, chemical modification and/or purification, formulation, dispensing of the pharmaceutical form, sterilisation, analytical control, packaging, labelling and release. Drawing patient doses for immediate application (e.g., from a multidose vial) is considered as part of clinical practice, and not part of the preparation of Radiopharmaceuticals."

As can be seen in the pharmacopoeia definition, the use of authorised materials and products is not a requirement. From this perspective, preparation and manufacturing processes could seem fairly similar, since purification and sterilisation steps are also encompassed within them. However, as it is stated in Pharmacopoeia European monograph (5.19), the manufacture of radiopharmaceuticals and investigational medicinal products should be covered by existing regulation (authorisation of any competent authority) and a pharmaceutical preparation definition would include all the preparations with licensed and non-licensed products. Additionally, the European Pharmacopoeia monograph 2619 [13] differences two categories, extemporaneous and stock preparations as it can be seen in the following extracts:

"Pharmaceutical preparations are medicinal products generally consisting of active substances that may be combined with excipients, formulated into a dosage form suitable for the intended use, where necessary after reconstitution, presented in a suitable and appropriately labelled container."

"Pharmaceutical preparations may be non-licensed by the competent authority, or unlicensed and made to the specific needs of patients according to legislation. There are 2 categories of unlicensed pharmaceutical preparations:

- extemporaneous preparations, i.e., pharmaceutical preparations individually prepared for a specific patient or patient group, supplied after preparation.
- stock preparations, i.e., pharmaceutical preparations prepared in advance and stored until a request for a supply is received."

On the other hand, we cannot overlook that most radiopharmaceutical preparations are used for parenteral administration, and therefore required to be sterile. Then, if we consider the *EMA guideline on the sterilisation of the medicinal product active substance, excipient, and primary container*, [14] it might seem that whenever a sterilisation procedure has to be applied, it will be considered as a manufacturing process according to the following extract:

"Sterility is a critical quality that cannot be assured by testing, it needs to be assured by the use of a suitably designed, validated and controlled manufacturing process".

Therefore, this consideration seems to contradict the previous pharmacopoeia extracts where the sterilisation process was included in the scope of the preparation definition.

Notwithstanding the difficulties to get an official consensus on the definitions of preparation and manufacturing, there should be an agreement on who bears the final responsibility in them:

- In the event licensed products were used, the responsibility would lie with the marketing authorisation holder (MAH) as long as the summary of product characteristics (SPC) instructions is followed. If these instructions include the need to apply sterilisation, the responsibility on the sterilisation process would also lie on the MAH.
- Otherwise, whenever non-licensed products or licensed products not compliant with SPC instructions were used, the final responsibility would always rest with the Chief Radiopharmacist who prepares/manufactures them.

6. Scientific guidelines

As is stated in the EMA website [8] "*The European Medicines Agency's Committee for Medicinal Products for Human Use prepares scientific guidelines in consultation with regulatory authorities in the European Union (EU) Member States, to help applicants prepare marketing authorisation applications for human medicines. Guidelines reflect a harmonised approach of the EU Member States and the Agency on how to interpret and apply the requirements for the demonstration of quality, safety and efficacy set out in the Community directives*".

These guidelines are complementary to European Pharmacopoeia monographs and chapters, since as detailed in the directive 2001/83 EC (annex I) [6] with respect to the quality part (chemical, pharmaceutical and biological) of the dossier, all monographs including general monographs and general chapters of the European Pharmacopoeia are applicable.

The catalogue of guidelines is categorised according to the Common Technical Document (CTD) [15] when they concern general issues and include the guidelines that are globally harmonised through the International Council on Harmonisation of Technical Requirements for Registration of Pharmaceuticals for Human Use (ICH).

The Guideline on Radiopharmaceuticals [16] issued by EMA Committee for human medicinal products provides information about specific requirements for radiopharmaceuticals in applications for both marketing and clinical trial authorisations.

Altogether, regulatory authorities and industry prepared ICH scientific guidelines as shown in **Table 2**.

However, CHMP scientific guidelines are just issued by the European Medicines Agency's Committee for Medicinal Products for Human Use.

In addition to the application of the mentioned guidelines, the manufacturing process shall comply with the requirements of Commission Directive 91/356/EEC, as amended by Directive 2003/94/EC, and 91/412/EEC respectively laying down the principles and guidelines of Good Manufacturing Practice (GMP) for medicinal products for human use and with the principles and guidelines on GMP, published by the commission in the rules governing medicinal products in the European Community, Volume 4 [17]. In particular, the EU GMP annex 3 [11] specifically addresses some of the practices, which may be specific for radiopharmaceuticals.

Furthermore, there are also other guidelines published whose main objective is to harmonise inspection procedures worldwide by developing common standards in the field of GMPs and by providing training opportunities to Inspectors. They are issued by The Pharmaceutical Inspection Co-operation Scheme (PIC/S) who is a non-binding, informal co-operative arrangement between Regulatory Authorities in the field of Good Manufacturing Practice (GMP) of medicinal products for human or veterinary use. Particularly, the annex 3 of PIC/S Guide to good practices for the preparation of medicinal products in healthcare establishments is devoted to Radiopharmaceuticals [10].

Similarly, EDQM has published in the European Pharmacopoeia, the monograph 5.19 Extemporaneous preparation of Radiopharmaceuticals [12]. Although this monograph is only for information, it covers guidance for preparing "kit-based preparations (from licensed and unlicensed kits) and unlicensed preparations containing radionuclides for positron emission tomography (PET), single photon emission computed tomography (SPECT) or for therapeutic applications".

In the USP several monographs can also be found regarding radiopharmaceuticals preparation, such as USP (825) [18] radiopharmaceuticals preparation, compounding, dispensing and repackaging or USP (823) [19] Positron emission tomography drugs for compounding, investigational, and research uses.

Besides, other "for information" guidelines can be mentioned. For instance, a guideline to achieve a good radiopharmacy practice for small-scale preparation was issued by The European Association of Nuclear Medicine (EANM) [20]. This is a professional non-profit medical association that facilitates communication worldwide among individuals pursuing clinical and research excellence in nuclear medicine.

In conclusion, many guidelines and guidance documents have been issued to foster good radiopharmacy practices for licensed or not licensed radiopharmaceuticals in both large and small-scale preparation.

Region	Regulatory authorities	Industry
Europe	EMA	EFPIA
USA	FDA	PhRMA
Japan	MHLW	JPMA

Table 2.
Summary of the parties involved in the ICH guidelines development.

7. Radiopharmaceuticals preparation outside the marketing track in the European Union

In the European Union (UE), the community code relating to medicinal products for human use is regulated by the Directive 2001/83/EC [6] as amended. This Directive has to be adopted by Member States. The rate and extent of adoption and interpretation of the Directive varies among countries. Each Member State may introduce changes, provided the general scope and limits of the directive is maintained.

In this way, several European Member States have set up a regulatory framework in which radiopharmaceuticals for routine use can be prepared on site without the requirements of a marketing authorization. These exemptions flow from the definitions in Article 3 of Directive 2001/83/EC [6], the so-called magistral and officinal formulae, and from Article 5(1) of Directive 2001/83/EC aimed to fulfil special needs.

The European Court of Justice. Document 62013CJ0544 and Judgement of the Court (Third Chamber) of 16 July 2015 has clarified both situations of Articles 3 and 5 [21].

Considering article 3, for "magistral formulae" defined as "any medicinal product prepared in a pharmacy in accordance with a medical prescription for an individual patient". The European Court of Justice specified that "[such a preparation] must of necessity be prepared on the basis of a prior prescription issued by a professional person qualified to do so". This prescription must, in addition "be 'for an individual patient'" and "that patient must be identified before the medicinal product is produced and it must be produced specifically for that patient". It was also stated that "the exception provided for in that provision can only concern situations in which the doctor considers that the state of health of his individual patients requires that a medicinal product be administered for which there is no authorised equivalent on the national market, or which is unavailable on that market", clearly excluding competition with licensed medicinal products.

Similarly, by virtue of Article 5(1) of Directive 2001/83 [6], to fulfil special needs, exclude from the provisions of that directive medicinal products supplied in response to a bona fide unsolicited order, formulated in accordance with the specifications of an authorised healthcare professional and for use by an individual patient under his direct personal responsibility. In that regard, the court has held that it is apparent from the conditions as a whole set out in that provision, read in the light of the fundamental objectives of that directive, and in particular the objective of seeking to safeguard public health, that the exception provided for in that provision can only concern situations in which the doctor considers that the state of health of his individual patients requires that a medicinal product be administered for which there is no authorised equivalent on the national market or which is unavailable on that market (see, to that effect, judgement in Commission v Poland, C-185/10, EU:C:2012:181, paragraphs 29 and 36).

United Kingdom (UK) is the clear example of applying the exception of art 5(1) of the Directive 2001/83/EC [6], despite after Brexit is no longer part of the European Union (UE). The regulation 167 of the Human Medicines Regulations 2012 sets out the exemption from the requirement for a medicinal product, placed on the market in the UK to hold a marketing authorisation. Additionally, the Medicines and Healthcare Products Regulatory Agency (MHRA) issued the MHRA Guidance Note 14 called "The supply of unlicensed medicinal products ("specials") [22].

In some Member States (Austria, Belgium etc..) the preparation of PET radiopharmaceuticals could be considered, in many situations, as magistral formulas since they are prepared in accordance with a medical prescription for an individual patient. The preparation of radiopharmaceuticals as magistral formulae is not covered under the Directive 2001/83/EC [6], therefore its legislation falls under the responsibility of each Member State.

In Germany, PET radiopharmaceuticals can be manufactured according to the requirements set in article 13(2b) of the Medicinal Products Act (Arzneimittelgesetz, AMG) where it is stated that "*a person who is a doctor or dentist or who is otherwise authorised to practise medicine on humans does not require a licence according to paragraph 1, insofar as the medicinal products are manufactured under his direct professional responsibility for the purpose of personal use on a specific patient*". However, it is important to note that the compliance with the Medicinal Products Act is controlled by the Federal States, coming along with the acceptance of varying practices by different state authorities. Hence, there is currently a lively discussion in the nuclear medicine community about minimum standards for this production, though the use of radiopharmaceuticals with marketing authorisation is preferential.

By contrast, in Spain, the preparation of radiopharmaceuticals cannot be considered as magistral formulae since they must be prepared with legally recognised action and indication substances as stated in Royal Legislative Decree RDL 1/2015. Therefore, the only way to prepare PET radiopharmaceuticals outside the marketing authorisation track would be under the regulatory framework of article 47.1c in Real Decree (RD) 1345/2007 on the marketing authorization procedure in medicines for human use [23]. This Decree completes the RDL 1/2015 [24], which is the transposition of Directive 2001/83/EC [6]. The article 47.1.c in the RD 1345/2007 [23] establishes the following criteria:

The marketing authorisation for PET radiopharmaceuticals will not be required, whenever they are prepared in an approved radiopharmaceutical unit under the supervision and control of a radiopharmaceutical specialist, provided that they meet the following requirements:

1. They are entirely prepared and used in the authorised radiopharmacy units with non-profit use and in centres linked to the National Health System.

2. They are substances used in clinical research, or medicines that the Spanish Agency for Medicines and Medical Devices (AEMPS) considers satisfying the guarantees of quality, safety, efficacy, identification, and information, and that are prepared in appropriate facilities.

Beyond the lack of alignment regarding the definition of radiopharmaceuticals preparations analysed above, differences can also be found with respect to the requirements that manufacturers have to comply with in their preparation. The following examples depict this situation:

- In United Kingdom as is stated in MHRA Guidance Note 14, [22] "the manufacturer or assembler of "specials" must hold a Manufacturer's "Specials" Licence granted by the Licencing Authority." Furthermore, it is also said that "the manufacturing/assembly site and its operations will be inspected for compliance with Good Manufacturing Practice (GMP) and the conditions of the licence".

- In Spain the situation seems to be fairly like UK, the manufacturer must apply the Spanish Medicines Agency (AEMPS) for a certificate of compliance with requirements and the sites operations will be inspected for compliance with Good Manufacturing Practices (GMPs).

- In the rest of the Member States there are different degrees of compliance with Good Manufacturing Practices (GMPs). In some countries as Germany full adherence to GMPs is required, while in other countries such as Italy special or adapted GMPs are enforced. Finally, there are other countries where this compliance is not clearly specified.

Summarising, there are different ways to carry out the radiopharmaceuticals small scale preparation outside the marketing authorisation track, depending on the national legislation in each Member State. Hence, a cornerstone of the radiopharmaceutical's preparation might currently be the lack of harmonisation at European level, especially regarding the quality standards applicable to these preparations.

Nevertheless, leaving aside the lack of harmonisation among countries, special attention shall be drawn to the achievement of the highest standard quality radiopharmaceutical preparations. It is a fact that, as a rule, this goal is accomplished in the manufacturing processes for medicinal products by applying GMPs. For sure, these practices should consider the special nature of radiopharmaceuticals balancing aseptic handling with radiation protection. Besides, authorities should ensure that manufacturers in their territory are subject to routine GMP inspections.

In the field of clinical trial this goal is on its way thanks to the new Regulation 536/2014 [25] repealing the Directive 2001/20/EC. This regulation will achieve the harmonisation between Member States, through the creation of a uniform regulatory framework for the authorization of clinical trials. It is to be noted that European Regulations are not transposed by the European Members but directly applied. Therefore, European Member States shall be compliant with this regulation.

The Regulation 536/2014 [25], in the case of radiopharmaceuticals used in clinical trials stablishes differences between therapeutic and diagnostic radiopharmaceuticals. While therapeutic radiopharmaceuticals are considered as any other medicinal product used in a Clinical Trial, regarding diagnostic radiopharmaceuticals substantial changes are introduced by the following article (Art. 61.5.b of Regulation 536/2014):

"preparation of radiopharmaceuticals used as diagnostic investigational medicinal products where this process is carried out in hospitals, health centers or clinics, by pharmacists or other persons legally authorized in the Member State concerned to carry out such process, and if the investigational medicinal products are intended to be used exclusively in hospitals, health centers or clinics taking part in the same clinical trial in the same Member State".

Based on the analysis of this article in conjunction with other relevant ones of this regulation it is observed that:

1. The authorization for manufacturing and import for the radiopharmaceuticals included in the art. 61.5.b is not needed.

2. GMPs to produce the Radiopharmaceuticals included in the exception of art. 61.5.b seems not to be needed. Because of Regulation 536/2014, two new legislation documents in relation to GMP have been released: (1) Directive 2017/1572 [26], the new GMP Directive that repeals the old GMP Directive 2003/94; and (2) Regulation 2017/1569 [27], a new GMP Regulation for IMPs (Investigational Medicinal Products) that does not apply to those radiopharmaceuticals included in art. 61.5.b of Regulation 536/2014. However, apparently contradicting the previous exception, this regulation remarks that Member States could carry on regular inspections to ensure subject safety and reliability and robustness of the data generated in the clinical trial, as detailed in the extract below of the Art. 61.6 in the mentioned Regulation 536/2014:

"Member States shall make the processes set out in paragraph 5 subject to appropriate and proportionate requirements to ensure subject safety and reliability and robustness of the data generated in the clinical trial. They shall subject the processes to regular inspections."

3. Simplified labelling of diagnostic radiopharmaceuticals used as investigational medicinal products (IMPs) and auxiliary medicinal products (AMPs)

It should be noted that this exception for diagnostic radiopharmaceutical is only in the context of a clinical trial where the number of patients and the length of study is limited. Moreover, art 61.6 of Regulation 536/2014 leaves open the possibility for each Member State of having regular inspections with their specific requirements.

This situation shall be seen as totally different from the small-scale radiopharmaceutical preparation on a routine basis, where bypassing the compliance with good manufacturing practices affecting the quality of the radiopharmaceuticals could have an impact on a much larger number of patients in the day-to-day usage.

8. Starting materials for the PET radiopharmaceuticals preparations

The definition of a starting material is depicted in part II of Good Manicuring Practices (GMPs) [28] as shown in the extract below:

"An Active Substance Starting Material is a raw material, intermediate, or an active substance that is used in the production of an active substance and that is incorporated as a significant structural fragment into the structure of the active substance. An Active Substance Starting Material can be an article of commerce, a material purchased from one or more suppliers under contract or commercial agreement or produced in-house. Active Substance Starting Materials normally have defined chemical properties and structure".

In case of the PET Radiopharmaceutical preparations, the main starting material is the chemical precursor whose definition is stated in the European Pharmacopoeia monograph 2902 named Chemical Precursors for Radiopharmaceuticals Preparations [29] as follows:

"Chemical precursors are non-radioactive substances obtained by chemical synthesis for combination with a radionuclide".

In this monograph a risk assessment is requested whenever the radiopharmaceutical preparation is required for special needs of individual patients, provided that non individual monograph for the precursor is available. Likewise, differences between diagnostic use versus therapeutic use as well as the frequency of use shall be taken into account for the risk assessment. These indications are fully described in the paragraph below extracted from monograph 2902:

"Where a chemical precursor not described in an individual monograph of the European Pharmacopoeia is used in a radiopharmaceutical preparation prepared for the special needs of individual patients, the need for compliance with this general monograph is decided in the light of a risk assessment.

This risk assessment takes account of:

- the quality of the chemical precursor and the information available for quality evaluation.
- any further processing after radiolabelling (which may or may not include purification before administration to the patient).
- the amount used to prepare a patient dose (e.g., diagnostic use versus therapeutic use) and the frequency of administration to the patient."

The quality of the chemical precursors is critical to ensure the final quality of the radiopharmaceutical product. These precursors are used in radiolabelling reactions for the preparation of the radioactive pharmaceutical ingredients (APIs) that are not isolated and/or fully analysed before incorporation in the final radiopharmaceutical preparation. For this reason, according to the Guideline on Radiopharmaceuticals [16] they should satisfy the Note for Guidance on Summary of Requirements for Active Substances in Part II of the Dossier [30].

It is relevant to remark that during the radiopharmaceutical quality dossier preparation to be submitted to the relevant authorities, the information on chemical precursors including those for synthesis of PET radiopharmaceuticals may be presented in a separate Section 3.2.S following the requirements of the Common Technical Document (CTD). This is stated in the European Commission Document Volume 2B Notice to Applicants Medicinal products for human use [15]. This approach must be followed for both marketing authorisation (MAA) and clinical trial authorization (CTA) applications.

In particular, the module 3 of the CTD covers chemical and pharmaceutical data including data for biological/ biotechnological products. This module has two parts: drug substance and drug product part. In the case of the chemical precursor of the radiopharmaceutical preparation, it should comply with the drug substance requirements section.

The Guideline on Radiopharmaceuticals [16] describes the specific additional information that needs to be submitted in relation to radiopharmaceuticals, when preparing the radiopharmaceutical quality dossier. The following sections included in **Table 3** should be completed:

The information depicted in **Table 3** can be submitted by the applicant to the regulatory authorities following two different procedures:

1. Firstly, according to the current EU Guideline on the ASMF procedure (Active Substance Master File Guideline [31]. The main objective of it, is to allow valuable confidential intellectual property or 'know-how' of the manufacturer of the active substance (ASM) to be protected, while at the same time allowing the Applicant or Marketing Authorisation (MA) holder to take full responsibility for the medicinal product and the quality and quality control of the active substance. In the case of radiopharmaceuticals preparation would be the chemical precursor manufacturer the ASMF holder.

2. Secondly, the applicant could submit the information included in **Table 3**, through the CEP procedure (certificate of suitability of the monograph of the European Pharmacopoeia) that is granted by the European Directorate for the Quality of Medicines (EDQM). It is stated in the Directive 2001/83/EC [6] amended by 2003/63/EC [32] as it is shown in the extract below:

"Where the active substance and/or a raw and starting material or excipient(s) are the subject of a monograph of the European Pharmacopoeia, the applicant can apply for a certificate of suitability that, where granted by the European Directorate for the Quality of Medicines, shall be presented in the relevant section of this Module. Those certificates of suitability of the monograph of the European Pharmacopoeia are deemed to replace the relevant data of the corresponding sections described in this Module. The manufacturer shall give the assurance in writing to the applicant that the manufacturing process has not been modified since the granting of the certificate of suitability by the European Directorate for the Quality of Medicines."

On the contrary, if the applicant did not want to use either of the two previous procedures, all sections could be submitted directly to the regulatory authorities.

3.2.S.1 General Information
• 3.2.S.1.1 Nomenclature
• 3.2.S.1.2 Structure
• 3.2.S.1.3 General Properties
3.2.S.2 Manufacture
• 3.2.S.2.1 Manufacturer(s)
• 3.2.S.2.2 Description of Manufacturing Process and Process Controls
3.2.S.2.3 Control of Materials
3.2.S.2.4 Controls of Critical Steps and Intermediates
3.2.S.2.5 Process Validation and/or Evaluation
3.2.S.2.6 Manufacturing Process Development
3.2.S.3 Characterisation
• 3.2.S.3.1 Elucidation of Structure and other Characteristics
• 3.2.S.3.2 Impurities
3.2.S.4 Control of Drug Substance
• 3.2.S.4.1 Specification
• 3.2.S.4.2 Analytical Procedures
• 3.2.S.4.3 Validation of Analytical Procedures
• 3.2.S.4.4 Batch Analyses
• 3.2.S.4.5 Justification of Specification
3.2.S.5 Reference Standards or Materials
3.2.S.6 Container Closure System
3.2.S.7 Stability
• 3.2.S.7.1 Stability Summary and Conclusions
• 3.2.S.7.2 Post-approval Stability Protocol and Stability Commitment
• 3.2.S.7.3 Stability Data

Table 3.
Module 3 of common technical document (CTD) drug substance part.

These requirements are mandatory for both clinical trial and marketing authorisation applications, however they should also be compulsory for radiopharmaceuticals prepared outside the marketing authorisation track, regardless of the category to which they belong (magistral formula, special product, etc...). A clear example where this information is required is Spain. Hence, to prepare PET radiopharmaceutical outside the marketing authorisation track under the regulatory framework of article 47.1c in RD 1345/2007 [23], it is always necessary to submit the previously mentioned module 3 of CTD to the regulatory authority (AEMPS). In this way, the quality of the preparation in both chemical precursor and final radiopharmaceutical would be ensured.

It is noteworthy that, as a general rule, the information provided by the chemical precursor manufacturers is very limited. It is usually only submitted the chemical precursor structure, the specification, and some batch results. Obviously, this information should not be considered as sufficient to guaranty the quality of the final product.

Regarding the stability studies, stress testing of the chemical precursor must be performed to identify the likely degradation products, as well as to complete stability studies to cover storage, shipment, and subsequent use, according to ICH Q 1 A (R2) Stability Testing of new Drug Substances and Products [33]. However, the chemical precursor manufacturer is not obliged to stablish a retest period, but in case no retest period is defined, a statement should be included that the precursor is tested immediately before the drug product manufacture. In case retest period had not been proposed, the radiopharmacy unit would test the chemical precursor before its use. The details on the retest period information should be considered by the drug product manufacturer, in the case under analyse, the radiopharmacy unit.

A relevant problem is that, in most cases, radiopharmacy units are not aware of this fact and even when they knew it, they would not be equipped for performing such tests.

Regarding compliance of GMPs, according to Good Manufacturing Practices Part II: Basic Requirements for Active Substances used as Starting Material [28] the following requirements should be complied:

- The identity of the chemical precursor should be verified at least of each batch.
- Full analyses on at least three batches should be conducted before reducing in-house testing.
- As a minimum, a full analysis should be performed at appropriate intervals and compared with the Certificates of Analysis.
- Reliability of Certificates of Analysis should be checked at regular intervals.

Considering that radiopharmacy units are not usually equipped to fulfil these requirements, the requested tests could be outsourced following the requirements of GMP Chapter 7 Outsourced Activities [34].

Hence, there should be written procedures describing the receipt, identification, quarantine, storage, handling, sampling, testing, and approval or rejection of materials. Additionally, for all starting materials and critical components, only qualified vendors should be used. Vendor qualification can be established by an audit, by responses to a Quality Assurance questionnaire, or simply based on experience with this supplier (e.g., the hospital pharmacy). In any case, vendor qualification should always be documented.

As we can see, special attention should be devoted to the purity and control methods for all starting materials, reactants, chemicals, reagents, and solvents used in synthesis and purification regardless they are licensed or unlicensed radiopharmaceuticals. Furthermore, it should be stressed that radiopharmaceuticals containing radionuclides of short physical half-life (e.g., PET radiopharmaceuticals), can be released before all results on finished product testing are available, therefore the consistency of all the steps in the production process has a crucial importance.

9. Conclusion

This text aimed to provide an overview on the radiopharmaceutical preparations in the European Union, focusing on the main differences between national laws regarding the non-licensed small-scale preparations, while analysing whether the quality expectations on them are really achieved or not. It went through a recap of the alternative methods to control sterility in radiopharmaceuticals, types of radiopharmaceutical marketing authorisations, differences between preparation and manufacturing of radiopharmaceuticals, available guidelines related to the quality in radiopharmaceuticals field, radiopharmaceuticals preparation outside the marketing track in the European Union and starting materials quality requirements for PET Radiopharmaceuticals preparations.

The intention was to raise some of the hot topics in the scientific community around the radiopharmaceutical compounds, considered a special group of medicines, that can be prepared outside the marketing authorisation track. In particular, small-scale preparations at non-commercial sites which represent an important segment, despite a lack of harmonisation in the regulation leads to extreme differences in the application and availability of radiopharmaceuticals across Europe.

It is noteworthy, that most radiopharmaceutical preparations are sterile injectable products. As developed along the text, the existing regulation on the manufacture of sterile medicines, shall imply the need of a harmonisation in the European Union regarding the requirements applicable in the small-scale preparation of radiopharmaceuticals, which are currently considered not clear enough. A possible way forward might be the compliance with Good Manufacturing Practices (GMPs) properly adapted to the special nature of small-scale preparation of radiopharmaceuticals.

Moreover, special attention should be put on the quality assurance process for non-licensed starting materials, given that the final radiopharmaceuticals quality chiefly depends on it.

To sum up, the radiopharmacists community should try to achieve a proven quality, efficacy, and safety for our radiopharmaceuticals, regardless if they are licensed or unlicensed products, both in large or small-scale preparations.

Abbreviation list

AIDS	Acquired Immune Deficiency Syndrome
AEMPS	Agencia Española del Medicamento y Productos Sanitarios
AMPs	Auxiliary Medicinal Products
ALARA	As Low As Reasonably Achievable
API	Active Pharmaceutical Ingredient
ASMF	Active Substance Master File Guideline
CEP	Certificate of suitability of the monograph of the European Pharmacopoeia
CHMP	Committee for Medicinal Products for Human Use
CTA	Clinical Trial Authorization
CTD	Common Technical Document
DEFT	Direct Epifluorescent Filter Technique
EANM	European Association of Nuclear Medicine
EDQM	European Directorate for the Quality of Medicines & HealthCare
EFPIA	European Federation of Pharmaceutical Industries Associations
EMA	European Medicines Agency
EU	European Union
FDA	Food and Drug Administration
GMPs	Good Manufacturing Practices
HIV	Human Immunodeficiency Virus
ICH	International Council for Harmonisation
IMPs	Investigational Medicinal Products
JPMA	Japan Pharmaceutical Manufacturers Association
MAA	Marketing Authorisation Application
MAH	Marketing Authorisation Holder
MHLW	The Ministry of Health, Labour and Welfare

MHRA	The Medicines and Healthcare Products Regulatory Agency (UK)
NAT	Nucleic Acid Amplification Techniques
PET	Positron emission tomography
PhRMA	Pharmaceutical Research and Manufacturers of America
PICs	Pharmaceutical inspection convention, pharmaceutical inspection co-operation scheme
SPC	Summary of Product Characteristics
SPECT	Single Photon Emission Computed Tomography

Author details

Estrella Moya Sánchez
Spanish Agency for Medicines and Health Products (AEMPS), Madrid, Spain

*Address all correspondence to: mmoya@aemps.es

References

[1] Council Directive 89/343/EEC of 3 May 1989 extending the scope of Directives 65/65/EEC and 75/319/EEC and laying down additional provisions for radiopharmaceuticals

[2] EDQM 0125 Radiopharmaceutical preparations. Available at: https://pheur.edqm.eu/app/10-5/content/default/0125E.htm

[3] EDQM 2.6.1 Sterility. Available at: https://pheur.edqm.eu/app/10-5/content/10-5/20601E.htm?highlight=on&terms=2.6.1

[4] EDQM 5.1.6 Alternative methods for control of microbiological quality. Available at: https://pheur.edqm.eu/app/10-5/content/10-5/50106E.htm?highlight=on&terms=5.1.6

[5] USP-NF ⟨1071⟩ Rapid Sterility Testing of Short Life Products A Risk Based Approach . Available at: https://online.uspnf.com/uspnf/document/1_GUID-EEDBFFA0-A579-4F26-ACFF-53248C30BFF6_2_en-US?source=Search%20Results&highlight=1071

[6] The European Parliament and the Council of the European Union. Directive 2001/83/EC of the European Parliament and the Council of 6 November 2001 on the Community code relating to medicinal products for human use. Available at: https://ec.europa.eu/health/sites/default/files/files/eudralex/vol-1/dir_2001_83_consol_2012/dir_2001_83_cons_2012_en.pdf

[7] Regulation (EC) No 726/2004 of the European Parliament and of the of 31 March 2004 laying down Community procedures for the authorisation and supervision of medicinal products for human and veterinary use and establishing a European Medicines Agency. Available at: https://ec.europa.eu/health/sites/default/files/files/eudralex/vol-1/reg_2004_726/reg_2004_726_en.pdf

[8] EMA website. Available at: https://www.ema.europa.eu/en/human-regulatory/marketing-authorisation

[9] EudraLex - Volume 10 - Clinical trials guidelines EudraLex - Volume 10 - Clinical trials guidelines | Public Health (europa.eu).

[10] Pharmaceutical Inspection Co-operation Scheme. Document PE 010-4, Annex 3: Good practices for the preparation of radiopharmaceuticals in healthcare establishments. 2014. Available at: Microsoft Word - PE 010-4 Guide to Good Practices for the Preparation of Medicinal Products in Healthcare Establishments (picscheme.org)

[11] Eudralex: The Rules Governing Medicinal Products in the European Union. Vol 4. EU Guidelines to Good Manufacturing Practice: Medicinal Products for Human and Veterinary Use. Annex 3: Manufacture of Radiopharmaceuticals. 2006. Available at: http://ec.europa.eu/enterprise/pharmaceuticals/eudralex/vol-4/pdfs-m/2006_10_10_annex3_consultation.pdf.

[12] EDQM. 5.19. Extemporaneous preparation of radiopharmaceutical preparations. Pharmeuropa [Internet] 2014;26(2):1-10. Available at: http://pharmeuropa.edqm.eu/TextsForComment/NetisUtils/srvrutiletdoc.aspx/0L3atCJKrELmrCJamC4KkQ7Hj//51900E.pdf.

[13] EDQM 2619 Pharmaceutical Preparations. Available at: https://pheur.edqm.eu/app/10-5/content/10-5/2619E.htm?highlight=on&terms=2619

[14] Guideline on the sterilisation of the medicinal product, active substance,

excipient and primary container 6 March 2019 EMA/CHMP/CVMP/QWP/850374/2015 Committee for Medicinal Products for Human use (CHMP). Available at: https://www.ema.europa.eu/en/documents/scientific-guideline/guideline-sterilisation-medicinal-product-active-substance-excipient-primary-container_en.pdf

[15] EudraLex - Volume 2 - Pharmaceutical legislation on notice to applicants and regulatory guidelines for medicinal products for human use. Available at: https://ec.europa.eu/health/documents/eudralex/vol-2_es

[16] Guideline on Radiopharmaceuticals. Available at: https://www.ema.europa.eu/en/radiopharmaceuticals

[17] Commission Directive 2003/94/EC of 8 October 2003 laying down the principles and guidelines of good manufacturing practice in respect of medicinal products for human use and investigational medicinal products for human use. Available at: https://eur-lex.europa.eu/LexUriServ/LexUriServ.do?uri=OJ:L:2003:262:0022:0026:en:PDF

[18] USP-NF ⟨825⟩ Radiopharmaceuticals—Preparation, Compounding, Dispensing, and Repackaging. Available at: https://online.uspnf.com/uspnf/document/1_GUID-4F561781-FBF6-4AF6-AF64-89A06583B7A1_4_en-US?source=Search%20Results&highlight=825

[19] USP-NF ⟨823⟩ Positron Emission Tomography Drugs for Compounding, Investigational, and research uses. Available at: https://online.uspnf.com/uspnf/document/1_GUID-D4D78DB7-60F3-4CA7-A792-E1F012A9A81B_1_en-US?source=Search%20Results&highlight=823

[20] Guidance on current good radiopharmacy practice (cGRPP) for the small-scale preparation of radiopharmaceuticals. Eur J Nucl Med Mol Imaging. Available at: https://eanm.org/publications/guidelines/5_EJNMMI_Guidance_cGRPPfulltext_05_2010.pdf

[21] The European Court of Justice. Document 62013CJ0544, Judgment of the Court (Third Chamber) of 16 July 2015. EUR-Lex - 62013CJ0544 - EN - EUR-Lex (europa.eu)

[22] The supply of unlicensed medicinal products ("specials") MHRA Guidance Note 14, Medicines and Healthcare Products Regulatory Agency. Available at: www.mhra.gov.uk

[23] Real Decreto 1345/2007, de 11 de octubre, por el que se regula el procedimiento de autorización, registro y condiciones de dispensación de los medicamentos de uso humano fabricados industrialmente. Available at: https://www.boe.es/buscar/doc.php?id=BOE-A-2007-19249

[24] Real Decreto Legislativo 1/2015, de 24 de julio, por el que se aprueba el texto refundido de la Ley de garantías y uso racional de los medicamentos y productos sanitarios. Available at: https://www.boe.es/buscar/doc.php?id=BOE-A-2015-8343

[25] European Parliament and Council of the European Union. Regulation (EU) No 536/2014 of the European Parliament and of the Council of 16 April 2014 on clinical trials on medicinal products for human use, and repealing Directive 2001/20/EC. Clinical trials - Regulation EU No 536/2014 | Public Health (europa.eu)

[26] Commission Directive (EU) 2017/1572 of 15 September 2017 supplementing Directive 2001/83/EC of the European Parliament and of the Council as regards the principles and guidelines of good manufacturing practice for medicinal products for

human use (Text with EEA relevance. Available at: https://eur-lex.europa.eu/eli/dir/2017/1572/oj

[27] Commission Delegated Regulation (EU) 2017/1569 of 23 May 2017 supplementing Regulation (EU) No 536/2014 of the European Parliament and of the Council by specifying principles of and guidelines for good manufacturing practice for investigational medicinal products for human use and arrangements for inspections (Text with EEA relevance). Available at: https://eur-lex.europa.eu/eli/reg_del/2017/1569/oj

[28] EudraLex: The Rules Governing Medicinal Products in the European Union Volume 4 Good Manufacturing Practice Medicinal Products for Human and Veterinary Use Part II: Basic Requirements for Active Substances used as Starting Materials. Available at: https://ec.europa.eu/health/sites/default/files/files/eudralex/vol-4/2014-08_gmp_part1.pdf

[29] EDQM 2902 Chemical Precursors for Radiopharmaceuticals Preparations. Available at: https://pheur.edqm.eu/app/10-5/content/10-5/2902E.htm?highlight=on&terms=precursors&terms=precursor

[30] Guidance on Summary of Requirements for Active Substances in Part II of the Dossier (CHMP/QWP/297/97 Rev. 1). Available at: https://www.ema.europa.eu/en/summary-requirements-active-substances-quality-part-dossier

[31] Active Substance Master File guideline (CHMP QWP/227/02). Available at: https://www.ema.europa.eu/en/documents/report/final-guideline-active-substance-master-file-procedure-revision-4_en.pdf

[32] Commission Directive 2003/63/EC of 25 June 2003 amending Directive 2001/83/EC of the European Parliament and of the Council on the Community code relating to medicinal products for human use. Available at: https://eur-lex.europa.eu/legal-content/EN/TXT/PDF/?uri=CELEX:32003L0063&from=en

[33] ICH Q 1 A (R2) Stability Testing of new Drug Substances and Products. Available at: https://www.ema.europa.eu/en/documents/scientific-guideline/ich-q-1-r2-stability-testing-new-drug-substances

[34] EudraLex The Rules Governing Medicinal Products in the European Union Volume 4 EU Guidelines for Good Manufacturing Practice for Medicinal Products for Human and Veterinary Use Chapter 7 Outsourced Activities. Available at: https://ec.europa.eu/health/sites/default/files/files/eudralex/vol-4/vol4-chap7_2012-06_en.pdf

Section 3

Radiopharmaceuticals Preclinical Studies Update

Chapter 8

Recent Advances in Biodistribution, Preclinical and Clinical Applications of Radiolabelled Iodine

Khaled Soliman, Ahmed Alenezi, Abdullah Alrushoud, Salman Altimyat, Mousa Bakkari, Hanaa Alshikh and Turki Alruwaili

Abstract

Adequate understanding of radiopharmaceutical distribution in the body of the patient has both spatial and temporal characteristics and they are the key factor to consider when planning successful radio pharmaceutical therapy, because they are an integral part of the radiation dosimetry calculations of any proposed personalized treatment. In this chapter we will focus on radioiodine therapy for thyroid cancer patients since it is a widely known practice in clinical oncology. Factors affecting the radioiodine organs' distribution will be examined in sufficient details using the available published research in the scientific literature. The literature will be reviewed extensively and summarized in this chapter. Another aim is to provide the medical practitioners with a quick reference guide to this clinically important area of expertise; often mastered by medical physicists with background in radiation physics, mathematics and medical imaging analysis. This chapter will cover recent advances in the area of radioiodine biodistribution modeling with applications in preclinical and clinical studies.

Keywords: radioactive iodine, biodistribution, clinical applications, recent advances

1. Introduction

This chapter will focus on presenting a review of the current situation regarding the use of radioiodine labeled agents in clinical and preclinical nuclear medicine imaging and radionuclide therapy. We will show the actual clinical applications and summarize the preclinical and clinical research efforts undergoing today in this dynamic field of medicine. These agents were found to be interesting since they can be applied to both imaging the disease and for therapy, by delivering a will localized radiation dose to a target tissues or tumor volume within the human anatomy. This delivery is carried out by the so called carrier systems such as, monoclonal antibodies or fragments of those and also by nanoparticles both inorganic and organic and microspheres. These carriers will carry the radioactivity of the radionuclide to the targeted biological site. There are two types of targeting the first is direct targeting, when the pharmaceutical accumulation in a tissue or site is done through inherent pathophysiological characteristics; or indirect which occurs if the used carries possess higher affinity to bind to a particular cell type or tissue. The good example of such radiopharmaceutical is tositumomab (131I-labeled anti-CD20 antibody), which received Food and Drug Administration (FDA) approval for the treatment of Non-Hodgkin's lymphoma in 2003.

2. Biodistribution modeling

Physical and temporal variability of the iodine −131 activity distributions in tissue constitute what is commonly called bio distribution models. The models are based on what is known in mathematics as compartmental modeling. For the sake of radiation dose calculations scientist may use different models to estimate the activity present in the patient body and the fraction of the radioactivity released from his or her body using simple two compartment model. More rigorous models also exist, having more than five compartments.

Biodistribution experiments are also published and new ones are still being published it is a dynamic field of research. The same apply for different radiopharmaceuticals. Organs Residence time is one important factors being measured while developing a bio distribution experiments leading to the proposal of a new bio distribution model.

Factors altering such models are very important to be aware of, because the alteration in the bio distribution will directly impact the radiation dose calculations and therefore the safety of the patients undergoing radioiodine therapy. To the best of our knowledge there are no general agreement on the methods or standards applied when reporting bio distribution studies. Therefore we will attempt to summarize the ones in the literature.

2.1 Biokinetic data

Biokinetic data are variables that describe the bio distribution space time functions.

Among the most common of these variables are: the uptake fraction by the organ example the thyroid, the excreted fraction as (urine or feces), the biological half-life or time in a specific organ or body tissues like blood, thyroid, and intestine for example. The fractions are mostly given as % and the time are often given in days most of the times in the case of radioactive iodine. Biokinetic data for radioactive iodine are reported in ICRP-30 [1].

2.2 Radionuclide delivery system

Radionuclide delivery systems are now as antibodies, nanoparticles both inorganic and organic and finally as Microspheres.

In this reference good information is given on targeted radionuclide therapy for the thyroid cancer treatment. Parallelism is shown between preclinical animal models in rats and mice versus humans [2].

Translation of the experimental findings and research results is an issue that warrants the attention of the researcher; in this case the range of radiation in tissues and the organ sizes needs to be considered. Also the difference among the metabolism and metabolism rate models used directly affects the biodistribution in the animal or the human under study.

2.3 Compartmental biological modeling

Compartmental models are used for internal radioisotope ingestions or injections dosimetry since the seventies. We are referring to the ICRP publication 30 published in 1979. In that documents several compartmental models are proposed, we focus on the model proposed for iodine metabolism in humans.

In order to apply the model a set of differential equations has to be solved simultaneously to obtain the biodistribution of iodine in human body. The equations can be solved numerically using algorithm included in software like Mathematica or Matlab.

Biokinetic models parameters are taken for healthy individuals. In order to apply the models to cancer patients for example, the metabolic data has to be customized to represent their actual metabolism status. Currently, scientists are recommending the use of personalized radiopharmaceutical therapy where each therapeutic procedures is planned based on the individual patient data and not using the generic data from reports like ICRP and others.

The following 4 differential equations are for the model in **Figure 1**:

$$dq_1 / dt = -(\lambda_p + \lambda_{12}) q_1 \tag{1}$$

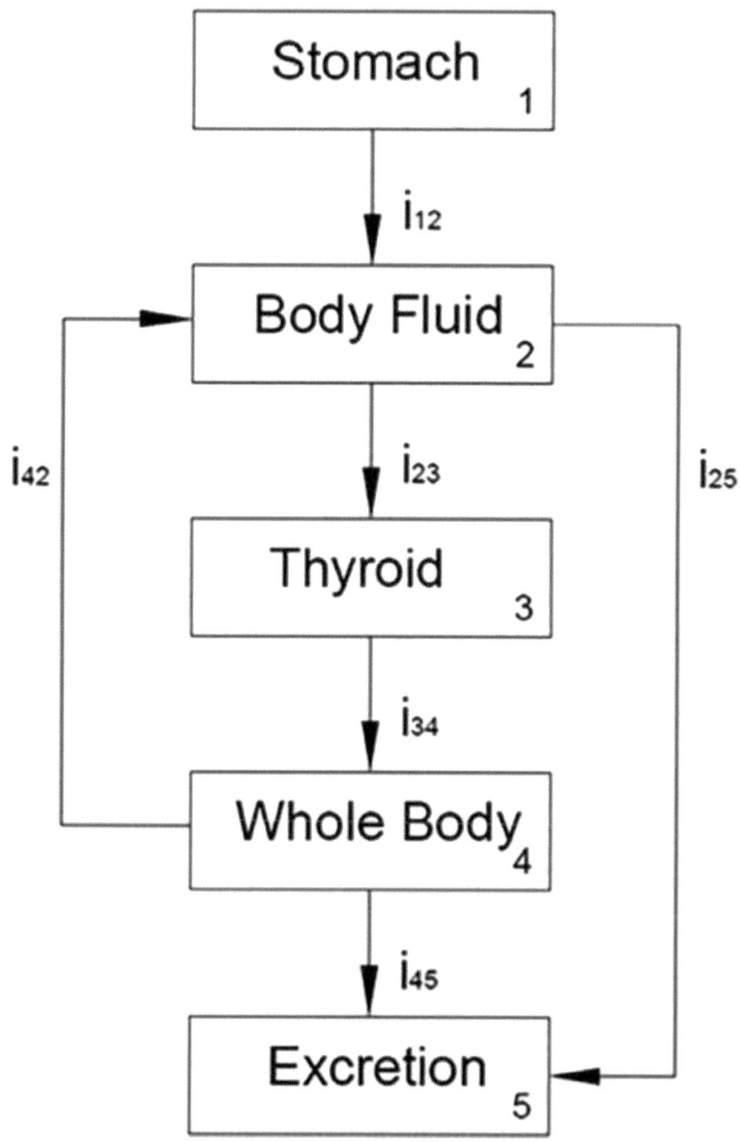

Figure 1.
Five compartments human body biokinetic model of iodine as per ICRP-30 report.

$$dq_2 / dt = \lambda_{12} q_1 - (\lambda_p + \lambda_{25} + \lambda_{23}) q_2 + \lambda_{42} q_4 \quad (2)$$

$$dq_3 / dt = \lambda_{23} q_2 - (\lambda_p + \lambda_{34}) q_3 \quad (3)$$

$$dq_4 / dt = \lambda_{34} q_3 - (\lambda_p + \lambda_{42} + \lambda_{45}) q_4 \quad (4)$$

This five compartment model is the one proposed by the −30 to represent the biokinetic model of iodine in healthy individuals.

After solving the system of simultaneous four differential equations above the solution yield the following.

$$T_{1/2}(thy) = 80\,d, T_{1/2}(Body\ Fluid) = 0.25\,d, i_{23}(thy) = 30\%, i_{25}(excretion) = 70\%.$$

These results are for the healthy individuals, solving the same system for thyroid cancer patients yields the following [3, 4]:

$$T_{1/2}(thy) = 0.66\,d, T_{1/2}(Body\ Fluid) = 0.52\,d, i_{23}(thy) = 12\%, i_{25}(excretion) = 88\%.$$

We can see that there is a significant difference in the values obtained. Where the importance of personalized dose estimates, the analysis of the results dictates the importance to take into account the pathology of the patients and his thyroid disease status and diagnosis before interpreting the results of any biokinetic experiment or data analysis.

2.4 Biodistribution studies and biokinetic models

The radiopharmaceutical kinetic data often known as Biodistribution is a function of space and time. Imaging the whole body or specific region using planar scintillation Gamma camera can be used to obtain the necessary data for the study. The accuracy of this method is better when the radiopharmaceutical is localized in a specific area of the body or organ and this region do not overlap with other uptake area in the planar projection.

A region of interest (ROI) is determined in order to estimate the absolute amount of radioactivity in the organ. Modern Gamma cameras provide capability to delineate ROI of nay shape and to perform statistical analysis on the pixels inside the ROI to obtain the number of counts per pixel inside the ROI and the count rate.

Sequential imaging as a function of time postadministration of the radiopharmaceutical provides the time dependence of activity (time-activity curve) [5]. In this reference a full description of the imaging based method using planar gamma camera, SPECT and PET are described in great details.

Clinical and preclinical imaging protocols are published by different groups of scientists worldwide. Imaging is the key part of the bio distribution data acquisition experiment and constitutes the primary data for the model that will be proposed based on the results obtained during the experiment.

Imaging acquisition at different times after oral administration of a known activity of I-131 1100 MBq is the most common used with human subjects. Using a clinical gamma camera scanned data form the organs of interest, example the stomach using an region of interest (ROI) is converted to counts per pixel per sec. Will be acquired and data will be extracted for further analysis.

2.5 Image- based, patient- specific dosimetry

Such technique will allow the distribution of the agent in tumors and normal organs to be quantified [6]. Dosimetry as implemented in RPT may be thought of as the ability to perform the equivalent of a pharmacodynamic study in treated patients in real time [7]. When patient dosimetry is performed it allow prediction of treatment success based on reported results in the literature, it is then possible to calculate both normal tissue and tumor doses.

Organ uptake, Reminder of body uptake, Assumed waste. Derivation of the biological half –life values in different organs: they are theoretical estimations of the time-dependent quantity of I-131 in various compartments.

In Ref. [7] the authors have found that estimated biological half-life's obtained via the biokinetic model of radioiodine for thyroid cancer patients was found to strongly deviate from those recommended by Eckerman's suggestion for healthy male.

2.6 Organs residence times

By definition lambda is given by:

$$\lambda = \text{Ln}(2) / T_{1/2} \tag{5}$$

Where $T_{1/2}$ is the half-life. it could be the biological (T_b), physical (T_p) or effective (T_{eff}) half-life depending on the application.

Knowing that:

$$1 / T_{eff} = 1 / T_b + 1 / T_p \tag{6}$$

The biological half-life of radiopharmaceuticals is organ dependents. We will observe dissimilar values for different organs.

Time integrated activity coefficients (TIAC) are known also as organs residence times. They are proportional to the radiation absorbed dose by the organ or body tissue.

The radiopharmaceutical effective half-life is different for each organ in the body. And they are dependent of the biodistribution or the individual organ uptake fraction of the total injected activity. The same applies to the tumor tissues targeted by the radiopharmaceutical therapy; in our case here it is the remaining of the post ablation thyroid tissues treated using I-131.

3. Radioactive iodine treatment for thyroid cancer patients

In many medical applications involving the administration of iodine-131 (^{131}I) in the form of iodide (I^-), most of the dose is delivered to the thyroid gland [3].

To reliably estimate the thyroid absorbed dose, the following data are required:

the thyroid gland size (i.e. mass), the fractional uptake of ^{131}I by the thyroid, the spatial distribution of ^{131}I within the thyroid, and the length of time ^{131}I is retained in the thyroid before it is released back to blood, distributed in other organs and tissues, and excreted from the body [4, 8–10].

Estimation of absorbed dose to non-thyroid tissues likewise requires knowledge of the time course of activity in each organ. Such data are rarely available, however, and therefore dose calculations are generally based on reference models. The MIRD and ICRP have published metabolic models and have calculated absorbed doses per unit intake for many nuclides and radioactive pharmaceuticals. Given the activity taken into the body, one can use such models and make reasonable calculations for average organ doses. When normal retention and excretion pathways are altered, the baseline models need to be modified, and the resulting organ dose estimates are subject to larger errors.

Even if the uptake of iodine is very specific to thyroid tissue, side effects from off-target accumulation are common. Frequent short-term side effects after 131I therapy of patients with differentiated thyroid cancer are gastrointestinal symptoms, pain or swelling in the neck or salivary glands, while frequent late effects are functional problems with salivary glands [11–15].

The hypothalamus-pituitary-thyroid (HPT) axis is an example of an endocrine feedback loop that is known to have a circadian rhythm [16].

Patients with chronic renal failure exhibited significant salivary gland, oral, nasal, and gastric activity 1 week after radioiodine administration [17].

3.1 Sodium/iodide symporter (NIS)

Active iodide (I^-) transport in both the thyroid and some extra-thyroidal tissues is mediated by the Na^+/I^- symporter (NIS).

The cDNA encoding NIS was isolated in 1996, marking a major breakthrough in thyroid research that led to the subsequent characterization of NIS at the molecular level. Functional NIS is found in several extra-thyroidal tissues, such as the salivary glands, stomach, and lactating breast, as well as in primary and metastatic breast cancers. The latter findings have raised the possibility that NIS-mediated $^{131}I-$ treatment may be effective in breast cancer. One of the most remarkable properties of NIS is that it transports different substrates with different stoichiometries. TSH is the primary regulator of NIS in the thyroid at both the transcriptional and post-transcriptional levels. At the molecular level, excess I− may have a deleterious effect on the thyroid by modifying NIS mRNA stability and increasing the production of reactive oxygen species. Thyroidal NIS function is also regulated by direct cross talk between NIS and a K^+ channel [18].

3.2 Future perspective and applications

In the last two decades, NIS has become an important player in the use and optimization of gene therapy owing to its capacity as a reporter and as a therapeutic gene. NIS could be introduced into virtually any cell or tissue for imaging and/or therapeutic purposes. NIS is becoming the counterpart for human studies of green fluorescent protein and luciferase, which have been used extensively in cells and other organisms.

NIS expression and activity correlate with cell viability because only living cells can accumulate I−. NIS also offers higher detection sensitivity, because it actively transports its substrates rather than simply binding a substrate stoichiometrically. Moreover, NIS can translocate a variety of substrates, which can be detected using different systems, such as gamma cameras, PET, and SPECT (single-photon emission computed tomography) combined with computed tomography (CT) [18].

4. Newly introduced I-131 labeled radiopharmaceutical therapy agents

Radiopharmaceutical therapy (RPT) is emerging as a safe and effective targeted approach to treating many types of cancer. In RPT, radiation is systemically or locally delivered using pharmaceuticals that either bind preferentially to cancer cells or accumulate by physiological mechanisms. Almost all radionuclides used in RPT emit photons that can be imaged, enabling non-invasive visualization of the biodistribution of the therapeutic agent. Compared with almost all other systemic cancer treatment options, RPT has shown efficacy with minimal toxicity. With the recent FDA approval of several RPT agents, the remarkable potential of this treatment is now being recognized [6]. We will mention a few emerging clinical development of radioiodine labeled RPT agents newly available or still under development at the present time. RPT development is a multidisciplinary endeavor, requiring expertise in radiochemistry, radiobiology, oncology, pharmacology, medical physics and radionuclide imaging and dosimetry.

Theranostic is the general concept of using a radionuclide- labeled agent that may be imaged to guide radiopharmaceutical therapy; a radionuclide that may be used for both imaging and therapy, and it is the new trend in RPT.

I-131 meta- iodobenzylguanidine (mIBG): for Adrenergic receptor tumors; the active uptake mechanism via the adrenaline transporter and storage in presynaptic neurosecretory granules. FDA approved but clinical trials are ongoing. This radiopharmaceutical can be used to treat patients with neuroblastomas [19].

mIBG radiolabelled with high- specific- activity iodine-131 was recently approved by the FDA for the treatment of adult and pediatric patients aged 12 years or older with unresectable metastatic phaeochromocytoma or paraganglioma.

I-131- labeled CLR131 for Pediatric cancer, head and neck cancer, multiple myeloma, leukemia, lymphoma. The radio-labeled phospholipid ether analogue targeting cancer cell- specific lipid raft microdomains. It is still undergoing the phase of clinical trials and testing.

I-131- labeled CLR1404 for unresponsive solid tumor, multiple myeloma. The radio-labeled phospholipid ether analogue targeting cancer cell-specific lipid raft microdomains. It is still undergoing the phase of clinical trials and testing.

4.1 Antibody based radionuclide therapy

Radiolabeled sdAbs prove to be promising vehicles for molecular imaging and targeted radionuclide therapy of metastatic lesions in the brain. Administration of [I-131]-2Rs15d and [Ac-225]-2Rs15d alone and in combination with trastuzumab showed a significant increase in median survival in 2 tumor models that remained largely unresponsive to trastuzumab treatment alone [20]. Puttemans et al. [21] have described the use of the anti-HER2 sdAb 2Rs15d, coupled to 111In or 131I for detection via PECT/CT, and coupled to 131I or 225Ac for targeted radionuclide therapy (TRNT) of $HER2^{pos}$ brain lesions and compare its therapeutic efficacy and systemic toxicity to that of trastuzumab, a clinically-approved anti-HER2 treatment. They have demonstrated that radiolabeled sdAbs are ideal vehicles for targeted radionuclide therapy and molecular imaging, not only for systemic disease, but also for metastatic lesions in the brain. Moreover, histopathological analysis after therapy revealed no significant early toxicity. Dosimetry based on ex vivo biodistribution data confirmed most activity is retained within the kidneys until 48 h after administration, however after extrapolation to therapeutic activities the cumulative absorbed dose (25 Gy) remains close to the considered toxicity threshold of 23 Gy to kidneys [21].

The amount of 131I- tositumomab prescribed to patients was determined by assessing the whole- body clearance rate, so that the amount administered was adjusted to deliver the same whole- body absorbed dose in all treated patients [21], making it the first RPT agent whose package insert specified an absorbed dose- based treatment planning procedure. Such an approach was, in part, necessitated because the radioiodine in iodine-131- labeled antibodies is cleaved (due to dehalogenation) from the antibody if the radiolabelled antibody construct is internalized.

4.2 Iodine-131 labeled Metuximab

Radioimmunotherpy using antibodies injection is another application of I-131 in oncology. Administered to patients suffering from hepatocellular carcinoma (HCC), the product will target the hepatic cancer cells while sparing other adjacent tissues. The whole body biodistribution is required in order to perform radiation dosimetry, evaluate the risk from the treatment and to ensure patient safety.

4.3 I-131 - labeled a CD45

I-131 - labeled a CD45 for Bone marrow transplant preparation.

The I-131 based antibody targeting CD45+ cells for bone marrow ablation before transplantation. It is still undergoing the phase of testing and planned clinical trials. Early studies showed the potential to image the radioiodinated antibodies using SPECT [22, 23].

The radiolabelled antibodies were used for total body irradiation in preparation for bone marrow transplantation (BMT). report results of a study on patients with acute myelogenous leukemia in a phase I clinical trial where results showed that it is possible while appending I-131 to M195 antibody to deliver beta emitter particles to the targeted cells in the bone marrow, it was also possible to image the disease in the bone marrow.

The tumor-homing property of mesenchyme stem cells (MSCs) allows targeted delivery of therapeutic genes into the tumor microenvironment. The application of sodium iodide symporter.

(NIS) as a theranostic gene allows noninvasive imaging of MSC biodistribution and transgene expression before therapeutic radioiodine application. Linking therapeutic transgene expression to induction of the chemokine CCL5/RANTES allows a more focused expression within primary tumors, as the adoptively transferred MSC develop carcinoma-associated fibroblast-like characteristics. Although RANTES/CCL5-NIS targeting has shown efficacy in the treatment of primary tumors, it was not clear if it would also be effective in controlling the growth of metastatic disease. To expand the potential range of tumor targets, we investigated the biodistribution and tumor recruitment of MSCs transfected with NIS under control of the RANTES/CCL5 promoter (RANTES-NIS-MSC) in a colon cancer liver metastasis mouse model established by intrasplenic injection of the human colon cancer cell line LS174t. Results show robust MSC recruitment with RANTES/CCL5-promoter activation within the stroma of liver metastases as evidenced by tumor-selective iodide accumulation, immunohistochemistry, and real-time polymerase chain reaction. Therapeutic application of 131I in RANTES-NIS-MSC–treated mice resulted in a significant delay in tumor growth and improved overall survival. Conclusion: This novel gene therapy approach opens the prospect of NIS-mediated radionuclide therapy of metastatic cancer after MSC-mediated gene delivery [24].

4.4 Newly introduced radioiodine labeled nanoparticles and microspheres

in the area of preclinical development regarding tumor targeted therapy using radioiodine labeled molecules an active research work is undergoing using Nano and microsphere technologies. The good example of such radiopharmaceutical is tositumomab (131I-labeled anti-CD20 antibody), which received Food and Drug Administration (FDA) approval for the treatment of Non-Hodgkin's lymphoma in 2003.

Initial clinical trials of 131I- labeled iodized oil (131I- labeled Lipiodol) were completed in the late 1980s/early 1990s (285–288), and clinical investigations of this treatment modality continued until 2013 (NCT00116454, NCT00870558 and NCT00027768).

Administration of 131I- labeled Lipiodol in the adjuvant setting, after resection or radiofrequency ablation for hepatocellular carcinoma, yielded a 6- month increase in recurrence free survival and a 24- month increase in median overall survival [25].

RPT has proven to be an effective cancer treatment when other standard therapeutic approaches have failed. However, despite more than 40 years of clinical investigation, RPT has not become a part of the cancer treatment armamentarium in the same way as other therapies. 'Targeted' cancer therapies are associated with clinical trial failure rates of 97% (ref. 1), partly because the agents targeted a pathway that was not involved in promoting the cancer phenotype2. By contrast, RPT has been unsuccessful owing to a failure to adopt and rigorously evaluate this treatment modality, which may be explained in part by the multidisciplinary nature of the treatment.

Additional challenges facing the development and application of RPT include public perception and fear of radioactivity as well as the perceived complexity of the treatment.

The need for a new specialty or subspecialty to provide the multidisciplinary training needed to safely and effectively administer RPT agents to patients and subsequently manage them. Such a specialty or subspecialty would require training in nuclear medicine, radiation oncology and also general oncology as delivery of radiation is involved, the participation of medical physicists familiar with both imaging and radionuclide dosimetry is important.

The article by Jongho Jeon [25], reviews recent progress in cancer therapy using radiolabeled nanomaterials including inorganic, polymeric, and carbon-based materials and liposomes. The article first provides an overview of radiolabeling methods for preparing anticancer agents that have been investigated recently in preclinical studies. Next, they discuss the therapeutic applications and effectiveness of beta or alpha emitter-incorporated nanomaterials in animal models and the emerging possibilities of these nanomaterials in cancer therapy [26].

In contrast to biologics or chemotherapeutics, both radiation delivery and the biological response to radiation may be mathematically modeled and used to understand the parameters of a treatment that are most important in influencing efficacy and toxicity. The capability to use multiple agents in one carrier is very unique about nanomaterials [27].

5. Conclusion

Unlike chemotherapy and external beam radiation therapy RPT has not yet been established as a treatment modality in oncology. Mainly because lots of suggested

RPT agents are still undergoing clinical trials and some are still in the preclinical stage. The known fact is that, the tumor response to RPT can be mathematically modeled and also the radiation dosimetry is well established [24, 25]. There are research projects underway that focus on the use of combination therapy using targeted RPT along with chemotherapy for example in the treatment of resistant tumors that cannot be treated uniquely by traditional therapy like chemotherapy, this area of research is also quit active at the present time [28].

One challenge is the validation studies and the regulatory approval of clinical software packages that need to be established prior to routine clinical use is still underway. Certainly this area of research and development is very dynamic and requires multidisciplinary team work including oncology, nuclear medicine, imaging sciences and medical physics; and clinically also it will probably require some kind of new medical subspecialty. The medical physicist should be trained in both imaging based and radionuclide dosimetry methods. As medical physicists we see this as an opportunity for future medical physicist starting his or her career to specialize in this new evolving area of clinical medical physics.

Conflict of interest

The authors declare no conflict of interest." or delete this entire section.

Author details

Khaled Soliman[1*], Ahmed Alenezi[2], Abdullah Alrushoud[1], Salman Altimyat[1], Mousa Bakkari[1], Hanaa Alshikh[1] and Turki Alruwaili[1]

1 Medical Physics Department, Prince Sultan Military Medical City, Riyadh, Saudi Arabia

2 College of Applied Medical Sciences, King Saud University Riyadh, Saudi Arabia

*Address all correspondence to: ksoliman@psmmc.med.sa

References

[1] ICRP 1979. Limits of intakes of Radionuclides by workers, ICRP Publication 30 (part 1). Ann. ICRP 2 (3-4).

[2] Spetz J, Rudqvist N, Forssell-Aronsson E. Biodistribution and dosimetry of free 211At, 125I- and 131I- in rats.Cancer Biother Radiopharm. 2013 Nov;28(9):657-664. doi: 10.1089/cbr.2013.1483. Epub 2013 Jun 22. PMID: 23789969.

[3] Brill, A. B., Stabin, M., Bouville, A. and Ron, E. Normal Organ Radiation Dosimetry and Associated Uncertainties in Nuclear Medicine, with Emphasis on Iodine-131. Radiat. Res. 166, 128-140 (2006).

[4] Chen CY, Chank PJ, Changlai SP, Pan LK. Effective half-life of iodine for five thyroidectomy patients using an in vivo Gamma Camera approach. L. Radiat. Res;48:4856-4493 (2007).

[5] Siegel JA, Thomas SR, Stubbs JB, Stabin MG, Hays MT et al. MIRD pamphlet No.16: Techniques for quantitative radiopharmaceutical biodistribution data acquisition and analysis for use in human radiation dose estimates. J Nucl Med 1999;40:37S-61S.

[6] Longcor, J. & Oliver, K. Phase 1, open- label, dose escalation study of I-131-CLR1404 (CLR 131) in patients with relapsed or refractory multiple myeloma. Blood **134**, 1864 (2019).

[7] Sgouros G, Bodei L, McDevitt MR, Nedrow JR. Radiopharmaceutical therapy in cancer: clinical advances and challenges. Nature Reviews 2020; 19: 589-608. https://doi.org/10.1038/s41573-020-0073-9.

[8] Charlotte K. Andersson1*, Mikael Elvborn1, Johan K. E. Spetz1, Britta Langen1 & Eva B. Forssell-Aronsson[1],[2] Biodistribution of 131I in mice is influenced by circadian variations. *Scientific reports, nature research open. 2020 10:15541.*

[9] Bolch, W. E., Eckerman, K. F., Sgouros, G. & Thomas, S. R. MIRD pamphlet N. 21:a generalized schema for radiopharmaceutical dosimetry–standardization of nomenclature. *J. Nucl. Med.* **50**, 477-484. https ://doi.org/10.2967/jnumed.108.056036 (2009).

[10] Huang C-C, Lin Y-H, Kittipayak S, Hwua Y-S, Wang S-Y, Pan L-K (2020) Biokinetic model of radioiodine I-131 in nine thyroid cancer patients subjected to in-vivo gamma camera scanning: A simplified five-compartmental model. PLoS ONE 15(5): e0232480. https://doi.org/10.1371/journal.pone.0232480

[11] Kolbert KS, Pentlow KS, Pearson JR, mSheikh A, Finn RD, Humm L, Larson SM. Prediction of absorbed dose to normal organs in thyroid cancer patients treated with ^{131}I by use of ^{124}I PET and 3-Dimensional internal dosimetry software. J NUcl Med 2007; 48:143-149.

[12] Lu, L., Shan, F., Li, W. & Lu, H. Short-term side effects after radioiodine treatment in patients with differentiated thyroid cancer. Biomed. Res. Int. **2016**,4376720. https://doi.org/10.1155/2016/43767 20 (2016).

[13] Almeida, J. P., Sanabria, A. E., Lima, E. N. & Kowalski, L. P. Late side effects of radioactive iodine on salivary gland function inpatients with thyroid cancer. *Head Neck* **33**, 686-690. https://doi.org/10.1002/hed.21520 (2011).

[14] Klein Hesselink, E. N. *et al.* Effects of radioiodine treatment on salivary gland function in patients with differentiated thyroid carcinoma: a prospective study. *J. Nucl. Med. Off. Publ. Soc. Nucl. Med.* **57**, 1685-1691.

https://doi.org/10.2967/jnume d.115.169888 (2016).

[15] Pashnehsaz, M. *et al.* Gastrointestinal side effects of the radioiodine therapy for the patients with differentiated thyroid carcinoma two days after prescription. *World J. Nucl. Med.* **15**, 173-178. https://doi.org/10.4103/1450-1147.17470 3 (2016).

[16] Philippe, J. & Dibner, C. Thyroid circadian timing: roles in physiology and thyroid malignancies. *J. Biol. Rhythms* **30**, 76-83. https://doi.org/10.1177/07487 30414 55763 4 (2015).

[17] Clement, S. C. *et al.* Intermediate and long-term adverse effects of radioiodine therapy for differentiated thyroid carcinoma—a systematic review. *Cancer Treat. Rev.* **41**, 925-934. https://doi.org/10.1016/j.ctrv.2015.09.001 (2015).

[18] Silvia Ravera, Andrea Reyna-Neyra, Giuseppe Ferrandino, L Mario Amzel, Nancy Carrasco Annual review of physiology 79, 261-289, 2017.

[19] Schoot, R. A. et al. The role of 131Imetaiodobenzylguanidine (MIBG) therapy in unresectable and compromising localized neuroblastoma. Eur. J. Nucl. Med. Mol. Imaging **40**, 1516-1522 (2013).

[20] Aktas A, Kazak K, Kocabas B, Aras M, Tutuncu NB, Gencoglu A. The biodistribution of radioiodine on posttherapy iodine-131 scanc in thyroid cancer patients with chronic renal failure. Nucl Med Commun. (2008) 29(11): 943-948 [DOI: 10.1097/MNM.0b013e32831089e0]. PMID: 18836371.

[21] Puttemans J, Dekempeneer Y, Eersels JL, Hanssens H, Debie P, Keyaerts M, Windhorst AD, van der Aa F, Lecocq Q, Breckpot K, Morgenstern A, Bruchertseifer F, Lahoutte T, Devoogdt N, D'Huyvetter M. Preclinical Targeted α- and β^--Radionuclide Therapy in HER2-Positive Brain Metastasis Using Camelid Single-Domain Antibodies. Cancers (Basel). 2020 Apr 21;12(4):1017. doi: 10.3390/cancers12041017. PMID: 32326199; PMCID: PMC7226418.

[22] Wahl, R. L. The clinical importance of dosimetry in radioimmunotherapy with tositumomab and iodine I 131 tositumomab. Semin. Oncol. **30**, 31-38 (2003).

[23] Larson, S. M. et al. Imaging of melanoma with I-131-labeled monoclonal antibodies. J. Nucl. Med. **24**, 123-129 (1983).

[24] Mach, J. P. et al. Tumor localization in patients by radiolabeled monoclonal antibodies against colon carcinoma. Cancer Res. **43**, 5593-5600 (1983).

[25] Jongho Jeon. Review of Therapeutic Applications of Radiolabeled Functional Nanomaterials. Int. J. Mol. Sci. **2019**, 20(9): 2323 [doi:10.3390/ijms20092323]. PMID: 31083402.

[26] Knoop K, chwenk N, Schmohl K, Müller A, Zach C, Cyran C, Carlsen J, Böning G, et Al. Mesenchymal Stem Cell–Mediated, Tumor Stroma–Targeted Radioiodine Therapy of Metastatic Colon Cancer Using the Sodium Iodide Symporter as Theranostic Gene. J Nucl Med 2015; 56:600-606 [DOI: 10.2967/jnumed.114.146662].

[27] Kim, D., Shin, K., Kwon, S.G., Hyeon, T. Synthesis and Biomedical Applications of Multifunctional Nanoparticles. Adv. Mater. **2018**, 30 (49), e1802309). PMID: 30133009.

[28] ICRP publication 140. Radiological protection in therapy with radiopharmaceuticals. (2019) ICRP. Published by SAGE.

Chapter 9

Radium-223 and Actinium-225 α-Emitter Radiopharmaceuticals in Treatment of Metastatic Castration-Resistant Prostate Cancer

Akbar Abbasi, Hesham M.H. Zakaly and Fatemeh Mirekhtiary

Abstract

In recent decades, multiple radiopharmaceutical conjugates have been tested and shown to be efficacious in treating metastasized castration-resistant prostate cancer (mCRPC). Several types of research have been published on the therapeutic use of α-emitter radiopharmaceuticals, and several authors suggested their treatment superiority. One of the suggested methods is targeted alpha therapy. In this method, alpha radiation delivers energy to cancer cells and the tumor microenvironment while minimizing toxicity to surrounding tissues. In this chapter, the alpha emitter radiopharmaceutical applications in castration-resistant prostate cancer patients were investigated. Hence, we studied the ^{223}Ra and ^{225}Ac α-emitter radiopharmaceuticals application method and distribution of dose throughout human body organs.

Keywords: radiopharmaceutical, treatment, alpha emitter, ^{223}Ra, ^{225}Ac, metastatic castration-resistant prostate cancer

1. Introduction

The prostate gland weighs around 20 g and is located at the base of the bladder, near the prostatic urethra. It is split into four zones: peripheral, central, transitional, and peri-urethral. The most frequent location of prostate cancer in the peripheral zone, and adenocarcinoma accounts for the majority of cases, generally arising from acinar cells in the prostate gland and accompanied by a rise in serum prostate-specific antigen (PSA). PSA is unaffected by some tumor forms, including neuro-endocrine tumors, small-cell carcinoma, and transitional cell carcinoma [1].

According to a study conducted in the United States, 241,740 men were diagnosed with prostate cancer in 2012, resulting in 28,170 fatalities. In the United States, about 160,000 men will be diagnosed with prostate cancer in 2017. Prostate cancer is the third largest cause of cancer mortality in males, despite its generally indolent course. Since 2011, there has been significant progress in finding treatment alternatives and defining illness risk [2].

IntechOpen

Prostate cancer is the third most common cancer worldwide among males and the fourth in terms of incidence worldwide [3]. Patients with PCa may be treated with radical prostatectomy or radiation as initial therapies, although disease recurrence is possible. A prostatic-specific antigen (PSA) in the clinical setting of PCa screening has resulted in earlier detection. The first symptom of disease recurrence is an increase in PSA levels, referred to as biochemical recurrence (BR). Early recurrence can be treated with potentially curative salvage treatments such as additional lymphadenectomy or targeted radiation, although both need the disease to be localized [4].

Several radiopharmaceutical conjugates have been tried and proved to be effective in treating bone metastases [5–7] and metastasized castration-resistant prostate cancer in recent decades (mCRPC). In addition, various research on the therapeutic use of α-emitter radiopharmaceuticals have been published, and several writers have indicated that they are preferable in terms of therapy [8–16]. Targeted alpha treatment targets cancer cells and the tumor microenvironment while limiting damage to adjacent organs. Radiopharmaceuticals are specific radioisotope formulations used for diagnosis and treatment in important clinical domains. ^{223}Ra and ^{225}Ac radionuclides are the major radiopharmaceuticals utilized in treating prostate cancer [17].

The linear energy transfer (LET) causes damage to the cell DNA owing to the movement of the α-particle into the tissue, but the shortened range of the α-particle restricts tumor damage to the adjacent healthy cells, decreasing the damage. However, α particles may cause serious harm at both cellular and genetic levels, if breathed or eaten. External body exposure to an α-particle is insignificant. The possible harmful kind of radiation is α-particles [2].

Routines throughout the world include systemic chemotherapy, hormone therapies, and targeted bone drugs such as radium-223 dichloride (^{223}Ra) and actinium-225 (^{225}Ac) for skeleton metastases [18].

2. Radium-223

^{223}Ra ($T_{1/2}$ = 11.43 day) is α-emitter radiopharmaceutical with an average energy of 5.78 MeV (accounting for 93.5 percent of emitted energy), 4% as particles, and 2% as radiation utilized in prostate cancer bone metastases. The dichloride-^{223}Ra is a targeted emitter that binds to accelerated bone turnover in bone metastases and releases high-energy alpha particles with a short-range (100 m) [19, 20]. ^{223}Ra treatment with a targeted-emitter provides radiation energy to cancer cells and tumor tissue while limiting damage to healthy tissues. **Table 1** shows ^{223}Ra

Radionuclide	Half-life (day)	Emission particles (parent and daughters)	E_{mean} (MeV) (%)	Tissue penetration average (mm)
Ac-225	10.0	α	5.8 (54%), 6.4 (82%), 7.1 (>99%), 5.7 (2%), 8.8 (100%)	0.051
		β	1.8 (98%), 1.4 (98%), 0.64 (100%)	11.21
Ra-223	11.4	α	5.7 (100%), 6.9 (100%), 7.5 (99%), 6.6 (99%), 7.4 (100%)	0.062
		β	0.47 (0.3%), 0.47 (100%), 0.35 (100%)	8.56

Table 1.
The properties of ^{223}Ra and ^{225}Ac radiopharmaceuticals in the treatment of bone metastases prostate cancer.

radiopharmaceutical characteristics. Also, the decay chain of ^{223}Ra radiopharmaceuticals is presented in **Figure 1**.

Radium-223 dichloride is a targeted alpha emitter that preferentially binds to regions where the bone turnover is enhanced in bones and produces short-range (<100 μm) high-energy alpha particulates. As osteoblastic calcium mimesis, ^{223}Ra is linked into newly developed osteoblast or sclerotic metastasis, especially in the microenvironment. The high-energy radiation of alpha-particles leads largely to dual-stranded DNA breaks with a powerful and highly localized cytotoxic impact on the target areas. The alpha particles' short distance also minimizes the harmful effects on nearby healthy tissue, especially bone marrow [21].

In phase I and phase II trials involving bone metastasis patients, radium-223 has been shown to have a good safety profile with little myelotoxicity [22]. Studies of Phase two showed the reduction of pain and improvement of biomarkers associated with diseases (e.g., bone-alkaline phosphatase and prostate-specific antigen [PSA]) and suggest a survival advantage among patients who have castration-resistant prostate cancer and bone metastases [23]. In order to investigate radium-223's survival impact, we conducted a Phase 3 randomized, two-blind multi-national research that compared ^{223}Ra effectiveness and safety to placebo in patients with

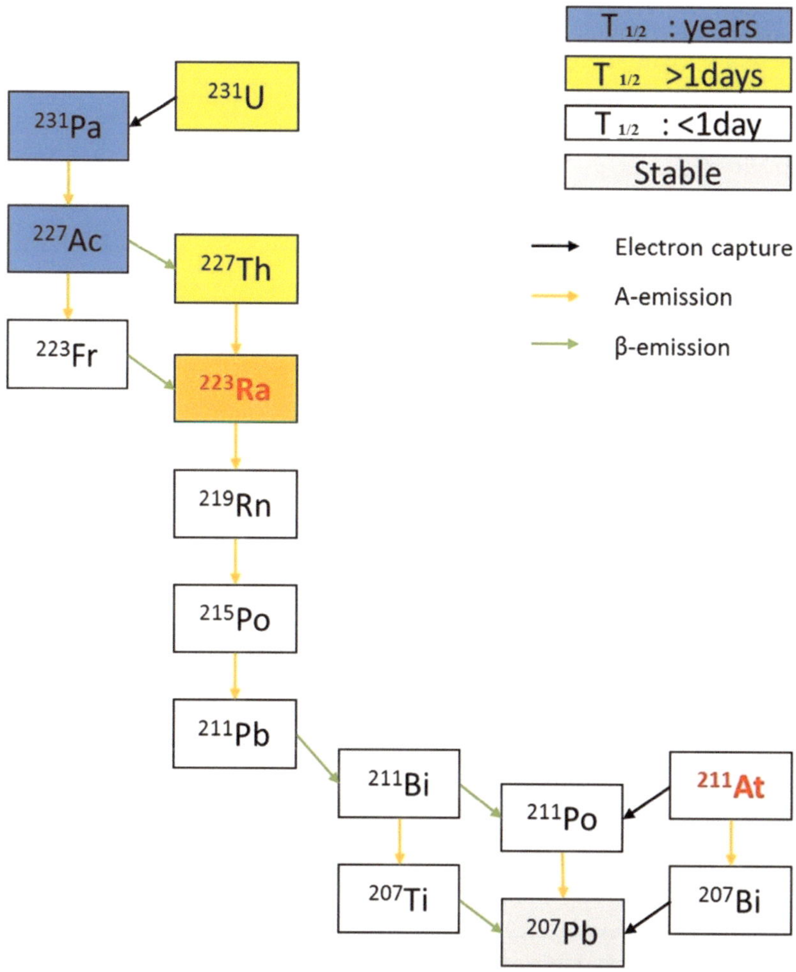

Figure 1.
The decay chain of ^{223}Ra radiopharmaceuticals.

castration-resistant prostate cancer and bone metastases in Symptomatic Prostate Cancer Painters (ALSYMPCA).

3. Actinium-225

^{225}Ac ($T_{1/2}$ = 10 days), like ^{223}Ra, is α-emitter radiopharmaceutical that decays to stable ^{209}Bi through six radionuclides [24]. The ^{225}Ac radioelement is a targeted alpha treatment that improves survival in individuals with metastatic castration-resistant prostate cancer. ^{225}Ac emits a particle with E_{α} = 6 MeV energy when it decays, yielding net four particles and three-particle disintegrations, the majority of which are high energy and useful gamma emissions, including ^{213}Bi ($T_{1/2}$ = 45.6 m; E_{α} = 6 MeV $E_{max(\beta)}$ = 444 keV and Eγ=440 keV), where this line has been used in imaging drug distribution [18]. Other daughters include ^{221}Fr ($T_{1/2}$ = 4.8 min; E_{α} = 5 Mev and 218 keV γ energy line emission), ^{217}At ($T_{1/2}$ = 32.3 ms; E_{α} = 7 MeV), ^{213}Po

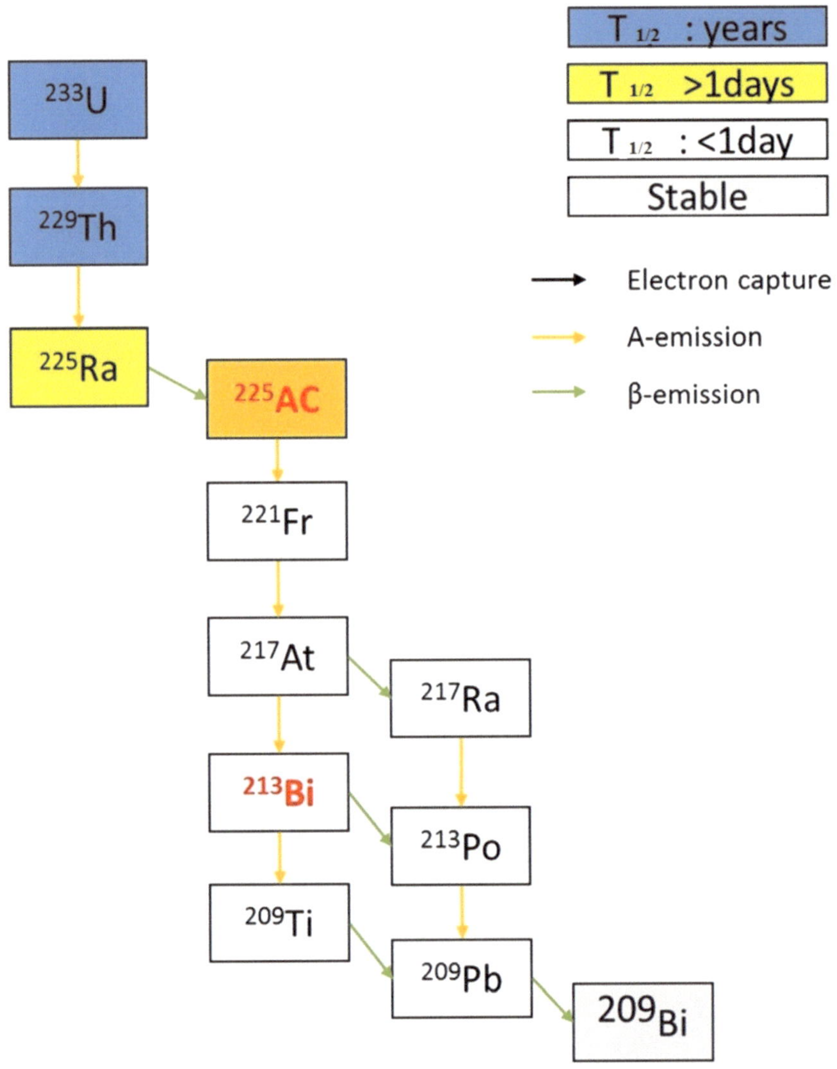

Figure 2.
The ^{225}Ac radiopharmaceuticals position in radioactive ^{233}U decay series.

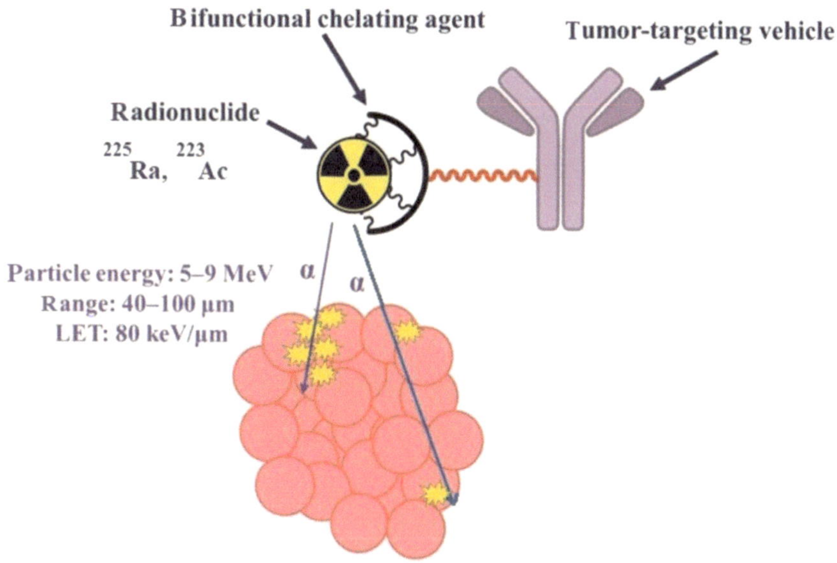

Figure 3.
Schematic diagram depicting the concept of targeted radionuclide therapy employing alpha (α) particles in a tumor-targeting construct. The high linear energy transfer (LET) and short-range of particles make them highly desirable for use in cancer therapy.

($T_{1/2}$ = 4.2 μs; E_α = 8 MeV), ^{209}Tl ($T_{1/2}$ = 2.2 m; $E_{max(\beta)}$ = 659 keV) (stable). Given ^{225}Ac with a 10 d half-life, the high emission of alpha particles, and the favorable, fast ^{209}Bi stable decay chain, this radionuclide is recognized to have a promising potential for cancer usage [2]. **Figure 2** illustrates the decay pattern for ^{225}Ac. Also, **Table 1** shows ^{225}Ac characteristics of radiopharmaceuticals. ^{225}Ac is a potential candidate among the α particle-producing ions with characteristics suited for usage in targeted α therapy (TAT) (**Figure 3**).

The radiological half-life of ^{225}Ac is 9.92 days, allowing it to be sent to clinics distant from the location of manufacture. Furthermore, this lengthy half-life is compatible with the use of macromolecular targeting vectors, such as antibodies or nanoparticles, which have long in-vivo circulation durations. As it decays to stable ^{209}Bi, ^{225}Ac produces eight short-lived progenies, producing a total of four high-energy a particle that kill cancer cells (**Figure 2**). Notably, in both in vitro and in vivo settings, ^{225}Ac is far more potent than its daughter nuclide, ^{213}Bi.

4. Dose calculations

The estimations of the doses were carried out with the application "Internal Computer Dose Assessment" (IDAC-Dose2.1). The dose coefficients of patients having radiopharmaceutical exams in nuclear medicine were calculated using this program by ICRP. In addition, dose estimates using the same ICRP computer architecture for the internal dose evaluation are the basis of the IDAC-Dose2.1 program.

For a time-independent system, the mean absorbed dose (D) to a target region (r_T) is calculated using the equation below [25]:

$$(r_T, T_D) = \sum_{r_S} \tilde{A}(r_S, T_D).S(r_T \leftarrow r_S) \tag{1}$$

where $\tilde{A}(r_S, T_D)$ is the cumulated activity (Bq) in source region r_S over the integration period T_D, and $S(r_T \leftarrow r_S)$ is the mean absorbed dose (Gy/Bq) in the

Organ	Dose coefficients				Absorbed dose (Gy/Bq)	
	Gy/Bq*		Sv/Bq**		^{223}Ra ($\times 10^{-9}$)	^{225}Ac ($\times 10^{-9}$)
	^{223}Ra ($\times 10^{-8}$)	^{225}Ac ($\times 10^{-9}$)	^{223}Ra ($\times 10^{-9}$)	^{225}Ac ($\times 10^{-9}$)		
Adrenals	2.06	4.14	8.24	1.65	41.2	8.27
Brain	0.471	0.945	1.88	0.378	9.41	1.89
Breast	0.477	0.955	1.91	0.382	9.54	1.91
Colon wall	2.65	5.35	10.6	2.14	52.9	10.7
Endosteum (bone surface)	0.660	1.31	2.64	0.524	13.2	2.62
Extra thoracic region	0.474	0.955	1.89	0.382	9.47	1.91
Eye lenses	0.0065	0.003	0.002	0.001	0.130	0.007
Gallbladder wall	0.478	9.55	1.91	0.382	9.55	1.91
Heart wall	1.57	3.11	6.28	1.24	31.4	6.21
Kidneys	2.81	0.056	11.2	2.26	56.2	11.3
Liver	2.52	5.05	10.1	2.02	50.4	10.1
Lung	3.40	6.85	13.6	2.74	67.9	13.7
Lymphatic nodes	0.635	1.27	2.54	0.506	12.7	2.53
Muscle	0.282	0.056	1.13	0.226	5.64	1.13
Esophagus	2.42	4.86	9.68	1.94	48.4	9.72
Oral mucosa	0.478	0.095	1.91	0.382	9.56	1.91
Pancreas	2.06	4.14	8.24	1.65	41.2	8.27
Prostate	0.475	0.095	1.89	0.382	9.47	1.91
Red (active) bone marrow	1.72	3.44	6.88	1.37	34.4	6.87
Salivary glands	0.474	0.955	1.89	0.382	9.47	1.91
Skin	0.515	1.04	2.06	0.414	10.3	2.07
Small intestine wall	2.61	5.25	10.4	2.10	52.2	10.5
Spleen	3.64	7.35	14.6	2.94	72.8	14.7
Stomach wall	2.42	4.86	9.68	1.94	48.4	9.72
Testes	0.63	1.29	2.54	0.514	12.7	2.57
Thymus	4.77	0.955	19.1	0.382	95.3	1.91
Thyroid	1.53	3.07	6.10	1.23	30.5	6.14
Urinary bladder wall	0.237	0.469	0.946	0.187	4.73	0.937
Total body	—	—	—	—	849	153

**Radiation weighting factor for α-radiation is 5, unit Gy/Bq as proposed by the ICRP [26].*

***Radiation weighting factor of 20 for α-radiation with unit Sv/Bq.*
ICRP = International Commission on Radiological Protection.

Table 2.
Intravenous ^{223}Ra and ^{225}Ac radiopharmaceutical doses and the doses absorbed (Gy/Bq) determined by computer-assessing computer-dose 2.1 in human body organs.

target tissue per nuclear transformation in the source region and defined by this Equation [26]:

$$S(r_T \leftarrow r_S) = \sum\nolimits_i \Delta_i . \varphi(r_T \leftarrow r_S, E_i) \quad (2)$$

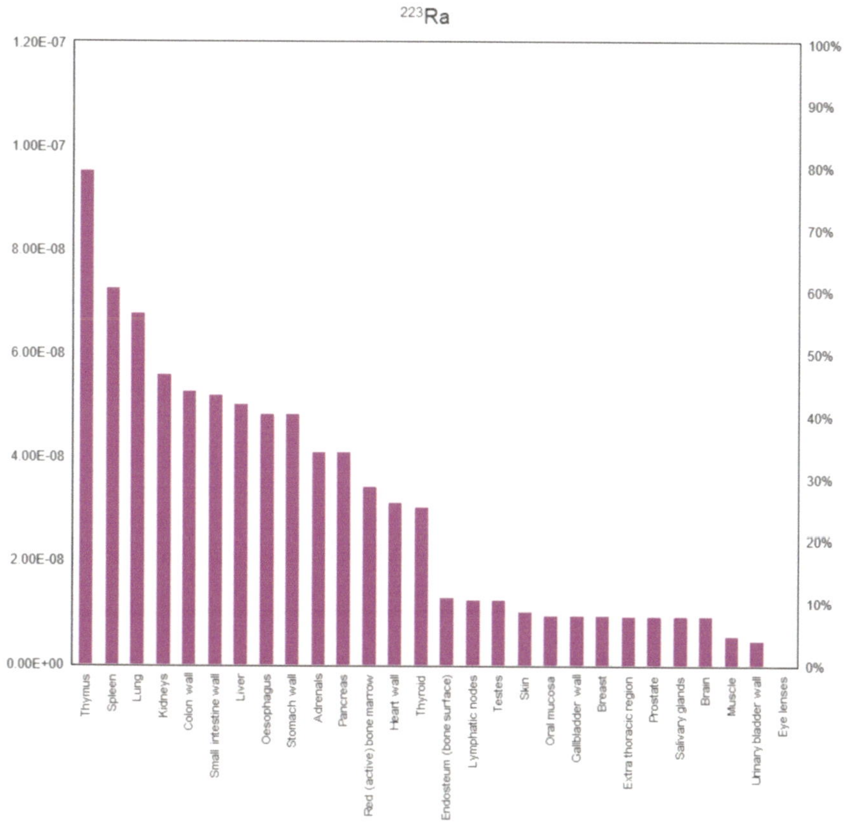

Figure 4.
The absorbed dose distribution of ^{223}Ra radiopharmaceutical in somebody organs.

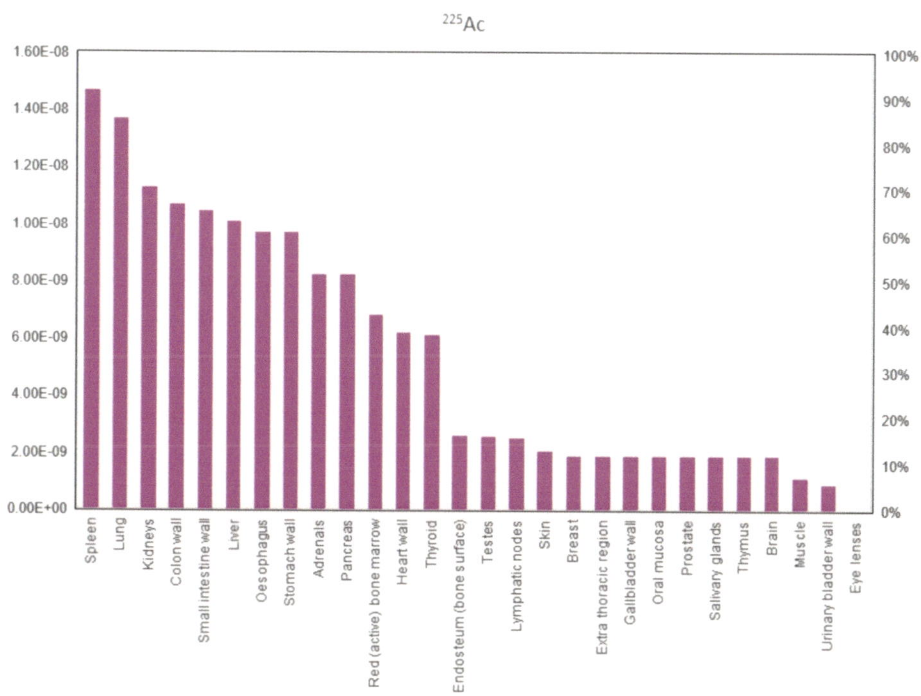

Figure 5.
The absorbed dose distribution of ^{225}Ac radiopharmaceutical in some body organs.

where $\varphi(r_T \leftarrow r_S, E_i)$ is the specific absorbed fractions (SAFs) value, and; $\Delta_i = E_i Y_i$ (where E_i is the yield and Y_i is the mean energy or part of the energy distribution for β-decay) of the $i - th$ the nuclear transition of the radionuclide in joules [27].

The absorbed dose of radiopharmaceuticals ^{223}Ra and ^{225}Ac was estimated with IDAC-Dose2.1 and given in **Table 2**. The findings were computed after one hour of intravenous doses. In the prostate organ, the absorbed doses of ^{223}Ra and ^{225}Ac radiopharmaceuticals were determined to be 9.47×10^{-9} Gy/Bq and 1.91E-9Gy/Bq, respectively. This number represents 1% of the total body dosage. The greatest and least absorbed doses of ^{223}Ra were observed in the Thymus (9.53×10^{-8} Gy/Bq) and Eye lenses (1.30×10^{-10} Gy/Bq) organs, respectively, according to biokinetics distribution. In addition, the ^{225}Ac distribution in bodily organs reveals that the Spleen (1.47×10^{-8} Gy/Bq) has the greatest concentration absorbed dosage and the Eye lenses have the lowest.

Figures 4 and **5** indicates doses taken in some human body organs by ^{223}Ra and ^{225}Ac radiopharmaceuticals, respectively. The histogram shows that 50 percent of the absorbed dosage is accumulated in six organs in both radiopharmaceuticals. These six organs are thymus, Spleen, lunge, kidney, colon wall, small intestine wall, Spleen, lung, kidney, colon wall, small intestine wall, and liver.

5. Conclusions

The alpha-emitting radionuclides of ^{223}Ra and ^{225}Ra are a targeted alpha emitter radiopharmaceutical used to treat prostate cancer. The properties and absorbed dose value of those radiopharmaceuticals in body organs are reviewed in this chapter. Total body absorbed dose value (Gy/Bq) per intravenous injections of ^{223}Ra was higher than ^{225}Ac radiopharmaceuticals. This difference is related to the energy of alpha particles and the half-life of the radiopharmaceuticals. The results of this study will assist in evaluating and analyzing human body organ doses from the application of ^{223}Ra and ^{225}Ac that are used in mCRPC patients. The main obstacles using of ^{223}Ra and ^{225}Ac radiopharmaceuticals are that the daughter nuclides will always dissociate from the targeting construct upon their formation. Therefore, they can make unwanted doses in other organs.

Conflict of interest

The authors declare no conflict of interest.

Author details

Akbar Abbasi[1*], Hesham M.H. Zakaly[2,3*] and Fatemeh Mirekhtiary[4]

1 Faculty of Engineering, University of Kyrenia, Kyrenia, North Cyprus, Turkey

2 Institute of Physics and Technology, Ural Federal University Named after the First President of Russia B.N. Yeltsin, Yekaterinburg, Sverdlovskaya Oblast, Russia

3 Department of Physics, Faculty of Science, Al-Azhar University, Assiut, Egypt

4 Faculty of Engineering, Near East University, Nicosia, North Cyprus, Turkey

*Address all correspondence to: akbar.abbasi@kyrenia.edu.tr; h.m.zakaly@azhar.edu.eg

References

[1] Pawson A, Ghumman Z, Kuo PH, Jadvar H, Bartel T, Shayegan B, et al. A review of prostate cancer imaging, positron emission tomography, and radiopharmaceutical-based therapy. Can Urol Assoc J. 2020;14(4):130.

[2] Abbasi A, Dadashpour M, Alipourfard I. Calculation of radium-223 and actinium-225 α-emitter radiopharmaceuticals dose rates in treatment of metastatic castration-resistant prostate cancer. 2020.

[3] Abbasi A, Sadikoglu F, Hassanzadeh M. Effect of Au-197 nanoparticles along with Sm-153 radiopharmaceutical in prostate cancer from simulation method. J Cancer Res Ther. 2019;15(8).

[4] Heidenreich A, Moul JW, Shariat S, Karnes RJ. Role of salvage lymph node dissection in prostate cancer. Curr Opin Urol. 2016;26(6):581–589.

[5] Zakaly HMH, Mostafa MYA, Deryabina D, Zhukovsky M. Comparative studies on the potential use of 177Lu-based radiopharmaceuticals for the palliative therapy of bone metastases. Int J Radiat Biol. 2020;96(6):779–789.

[6] Zakaly HMH, Mostafa MYA, Zhukovsky M. Biokinetic modelling of 89Zr-labelled monoclonal antibodies for dosimetry assessment in humans. Int J Radiat Res. 2020;18(4):825–833.

[7] Zakaly HMH, Mostafa MYA, Dzholumbetov S, Issa SAM, Tekin HO, Erdemir RU, et al. Comparative study on application of 177Lu-labeled rituximab, tetulomab, cetuximab and huA33 monoclonal antibodies to targeted radionuclide therapy. Biomed Phys Eng Express. 2020 Nov;7(1):15015.

[8] Banerjee SR, Minn IL, Kumar V, Josefsson A, Lisok A, Brummet M, et al. Preclinical evaluation of 203/212Pb-labeled low-molecular-weight compounds for targeted radiopharmaceutical therapy of prostate cancer. J Nucl Med. 2020;61(1):80–88.

[9] Patel CM, Wadas TJ, Shiozawa Y. Progress in targeted alpha-particle-emitting radiopharmaceuticals as treatments for prostate cancer patients with bone metastases. Molecules. 2021; 26(8):2162.

[10] Lin M, Ta RT, Kairemo K, Le DB, Ravizzini GC. Prostate-specific membrane antigen-targeted radiopharmaceuticals in diagnosis and therapy of prostate cancer: Current status and future perspectives. Cancer Biother Radiopharm. 2021;36(3): 237–251.

[11] Okarvi SM. Recent developments of prostate-specific membrane antigen (PSMA)-specific radiopharmaceuticals for precise imaging and therapy of prostate cancer: An overview. Clin Transl Imaging. 2019;7(3):189–208.

[12] Nonnekens J, Chatalic KLS, Molkenboer-Kuenen JDM, Beerens CEMT, Bruchertseifer F, Morgenstern A, et al. 213Bi-labeled prostate-specific membrane antigen-targeting agents induce DNA double-strand breaks in prostate cancer xenografts. Cancer Biother Radiopharm. 2017;32(2):67–73.

[13] Kesavan M, Turner JH, Meyrick D, Yeo S, Cardaci G, Lenzo NP. Salvage radiopeptide therapy of advanced castrate-resistant prostate cancer with Lutetium-177-labeled prostate-specific membrane antigen: Efficacy and safety in routine practice. Cancer Biother Radiopharm. 2018;33(7):274–281.

[14] Sartor O, Sharma D. Radium and other alpha emitters in prostate cancer. Transl Androl Urol. 2018;7(3):436.

[15] Mostafa MYA, Zakaly HMH, Zhukovsky M. Assessment of exposure after injection of 99m Tc-labeled intact monoclonal antibodies and their fragments into humans. Radiol Phys Technol. 2019 Mar;12(1):96–104.

[16] Zakaly HMH, Mostafa MYA, Zhukovsky M. Dosimetry assessment of injected 89Zr-labeled monoclonal antibodies in humans. Radiat Res. 2019 May;191(5):466–474.

[17] Du Y, Carrio I, De Vincentis G, Fanti S, Ilhan H, Mommsen C, et al. Practical recommendations for radium-223 treatment of metastatic castration-resistant prostate cancer. Eur J Nucl Med Mol Imaging. 2017;44:1671–1678.

[18] Mangano AM, Pacilio M, Ialongo P, Semprebene A, Ventroni G, Mango L. Dosimetry-based consideration on remission and relapse after therapy with 223Ra-dichloride in castration-resistant prostate cancer (CRPC) with bone metastases. A case report. Diagnostics. 2018;8:18.

[19] Tagawa ST, Vallabhajosula S, Jhanwar Y, Ballman K V, Hackett A, Emmerich L, et al. Phase I dose-escalation study of 225Ac-J591 for progressive metastatic castration resistant prostate cancer (mCRPC). American Society of Clinical Oncology; 2018.

[20] Osvaldo G-PF, Salvador M-OS, Zael S-R, Nora S-M. Radium-223 in metastatic hormone-sensitive high-grade prostate cancer: Initial experience. Am J Nucl Med Mol Imaging. 2017;7(5): 236.

[21] Parker C, Nilsson S, Heinrich D, Helle SI, O'sullivan JM, Fosså SD, et al. Alpha emitter radium-223 and survival in metastatic prostate cancer. N Engl J Med. 2013;369:213–223.

[22] Nilsson S, Larsen RH, Fosså SD, Balteskard L, Borch KW, Westlin J-E, et al. First clinical experience with α-emitting radium-223 in the treatment of skeletal metastases. Clin cancer Res. 2005;11(12):4451–4459.

[23] Nilsson S, Franzén L, Parker C, Tyrrell C, Blom R, Tennvall J, et al. Bone-targeted radium-223 in symptomatic, hormone-refractory prostate cancer: A randomised, multicentre, placebo-controlled phase II study. Lancet Oncol. 2007;8(7):587–594.

[24] Jurcic JG. Targeted alpha-particle therapy for hematologic malignancies. J Med imaging Radiat Sci. 2019;50(4): S53–S57.

[25] Andersson M, Johansson L, Eckerman K, Mattsson S. IDAC-dose 2.1, an internal dosimetry program for diagnostic nuclear medicine based on the ICRP adult reference voxel phantoms. EJNMMI Res. 2017;7:88.

[26] Bolch WE, Jokisch D, Zankl M, Eckerman KF, Fell T, Manger R, et al. ICRP publication 133: The ICRP computational framework for internal dose assessment for reference adults: Specific absorbed fractions. Ann ICRP. 2016;45:5–73.

[27] Protection IC On R. nuclear decay data for dosimetric calculations. ICRP Publ 107, Ann ICRP. 2008;38.

Section 4

Radiopharmaceuticals Applications in Diagnosis and Therapy

Chapter 10

Molecular Imaging with Genetically Programmed Nanoparticles

Donna E. Goldhawk

Abstract

Nanoparticle research has greatly benefitted medical imaging platforms by generating new signals, enhancing detection sensitivity, and expanding both clinical and preclinical applications. For magnetic resonance imaging, the fabrication of superparamagnetic iron oxide nanoparticles has provided a means of detecting cells and has paved the way for magnetic particle imaging. As the field of molecular imaging grows and enables the tracking of cells and their molecular activities so does the possibility of tracking genetically programmed biomarkers. This chapter discusses the advantages and challenges of gene-based contrast, using the bacterial magnetosome model to highlight the requirements of *in vivo* iron biomineralization and reporter gene expression for magnetic resonance signal detection. New information about magnetosome protein interactions in non-magnetic mammalian cells is considered in the light of design and application(s) of a rudimentary magnetosome-like nanoparticle for molecular imaging. Central to this is the hypothesis that a magnetosome root structure is defined by essential magnetosome genes, whose expression positions the biomineral in a given membrane compartment, in any cell type. The use of synthetic biology for programming multi-component structures not only broadens the scope of reporter gene expression for molecular MRI but also facilitates the tracking of cell therapies.

Keywords: magnetosome, iron biomineral, reporter gene expression, iron contrast, magnetic resonance imaging

1. Introduction

With over a 20-year history, the field of molecular imaging is now well-entrenched [1–3] and continuing to expand its influence over multiple imaging modalities, including optical [4], nuclear [5], magnetic resonance (MR) [6] and acoustic [7]. In all these platforms, the use of contrast agents is a central theme, to enhance tissue structure and differentiate between healthy and diseased cells. Image-guidance has been achieved with simple molecules like the fluorophore indocyanin green [8], with macromolecules like antibodies [9], and with synthetic particles like superparamagnetic iron oxides (SPIO) [10] or perfluorocarbon emulsions [11]. Moreover, by adding targeting groups to these contrast agents, additional tissue specificity and/or image resolution may be obtained.

Despite these attributes, there are challenges in biomarker development for medical imaging, such as longevity of the signal and intrinsic biological activity.

IntechOpen

Exogenous contrast agents that reach their cellular targets may still be lost during cell division, metabolized, or decay too rapidly for effective longitudinal study. In addition, their role as beacon does not necessarily provide a measure of inherent biological activity. One solution is to adopt a gene-based approach in which contrast is synthesized by the cell and thus remains with it throughout its life cycle. Not only does this type of endogenous contrast get passed to daughter cells, it also permits reporter gene expression in response to biological cues. In this way, using the tools of molecular biology, cellular contrast may be directly linked to the presence of proteins (*i.e.* transcription factors, TF) that regulate genetically programmed contrast gene expression [12]. This approach has been tremendously effective with fluorescent proteins and the optical detection of cells and tissues, where depth of penetration is low enough to avoid losses in sample resolution from the scatter of light. Addressing gene-based contrast for other types of non-invasive detection systems is, in general, still a work in progress.

In this chapter, the development of gene-based contrast for MR detection will be described using the bacterial magnetosome as a model for biogenic iron biominerals. Integral to this discussion are the factors that regulate gene expression, determine protein localization, guide macromolecular assembly, and permit iron crystal formation without the need for exogenous contrast agent.

2. Magnetosome model

The magnetosome is a remarkable structure synthesized by magnetotactic bacteria (MTB) [13]. These micron size cells produce nanometer size iron crystals for magnetotaxis, responding to the earth's magnetic field through the creation of a single magnetic dipole within each biomineral. Ingeniously, to avoid cytotoxicity associated with the oxidation and reduction of iron, crystallization proceeds within a protective compartment, *i.e.* a vesicle invaginated from the cell's innermost plasma membrane [14]. Arguably one of the earliest examples of a subcellular organelle [15, 16], magnetosomes are typically arranged in a defined pattern within the cell and connected to cytoskeletal protein (**Figure 1**) [17]. Importantly, various magnetosome membrane (Mam) proteins and magnetosome membrane specific (Mms) proteins enable the compartment to carry out its functions [18]: recruiting the necessary activities to define the vesicle, connecting the magnetosomes to cytoskeletal elements, concentrating iron, defining the crystal, and assembling individual magnetosomes into an effective magnet.

In MTB, magnetosome biosynthesis is thus a protein-directed process, genetically encoded by structural genes arranged in units, termed operons, and located largely in a gene cluster, termed the magnetosome genomic island. Of the approximately 30 genes involved in magnetosome formation, roughly one third are located elsewhere in the bacterial genome, possibly indicative of magnetosome protein interactions with common cellular components. In support of this, mammalian cation diffusion facilitator protein complements bacterial MamM function [19]. In addition, mammalian molecular motors appear to interact with MamL [20]. While more studies are required to fully elucidate magnetosome structure, and potentially reproduce it in other cell types, the following functional categorization may prove useful for dissecting the steps and partners involved in magnetosome formation.

2.1 Membrane designation

Mutations designed to delete individual magnetosome genes from MTB have exposed the absolute requirement of a select few genes for magnetosome

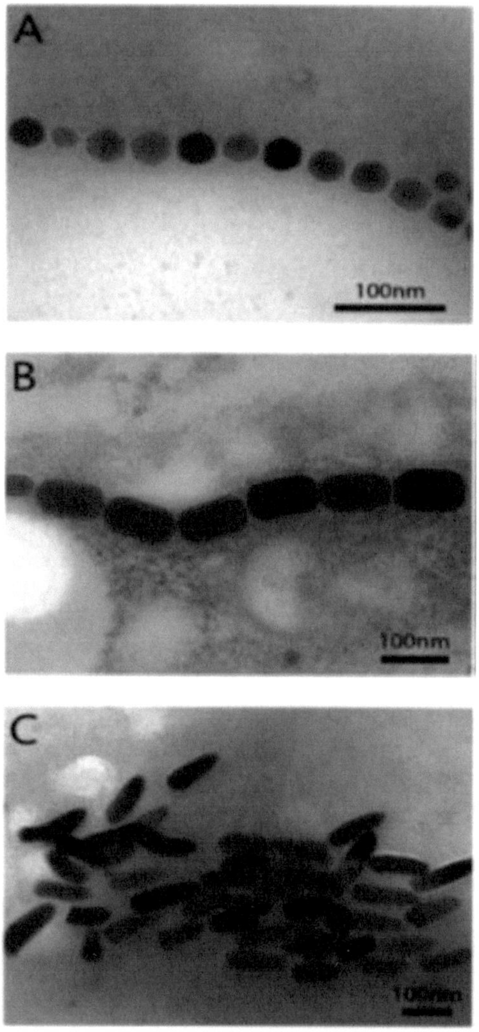

Figure 1.
Magnetosome crystal morphologies. Transmission electron microscopy of MTB shows three types of magnetite crystal: cubooctahedral (A), prismatic (B) and bullet-shaped (C). Size, shape, composition, and subcellular arrangement of magnetosomes is generally species-specific. Adapted from Vargas et al. [17].

production. When anyone of these essential genes is missing, there is either no magnetosome vesicle and/or no biomineral [21]. Among these genes are *mamB*, *mamE*, *mamI* and *mamL*. Numerous other genes may be selectively deleted without damaging the entire magnetosome structure [13]. In this case, what results is a compromised biomineral with a less than perfect crystal, altered size or disruption in cellular location. As the genes responsible for various magnetosome attributes become clearer so does the opportunity for designing nanoparticles that are not only compatible with a given intracellular environment but also impart desirable magnetic properties [22, 23]. For magnetic resonance imaging (MRI), subcellular arrangement of magnetosomes through MamJ-MamK interactions [24] may be a dispensable feature. Likewise, in magnetic particle imaging (MPI) individual magnetosomes constitute an ideal tracer owing to their perfect crystal morphology [25].

With a view to forming a rudimentary magnetosome-like nanoparticle in any cell type, we have proposed that essential magnetosome genes constitute a common base upon which diverse biominerals are synthesized [22]. This notion is predicated on the specificity of certain protein–protein interactions, needed to establish the magnetosome as a distinct structure. Plausibility is evident based on genomic sequencing and the commonality of sequence across diverse classes of MTB [26]. Likewise, large scale magnetosome gene expression has been successfully tested in a non-magnetic bacterium [27]. In this work, magnetosome related operons from the magnetotactic bacterium *Magnetospirillum gryphiswaldense* were transferred to the non-magnetic bacterium *Rhodospirillum rubrum.* Characterization of newly imparted magnetic properties included the appearance of intracellular, electron dense particles by transmission electron microscopy, with Fourier transforms in high-resolution images displaying intensity maxima typical of magnetite. In addition, magnetically transformed *R. rubrum* continued to perform photosynthesis, indicating compatibility between magnetosome-like nanoparticles and normal cellular function. Nevertheless, the minimum number of magnetosome genes required to build the basic magnetosome unit has not been clearly defined. Moreover, this knowledge would greatly enable the rational use of synthetic biology aimed at tailoring magnetosome-like nanoparticles for multiple purposes, above and beyond magnetotaxis, and in a wider variety of cell types.

Toward understanding the genetic make-up of a rudimentary magnetosome-like nanoparticle, MamI-MamL interactions have recently been described in a mammalian cell system [28]. This work showed that (1) MamI and MamL are compatible with a mammalian cell expression system; (2) MamL specifically recruits MamI to the same intracellular location despite co-expression in the complex intracellular environment of the mammalian host; and (3) MamL particles, alone and in the presence of MamI, also interact with putative mammalian molecular motors. These findings suggest that MamL may have a role in anchoring magnetosome assembly within a given membrane and raises the possibility that MamL also forms previously unrecognized cytoskeletal connections in MTB. Such a dual function further implies that membrane localization and magnetosome assembly may be initiated simultaneously, accounting for the essential role of MamL in both vesicle formation and subsequent biomineralization.

2.2 Protein recruitment

There are numerous corollaries to be considered for optimal expression of magnetosome-like nanoparticles in foreign non-magnetic cells. If the role of MamL is indeed to designate the membrane compartment, then eukaryotic cells equipped with vesicles may yet form magnetosomes by drawing on only those genes that attract biomineralizing activities (**Figure 2**). This would simplify magnetosome biosynthesis in eukaryotic cells. This is not to say that genetic encoding of vesicle formation should be ignored. A fuller understanding of how magnetosome vesicles form may be useful for ultrasound technologies that would benefit from reporter gene expression (discussed below). If the role of MamL lies in recruitment of magnetosome proteins involved in iron crystallization, then perhaps vesicle formation is largely carried out by other magnetosome proteins that shape the vesicle and accommodate biominerals of varying dimensions and morphologies [13, 21]. To this point, seven *mam* genes, including the essential ones (*mamB, mamE, mamI* and *mamL*) have been implicated in magnetosome membrane formation in MTB [29].

Interestingly, there may be a dual role for MamI in both iron crystal nucleation [30] and size of the magnetosome vesicle [31]. Using a mammalian expression system to substantiate this hypothesis, we showed that MamI-derived contrast significantly increases MRI transverse relaxivity over the parental control, when cells are cultured in the presence of an iron supplement [32]. In this work, cells were mounted in a spherical gelatin phantom and placed in a knee coil for scanning

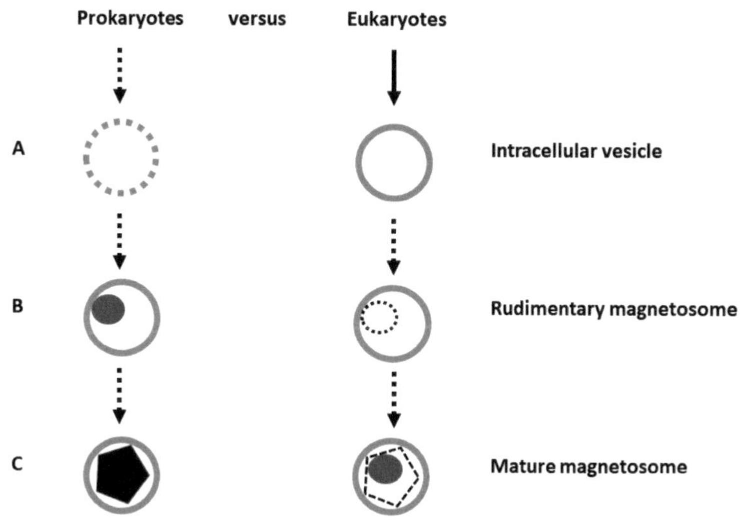

Figure 2.
Modelling magnetosome formation in prokaryotes and eukaryotes. In MTB, genetic encoding of magnetosomes begins with plasma membrane invagination to form an intracellular vesicle (A). Once formed, magnetosome membrane proteins located in this subcellular compartment initiate iron crystal formation (B). The full complement of magnetosome genes specifies the final composition, size, shape, and arrangement of mature biominerals (C). Unlike these prokaryotes, eukaryotic cells readily synthesize intracellular vesicles (denoted in A with a solid line). To designate a magnetosome-like compartment requires a subset of magnetosome genes, providing genetic information for the initiation of biomineralization (outlined in B with stipple). The transition from rudimentary magnetosome to mature nanoparticle (outlined in C with stipple) has not been fully elucidated in non-magnetic (e.g. mammalian) cells.

at 3 Tesla using previously described MR sequences [33]. With this experimental setup, measurements obtained from a compact layer of cells can be assessed in any cell type, expression system and treatment condition. Using the same expression system and human melanoma cell line, the motility of fluorescent MamL particles increased in the presence of MamI, influencing both directed and Brownian motion and suggesting that particle size may be more compact in the presence of MamI [20]. These unexpected findings, from two small but essential magnetosome genes, reflect at once the beauty and simplicity of the MTB genome in its capacity to streamline the formation of magnetosomes using a minimum of genetic encoding.

2.3 Rudimentary nanoparticle

Given these findings, we might expect that the distinction between magnetosome vesicle formation and iron biomineralization is not so clear-cut. A subset of magnetosome genes, perhaps the essential genes, may link the two fundamental processes that define the magnetosome, *i.e.* vesicle and biomineral, by recruiting proteins to a designated site on the membrane and establishing the base structure upon which the magnetosome is elaborated. In cells where the vesicle is otherwise formed, the key challenge is deciphering biomineralization. To this point, the reported activity of MamE fits into this framework [34, 35]. Also provisionally defined as a bifunctional protein, in the absence of MamE there is no biomineral, although, vesicle formation proceeds [21].

There is still much to learn about magnetosome assembly. Ideally, its formation in any cell can be accomplished by adapting the needed set of instructions from MTB. Toward this goal, the emerging picture of magnetosome assembly indicates that bifunctional proteins link one magnetosome component to the next, progressively defining the magnetosome compartment and biomineral. Until we can properly define how each genetic feature fits together, a rudimentary magnetosome-like nanoparticle is likely to bridge the gap created by our partial understanding of magnetosome biology. Since different cell types have different abilities for building and tolerating membrane-enclosed vesicles, research in this area should continue to expose fundamental processes involved in both magnetosome vesicle formation and iron biomineralization.

3. Iron biomineralization

Virtually all cells regulate iron carefully to prevent cellular damage from free radical formation all the while retaining access to a pool of iron co-factor, needed to drive vital cellular processes [36]. The magnetosome is a fine example of iron sequestration for the purpose of magnetite formation. This iron oxide (Fe_3O_4) has the necessary superparamagnetic properties for effective MRI detection [37]. Indeed, theoretical calculations indicate that approximately 3000 cells/voxel could be detected on large animal/human scanners at 3 Tesla if mammalian cells could be engineered to express the same magnetosomes as found in MTB [22]. On small animal scanners, this improves to as few as 3 cells/voxel. Therefore, a fuller understanding of how to regulate magnetosome formation will ultimately provide MR platforms with a sensitive and versatile method for long-term tracking of cells and their molecular activities.

Use of the magnetosome for this purpose in mammalian cells requires that some iron be diverted from its usual pathways of distribution, namely iron uptake, storage and export [38]. Little is known about how iron uptake into a magnetosome-like vesicle will compete for the available cellular iron. Factors to consider include the cell's labile iron pool and response to shifts in iron homeostasis. For example, the mouse, multi-potent P19 embryonic carcinoma cell line is an iron exporting cell type, with high iron import and export activities similar to alternatively activated macrophages [39]. This cell type is programmed to recycle iron and, as such, retains very low levels of iron storage. Furthermore, P19 iron export is hormonally regulated by hepcidin, which induces a transient decrease in iron export protein (ferroportin) and an increase in the relationship between MR transverse relaxation rates and total cellular iron. In addition to this endocrine response, P19 cells secrete hepcidin activity that effectively decreases ferroportin levels in human THP-1 monocytes, indicating the ability for paracrine and/or autocrine regulation of cellular iron content [40]. How will the formation of magnetosome-like particles affect iron homeostasis in multi-potent cells like P19?

Despite the complexity of P19 iron metabolism, we know the cell's capacity for iron retention is increased by expression of the MTB gene *magA* [41]. This putative iron transporter [42, 43] has been localized to Golgi vesicles and sequesters iron in P19 cells regardless of competing iron export activity. In culture, MagA-derived activity depends on extracellular iron supplementation, potentially rerouting iron that is imported through the transferrin receptor and deposited in the labile iron pool, into a magnetosome-like storage vesicle. Presumably, this is indicative of the rudimentary magnetosome-like nanoparticle and the unique manner in which it may compartmentalize iron when further defined by the expression of essential magnetosome genes.

Early results with mammalian MamI-expressing cells indicate the same capacity for enhancing the iron-related MR transverse relaxation rates as MagA-expressing cells [32, 33]. In a direct comparison, using the same MDA-MB-435 host cell, both irreversible R_2 and reversible R_2' components of the total R_2^* transverse relaxation rate ($R_2^* = R_2 + R_2'$) were affected. This is a remarkable result, considering how different these two MTB proteins are. Apart from being integral membrane proteins, they are vastly different sizes, have distinct genomic localization, and are opposites in terms of their supporting role in magnetosome biosynthesis. While MamI is essential, MagA is nonessential [44] as are the majority of magnetosome gene products [45], including the iron crystallizing protein Mms6 [21]. These results confirm that no one MTB or magnetosome-specific gene is sufficient for recreating the magnetosome structure. The iron biomineral is shaped within a membrane-enclosed compartment that not only imports iron but also creates the necessary environment for crystal formation, including maintaining the appropriate pH and oxygen concentration for nucleation and crystallization. Once assembly of the basic magnetosome unit is understood, the possibility of genetically regulating crystal size, shape and composition [22] will have broad implications. Below, we identify features that impinge upon molecular imaging.

4. Applications in molecular imaging

The use of reporter genes to track molecular activity, and therefore cellular activity, is well known in biology. Reporter genes have provided all sorts of signals that may be detected optically under a microscope in cells or histological sections, or by using luminometry or chromatography on tissue extracts. Adapting reporter genes for non-invasive molecular imaging is an enabling technology that adds spatial information in the context of a living subject as well as the possibility of repetitive imaging for longitudinal study of *in vivo* processes. In addition, medical imaging is typically tomographic and may account for motion like heartbeat and respiration. On the other hand, there are added challenges for *in vivo* imaging, not the least of which involves reconciling cellular signals and tissue motion. Molecular signals are also frequently lost within large imaging volumes. While greater detail from smaller voxels may be resolved on scanners designed for small animals, these detection methods do not always scale up on large animal and human scanners, making translation from preclinical to clinical applications an ongoing challenge.

Nevertheless, the magnetosome is an interesting nanoparticle with multiple possible applications in molecular imaging. Magnetosomes may serve as a gene-based, contrast agent for tracking cell therapies without the need for exogenous substrate. By sequestering iron, the magnetosome is ideal for MR signal detection on various modalities, including MRI, hybrid imaging with positron emission tomography (PET)/MRI and MPI. The nature of the magnetosome biomineral may also be used to amplify and manipulate MR signals, by varying iron content and form [39]. For instance, in cultured P19 cells the negative regulation of iron export by hepcidin does little to increase total cellular iron; however, R_2 is nevertheless more sensitive to hepcidin treatment than the untreated control. This study implicated changes in the form of intracellular iron (upon ferroportin degradation) and its influence on MR signal detection. Genetically encoded magnetosome components may also have yet unexplored applications, like using magnetosome vesicles as liposomes for ultrasound or for regulating iron overload by sequestering the excess mineral. Just as hybrid imaging combines more than one type of signal, *e.g.* co-localizing radiotracer and anatomical position [46], image-guidance may influence many aspects of medical care, *e.g.* delivering therapy and monitoring treatment [47]. It should be noted that MRI is a particularly versatile modality, with the capacity for multiparametric imaging [48, 49].

Adding gene-based contrast to this mix widens the scope of MR detection even further. Genetic regulation of nanoparticles [50] means that expression of the magnetosome can be tailored to include desirable features or exclude what is not needed.

For example, magnetosomes with genetically programmed, cell surface modifications have been prepared for a variety of applications from magnetic separation [51] to cancer diagnosis [52] and therapy [53]. In these examples, modified magnetosomes are isolated from MTB, ensuring the biomineral is fully formed and has the expected magnetic properties. A breast cancer model was used to compare isolated magnetosomes with chemically synthesized SPIO coated with serum albumin [54]. Both types of nanoparticle were crosslinked with fluorescent-labelled antibody to the epidermal growth factor receptor and examined in cultured MDA-MB-231 cells and their tumour xenografts. The modified magnetosomes outperformed SPIO with respect to MR signal and tumour distribution. At high field strength, low doses of iron in purified magnetosomes gave higher R_2 than an equivalent dose of the commercial SPIO, ferumoxide, and were suitable for MRI detection of rodent brain vasculature [55]. Following on this, genetically modified magnetosomes were used to locate glioblastoma in the rodent brain using purified magnetosomes expressing the RGD peptide fused to yellow fluorescent protein and MamC [52]. Others have successfully used purified magnetosomes for direct injection into rodent glioblastoma, at once treating with magnetic hyperthermia and monitoring tumour shrinkage by MRI [56]. The strategy of using modified magnetosomes as exogenous contrast agents for molecular imaging has gained a measure of commercial success with the Magnelle reagent [57]. In all these examples, subcellular arrangement of the magnetosome is an unnecessary feature since the iron biomineral is isolated from the bacterium. As such, the modified particles could be produced by mutant MTB that harbour only enough genetic information to recreate individual membrane-enclosed biominerals, devoid of attachments to cytoskeletal elements and each other. These modifications may facilitate purification and uptake of magnetosome-like nanoparticles into foreign hosts while reducing the possibility of unwanted immune response(s) in animal models, by limiting the number of exposed magnetosome proteins.

A compelling future strategy entails direct expression of rudimentary magnetosome-like nanoparticles in any cell type. Envisioning gene-based contrast of this nature for molecular imaging, using essential magnetosome genes to produce partially formed magnetosomes, is still under development (**Figure 3**). Clearly, MRI detects significant increases in mammalian cell contrast derived from single,

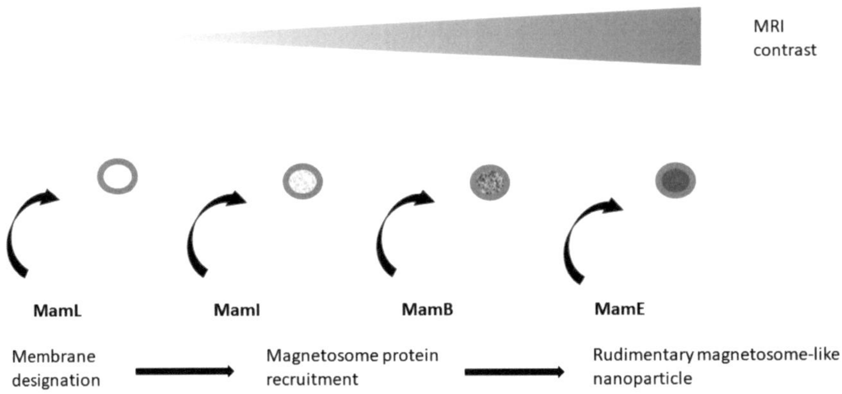

Figure 3.
Envisioning the rudimentary magnetosome-like nanoparticle. In any cell, essential magnetosome genes are expected to perform a central role in designating the point at which iron biomineralization will be initiated. The diagram depicts MamL in the role of magnetosome membrane designation, consistent with its ability to recruit MamI to the same intracellular particle. Incorporation of MamI initiates iron-handling activity, measured as an increase in MRI transverse relaxivity in iron-supplemented cells. Further MRI contrast enhancement is anticipated secondary to the recruitment of MamB and MamE iron-handling activities.

MTB and magnetosome gene expression systems, including *magA* [58, 59], *mms6* [60, 61], and now the essential gene *mamI* [32]. MagA-derived MR contrast has also been studied in several rodent models, providing a measure of contrast enhancement in xenografts of both tumour [62, 63] and stem [64] cells. Nevertheless, these single magnetosome gene expression systems fall short of the MR detection sensitivity promised by a more mature nanoparticle. In addition, by underestimating the value of critical interactions between combinations of magnetosome proteins, there is not only the risk of losing iron biomineral fidelity but also encouraging unintended interactions with the foreign host. At present, what limits this technology the most is our lack of appreciation for the fundamental magnetosome protein interactions that underlie the basic unit upon which the biomineral is structured. Noting the faithful interactions of MamI and MamL in mammalian cells, we expect that a minimum set of indispensable genes is involved in the biosynthesis of any magnetosome-like nanoparticle.

The combination of magnetosome genes that further elevates the MR signal is anxiously anticipated. Can we use the rudimentary magnetosome-like particle, consisting of essential magnetosome genes, to fashion nanoparticles that are MR silent until complemented by the protein(s) that trigger assembly of the complex or activation of biomineralization? Will subcellular arrangement of nanoparticles be sufficient to alter the MR signal? To what degree will changes in iron form or content alter MR detection? What types of cellular activity could be programmed to modulate magnetosome-like nanoparticle expression in mammalian cells?

4.1 Reporter gene expression

A special application of gene-based contrast is referred to as reporter gene expression. Basically, this is the difference between constant expression of the reporter gene versus its selective expression. Regions on DNA that promote gene expression (*i.e.* promoters, response elements, activating sequences) do so in response to protein-DNA interactions orchestrated by the cell. These transcription factors (TF) may vary from cell type to cell type; however, the factors that stimulate common functions across all cells are often continually present and drive expression of vital functions. As such, expression constructs driving reporter gene transcription in response to ever present TF, provide constitutive expression of the reporter gene, which is akin to a cell label. The protein encoded by that reporter gene will label the cell throughout its life cycle and be faithfully reproduced in daughter cells. On the contrary, TF that distinguish one cell type from another are selectively expressed. These TF often drive expression of developmental genes that determine the stage of cellular differentiation and ultimate phenotype. These TF are neither active in every cell nor at all times in the cell's history. For example, there are multiple TF that carry pluripotent stem cells toward terminal differentiation [12]. The phrase "reporter gene expression" was intended for this type of selective expression, which is often a defining feature of cellular activity in both health and disease and a valuable biomarker for molecular imaging.

Historically, most reporters are single gene expression systems that encode any protein for which there is a suitable means of detection. Of course, how the reporter signal is detected is intrinsically connected to the type of sample used for measurement and the available equipment. Luminometry using the reporter gene firefly luciferase, for example, began as a routine tool for the analysis of cell extracts but expanded to include small animal bioluminescence imaging once these scanners became available. For MR applications, however, single iron-handling reporter genes do not afford a large enough signal to be competitive with chemically synthesized SPIO. Since the evidence in MTB indicates that iron biomineralization *in vivo* is a multi-step multi-component process, some consideration of multi-gene structures like the magnetosome is warranted. With this complexity, there may potentially be several types of reporter gene expression constructs that prove useful. For example, in mammalian cells, selective expression of anyone of the essential magnetosome genes could theoretically be used to regulate assembly of the magnetosome-like particle. Recently, a multi-component reporter gene construct has been described that is patterned on bacterial gas vesicles, to create an acoustic signal for ultrasound imaging [65]. A polycistronic DNA construct was subsequently prepared for mammalian cell expression, demonstrating the feasibility of replicating a facsimile of the bacterial structure for small animal imaging [66].

The unique protein–protein interactions found in single-cell organisms like prokaryotes offer a unique opportunity to build reporter gene expression systems in eukaryotes that faithfully reproduce complex structures for non-invasive imaging modalities. The magnetosome is easily such a candidate, well-suited to MR signal detection platforms by virtue of its iron biomineral. Just what facsimile of this nanoparticle is required for a given application still needs to be properly defined. For MPI, uniform, well-formed iron crystals are required; however, genetically programming variations in biomineral size would provide distinct signals for reporter gene expression [22]. For MRI, there is a great deal of latitude in magnetosome-like particle detection, given the sensitivity of transverse relaxation rates to both the quantity and form of iron. Building reporter gene expression around multiple TF signals that successively add desirable features to the magnetosome-like particle, enhancing MR detection at each step, opens a new frontier in non-invasive imaging. This vision begins with the understanding of magnetosome root structure.

5. Conclusions

Medical imaging has transformed medical care: guiding diagnosis and the timely delivery of therapy, monitoring treatment success and avoiding unnecessary procedures. MRI, with its superior soft tissue resolution and depth of penetration in a non-ionizing form of radiation, is continually expanding its reach. To keep up with inroads in pre- and post-natal care [67, 68], pediatric MRI [69], specialty coils for the brain and cardiac imaging [46], as well as inserts for hybrid PET/MRI [70], there is a continuing need to foster technological developments in MR-sensitive contrast agents. Cellular imaging is enabled by magnetic nanoparticles. Furthermore, molecular imaging successes achieved with exogenous SPIO [47] indicate that future imaging with gene-based contrast is a realistic expectation. To this end, the magnetosome offers the necessary blueprint for patterning iron biomineralization in a safe and effective way.

Gene-based contrast permits greater understanding of a given disease process because it can be tied to the gene expression responsible for the cell's behaviour, be this oncogenic, inflammatory, fibrotic, infectious, apoptotic, or the lack of appropriate signal transduction. While genetic regulation of contrast gene expression will initially pertain to preclinical research in animal models, many learnings will benefit clinically useful cell therapies either directly or indirectly. Microbiome research, for example, has already led to widely accepted probiotic supplements and experimental procedures like fecal microbiota transplantation [71]. Stem cell therapies are likewise destined to become mainstream. Developing the methods to visualize these therapies, deep within the body, is of paramount importance [72]. Holding back both microbial and mammalian cell therapies is an understanding of where these cells disseminate once introduced, how long they remain in the body, and how well they function. Molecular imaging of cellular activity holds the answer to many of these questions.

The introduction of multi-component assemblies as contrast agents for molecular imaging is an exciting new direction in nanoparticle research. Compared to single gene expression with injected contrast agent as substrate [73], multi-gene complexes offer a wider variety of imaging opportunities. For example, there may be no need for exogenous substrate, as assembly of the structure itself provides the imaging signal. In addition, there may be multiple levels of regulation, permitting finer control of assembly, disassembly and perhaps reassembly under the correct circumstances. This opens the possibility of creating suboptimal structures that are imaging silent until complemented by gene expression that switches on a detectable signal. Developing such structures could involve a role for constitutive and reporter gene expression. Further, by augmenting contrast incrementally, different stages of development could be monitored in (stem) cells that fulfill their therapeutic mission by reaching a terminally differentiated phenotype. This would also permit troubleshooting cell therapies that fall short, including (re)programming the timing of signal detection to validate stages where therapeutic function was successfully delivered.

The magnetosome is formed in a multi-step process that is regulated by a cohort of essential and auxiliary proteins. The genes that encode this process sequester iron in a membrane-enclosed compartment, shaping the biomineral while protecting the cell from iron toxicity. Can other cells be taught how to synthesize a magnetosome-like nanoparticle? Research is steadily showing this is the case. What then are the essential components required in any cell to reproduce the main structure? The notion that a minimal root structure underlies magnetosome formation has been advanced. Are all features of the bacterial magnetosome necessary? The MR evidence indicates that select magnetosome genes provide a measure of contrast enhancement when individually expressed in mammalian cells. What then are the protein(s) required for biosynthesis of the most desirable MR signal(s)? As outlined in this chapter, the magnetosome genes that define this compartment are steadily being elucidated, demonstrating that iron biomineralization can be programmed in all types of cells.

Acknowledgements

DEG is supported by a grant from the Ontario Research Fund Research Excellence program, ORF-RE07-021, in partnership with Multi-Magnetics Inc.

Conflict of interest

The use of magnetosome genes in mammalian systems is patented technology assigned to Multi-Magnetics Inc.

Appendices and nomenclature

MPI	magnetic particle imaging
Mms	magnetic particle membrane specific
MR	magnetic resonance
Mam	magnetosome membrane
MTB	magnetotactic bacteria
SPIO	superparamagnetic iron oxides

Author details

Donna E. Goldhawk
Lawson Health Research Institute, Western University, London, Canada

*Address all correspondence to: dgoldhawk@lawsonimaging.ca

References

[1] James M, Gambhir S. A molecular imaging primer: modalities, imaging agents, and applications. Physiol Rev. 2012;92:897-965.

[2] Massoud T, Gambhir S. Molecular imaging in living subjects: seeing fundamental biological processes in a new light. Genes Dev. 2003;17:545-580.

[3] Matsuura N, Rowlands J. Towards new functional nanostructures for medical imaging. Med Phys. 2008;35:4474-4487.

[4] Milej D, Abdalmalak A, Desjardins L, Ahmed H, Lee T-Y, Diop M, et al. Quantification of blood-brain barrier permeability by dynamic contrast-enhanced NIRS. Sci Rep. 2017;7:1702.

[5] Al-Khishman N, Qi Q, Roseborough A, Levit A, Allman B, Anazodo U, et al. TSPO PET detects acute neuroinflammation but not diffuse chronically activated MHCII microglia in the rat. EJNMMI Res. 2020;10:113.

[6] Broeke N, Peterson J, Lee J, Martin P, Farag A, Gomez J, et al. Characterization of clinical human prostate cancer lesions using 3.0-T sodium MRI registered to Gleason-graded whole-mount histopathology. J Magn Reson Imaging. 2019;49:1409-1419.

[7] Sheeran P, Matsuura N, Borden M, Williams R, Matsunaga T, Burns P, et al. Methods of Generating Submicrometer Phase-Shift Perfluorocarbon Droplets for Applications in Medical Ultrasonography. IEEE Trans Ultrason Ferroelectr Freq Control. 2017;64:252-263.

[8] Dip F, LoMenzo E, Sarotto L, Phillips E, Todeschini H, Nahmod M, et al. Randomized Trial of Near-infrared Incisionless Fluorescent Cholangiography. Ann Surg. 2019;270:992-999.

[9] England C, Ehlerding E, Hernandez R, Rekoske B, Graves S, Sun H, et al. Preclinical Pharmacokinetics and Biodistribution Studies of 89 Zr-Labeled Pembrolizumab. J Nucl Med. 2017;58:162-168.

[10] Cromer Berman S, Walczak P, Bulte J. Tracking stem cells using magnetic nanoparticles. WIREs Nanomedicine and Nanobiotechnology. 2011;3:343-355.

[11] Xiang Y, Bernards N, Hoang B, Zheng J, Matsuura N. Perfluorocarbon nanodroplets can reoxygenate hypoxic tumors in vivo without carbogen breathing. Nanotheranostics. 2019;3:135-144.

[12] Goldhawk D, Rohani R, Sengupta A, Gelman N, Prato F. Using the magnetosome to model effective gene-based contrast for magnetic resonance imaging. WIRES Nanomed Nanobiotechnol. 2012;4:378-388.

[13] Uebe R, Schuler D. Magnetosome biogenesis in magnetotactic bacteria. Nat Rev Microbiol. 2016;14:621-637.

[14] Komeili A, Li Z, Newman DK, Jensen GJ. Magnetosomes are cell membrane invaginations organized by the actin-like protein MamK. Science. 2006;311(5758):242-245.

[15] Lin W, Zhang W, Paterson G, Zhu Q, Zhao X, Knight R, et al. Expanding magnetic organelle biogenesis in the domain Bacteria. Microbiome. 2020;8:152.

[16] Lower B, Bazylinski D. The bacterial magnetosome: a unique prokaryotic organelle. J Mol Microbiol Biotechnol. 2013;23:63-80.

[17] Vargas G, Cypriano J, Correa T, Leao P, Bazylinski D, Abreu F. Applications of magnetotactic bacteria, magnetosomes and magnetosome crystals in biotechnology and nanotechnology: mini-review. Molecules. 2018;23:2438.

[18] Silva K, Schüler M, Mickoleit F, Zwiener T, Müller F, Awal R, et al. Genome-Wide Identification of Essential and Auxiliary Gene Sets for Magnetosome Biosynthesis in Magnetospirillum gryphiswaldense. mSystems. 2020;5:e00565–e00520.

[19] Zeytuni N, Uebe R, Maes M, Davidov G, Baram M, Raschdorf O, et al. Bacterial Magnetosome Biomineralization - A Novel Platform to Study Molecular Mechanisms of Human CDF-Related Type-II Diabetes. PLoS ONE. 2014;9:e97154.

[20] Sun Q, Fradin C, Thompson R, Prato F, Goldhawk D. Developing Magnetic Resonance Reporter Gene Imaging: Trajectory Analysis of Co-expressed Magnetosome Genes mamI and mamL. World Molecular Imaging Congress; Online 2020.

[21] Nudelman H, Zarivach R. Structure prediction of magnetosome-associated proteins. Front Microbiol. 2014;5:article 9.

[22] Goldhawk D, Gelman N, Thompson R, Prato F. Forming magnetosome-like nanoparticles in mammalian cells for molecular MRI. In: Bulte J, Modo M, editors. Design and Applications of Nanoparticles in Biomedical Imaging. Switzerland: Springer International Publishing; 2017. p. 187-203.

[23] Staniland S, Williams W, Harrison A, Ward B, Telling N, Van Der Laan G. Controlled cobalt doping of magnetosomes in vivo. Nat Nanotech. 2008;3:158-162.

[24] Draper O, Byrne M, Li Z, Keyhani S, Cueto Barrozo J, Jensen G, et al. MamK, a bacterial actin, forms dynamic filaments in vivo that are regulated by the acidic proteins MamJ and LimJ. Mol Microbiol. 2011;82:342-354.

[25] Kraupner A, Eberbeck D, Heinke D, Uebe R, Schüler D, Briel A. Bacterial magnetosomes - nature's powerful contribution to MPI tracer research. Nanoscale. 2017;9:5788-5793.

[26] Lefevre C, Trubitsyn D, Abreu F, Kolinko S, Jogler C, Gonzaga Paula de Almeida L, et al. Comparative genomic analysis of magnetotactic bacteria from the Deltaproteobacteria provides new insights into magnetite and greigite magnetosome genes required for magnetotaxis. Env Microbiol. 2013;15:2712-2735.

[27] Kolinko I, Lohße A, Borg S, Raschdorf O, Jogler C, Tu Q, et al. Biosynthesis of magnetic nanostructures in a foreign organism by transfer of bacterial magnetosome gene clusters. Nature Nanotechnology. 2014;9:193-197.

[28] Sun Q, Fradin C, Tahir M, Thompson R, Prato F, Goldhawk D. Interaction of Essential Magnetosome Genes in Mammalian Cells. Magnetotactic Bacteria; Kanazawa 2018.

[29] Raschdorf O, Forstner Y, Kolinko I, Uebe R, Plitzko J, Schüler D. Genetic and Ultrastructural Analysis Reveals the Key Players and Initial Steps of Bacterial Magnetosome Membrane Biogenesis. PLoS Genet. 2016;126:e1006101.

[30] Bereczk-Tompa E, Posfai M, Toth B, Vonderviszt F. Magnetite-Binding Flagellar Filaments Displaying the MamI Loop Motif. ChemBioChem. 2016;17:2075-2082.

[31] Barber-Zucker S, Zarivach R. A Look into the Biochemistry of

Magnetosome Biosynthesis in Magnetotactic Bacteria. ACS Chem Biol. 2017;12:13-22.

[32] Vivekanantha P, Sun Q, Thompson R, Prato F, Goldhawk D. Magnetic Resonance Image Analysis of Mammalian Cells Expressing Essential Magnetosome Genes mamI and mamL. Imaging Network of Ontario; Toronto 2021.

[33] Sengupta A, Quiaoit K, Thompson R, Prato F, Gelman N, Goldhawk D. Biophysical features of MagA expression in mammalian cells: implications for MRI contrast. Front Microbiol. 2014;5:29.

[34] Quinlan A, Murat D, Komeili A. The HtrA/DegP family protease MamE is a bifunctional protein with roles in magnetosome protein localization and magnetite biomineralization. Mol Microbiol. 2011;80:10-75-1087.

[35] Yang W, Li R, Peng T, Zhang Y, Jiang W, Li Y, et al. mamO and mamE genes are essential for magnetosome crystal biomineralization in Magnetospirillum gryphiswaldense MSR-1. Res Microbiol. 2010;161:701-705.

[36] Lane D, Merlot A, Huang M, Bae D, Jansson P, Sahni S, et al. Cellular iron uptake, trafficking and metabolism: Key molecules and mechanisms and their roles in disease. Biochim Biophys Acta-Mol Cell Res. 2015;1853:1130-1144.

[37] Brown R, Cheng Y-C, Haacke E, Thompson M, Venkatesan R. Magnetic resonance imaging: physical principles and sequence design. Second Edition ed: Wiley; 2014.

[38] Goldhawk D, Gelman N, Sengupta A, Prato F. The interface between iron metabolism and gene-based iron contrast for MRI. Magnetic Resonance Insights. 2015;8(S1):9-14.

[39] Alizadeh K, Sun Q, McGuire T, Thompson R, Prato F, Koropatnick J, et al. Hepcidin-mediated Iron Regulation in P19 Cells is Detectable by Magnetic Resonance Imaging. Sci Rep. 2020;10:3163.

[40] Prajapati R, Sun Q, Prato F, Goldhawk D, editors. Modelling Cellular Iron-handling in Inflammation: P19 Cells Secrete Biologically-active Hepcidin. Imaging Network of Ontario; 2021; Toronto.

[41] Liu L, Alizadeh K, Donnelly S, Dassanayake P, Hou T, McGirr R, et al. MagA expression attenuates iron export activity in undifferentiated multipotent P19 cells. PLOS ONE. 2019;14:e0217842.

[42] Nakamura C, Burgess JG, Sode K, Matsunaga T. An iron-regulated gene, *magA*, encoding an iron transport protein of *Magnetospirillum* sp. Strain AMB-1. J Biol Chem. 1995;270:28392-28396.

[43] Nakamura C, Kikuchi T, Burgess JG, Matsunaga T. Iron-regulated expression and membrane localization of the MagA protein in *Magnetospirillum* sp. Strain AMB-1. J Biochem. 1995;118:23-27.

[44] Uebe R, Henn S, Schuler D. The MagA protein of Magnetospirilla is not involved in bacterial magnetite biomineralization. J Bacteriol. 2012;194:1018-1023.

[45] Scheffel A, Gardes A, Grunberg K, Wanner G, Schuler D. The major magnetosome proteins MamGFDC are not essential for magnetite biomineralization in Magnetospirillum gryphiswaldense but regulate the size of magnetosome crystals. J Bacteriol. 2008;190(1):377-386.

[46] Wilk B, Wisenberg G, Dharmakumar R, Thiessen J, Goldhawk D, Prato F. Hybrid PET/MR imaging in myocardial inflammation

post-myocardial infarction. J Nucl Cardiol. 2020;27:2083-2099.

[47] Murrell D, Zarghami N, Jensen M, Dickson F, Chambers A, Wong E, et al. MRI surveillance of cancer cell fate in a brain metastasis model after early radiotherapy. Magn Reson Med. 2017;78:1506-1512.

[48] Manning K, Llera A, Dekaban G, Bartha R, Barreira C, Brown A, et al. Linked MRI signatures of the brain's acute and persistent response to concussion in female varsity rugby players. NeuroImage Clin. 2019;21:101627.

[49] Manning K, Schranz A, Bartha R, Dekaban G, Barreira C, Brown A, et al. Multiparametric MRI changes persist beyond recovery in concussed adolescent hockey players. Neurology. 2017;89:2157-2166.

[50] Arakaki A, Goto M, Maruyama M, Yoda T, Tanaka M, Yamagishi A, et al. Restoration and Modification of Magnetosome Biosynthesis by Internal Gene Acquisition in a Magnetotactic Bacterium. Biotechnol J. 2020;15:e2000278.

[51] Yoshino T, Maeda Y, Matsunaga T. Bioengineering of bacterial magnetic particles and their applications in biotechnology. Recent Pat Biotechnol. 2010;4:214-225.

[52] Boucher M, Geffroy F, Preveral S, Bellanger L, Selingue E, Adryanczyk-Perrier G, et al. Genetically tailored magnetosomes used as MRI probe for molecular imaging of brain tumor. Biomaterials. 2017;121:167-178.

[53] Howard F, Muthana M. Designer nanocarriers for navigating the systemic delivery of oncolytic viruses. Nanomed. 2020;15:93-110.

[54] Erdal E, Demirbilek M, Yeh Y, Akbal O, Ruff L, Bozkurt D, et al. A Comparative Study of Receptor-Targeted Magnetosome and HSA-Coated Iron Oxide Nanoparticles as MRI Contrast-Enhancing Agent in Animal Cancer Model. Appl Biochem Biotechnol. 2018;185:91-113.

[55] Mériaux S, Boucher M, Marty B, Lalatonne Y, Préveral S, Motte L, et al. Magnetosomes, biogenic magnetic nanomaterials for brain molecular imaging with 17.2 T MRI scanner. Adv Healthc Mater. 2015;4:1076-1083.

[56] Mannucci S, Tambalo S, Conti G, Ghin L, Milanese A, Carboncino A, et al. Magnetosomes Extracted from Magnetospirillum gryphiswaldense as Theranostic Agents in an Experimental Model of Glioblastoma. Contrast Media Mol Imaging. 2018;2018:2198703.

[57] Brewer K, Spitler R, Lee K, Chan A, Barrozo J, Wakeel A, et al. Characterization of Magneto-Endosymbionts as MRI Cell Labeling and Tracking Agents. Mol Imaging Biol. 2018;20:65-73.

[58] Goldhawk D, Lemaire C, McCreary C, McGirr R, Dhanvantari S, Thompson R, et al. Magnetic resonance imaging of cells overexpressing MagA, an endogenous contrast agent for live cell imaging. Mol Imaging. 2009;8:129-139.

[59] Zurkiya O, Chan AW, Hu X. MagA is sufficient for producing magnetic nanoparticles in mammalian cells, making it an MRI reporter. Magn Reson Med. 2008;59(6):1225-1231.

[60] Elfick A, Rischitor G, Mouras R, Azfer A, Lungaro L, Uhlarz M, et al. Biosynthesis of magnetic nanoparticles by human mesenchymal stem cells following transfection with the magnetotactic bacterial gene mms6. Scientific Reports. 2017;7:39755.

[61] Zhang X-Y, Robledo B, Harris S, Hu X. A Bacterial Gene, mms6, as a New

Reporter Gene for Magnetic Resonance Imaging of Mammalian Cells. Mol Imaging. 2014:1-12.

[62] Guan X, Yang B, Xie M, Kumar Ban D, Zhao X, Lal R, et al. MRI reporter gene MagA suppresses transferrin receptor and maps Fe2+ dependent lung cancer. Nanomed. 2019;21:102064.

[63] Rohani R, Figueredo R, Bureau Y, Koropatnick J, Foster P, Thompson R, et al. Imaging tumor growth non-invasively using expression of MagA or modified ferritin subunits to augment intracellular contrast for repetitive MRI. Mol Imaging Biol. 2014;16:63-73.

[64] Cho I, Moran S, Paudya R, Piotrowska-Nitsche K, Cheng P-H, Zhang X, et al. Longitudinal Monitoring of Stem Cell Grafts In Vivo Using Magnetic Resonance Imaging with Inducible Maga as a Genetic Reporter. Theranostics. 2014;4:972-989.

[65] Bourdeau R, Lee-Gosselin A, Lakshmanan A, Farhadi A, Kumar S, Nety S, et al. Acoustic reporter genes for noninvasive imaging of microorganisms in mammalian hosts. Nature. 2018;553:86-90.

[66] Farhadi A, Ho G, Sawyer D, Bourdeau R, Shapiro M. Ultrasound imaging of gene expression in mammalian cells. Science. 2019;365:1469-1475.

[67] Kazan-Tannus J, Levine D, Mckenzie C, Lim K-H, Cohen B, Farrar N, et al. Real-time Magnetic Resonance Imaging Aids Prenatal Diagnosis of Isolated Cleft Palate. J Ultrasound Med. 2005;24:1533-1540.

[68] Sinclair K, Friesen-Waldner L, McCurdy C, Wiens C, Wade T, de Vrijer B, et al. Quantification of fetal organ volume and fat deposition following in utero exposure to maternal Western Diet using MRI. PLoS One. 2018;13:e0192900.

[69] Tan K, Meiri A, Mowrey W, Abbott R, Goodrich J, Sandler A, et al. Diffusion tensor imaging and ventricle volume quantification in patients with chronic shunt-treated hydrocephalus: a matched case-control study. J Neurosurg. 2018;129:1611-1622.

[70] Farag A, Thompson R, Thiessen J, Biernaski H, Prato F, Théberge J. Evaluation of 511 keV photon attenuation by a novel 32-channel phased array prospectively designed for cardiovascular hybrid PET/MRI imaging. Eur J Hybrid Imaging. 2020;4:7.

[71] Craven L, Rahman A, Parvathy S, Beaton M, Silverman J, Qumosani K, et al. Allogenic fecal microbiota transplantation in patients with non-alcoholic fatty liver disease improves abnormal small intestinal permeability: a randomized control trial. Am J Gastroenterol. 2020;115:1055-1065.

[72] Bulte J, Daldrup-Link H. Clinical Tracking of Cell Transfer and Cell Transplantation: Trials and Tribulations. Radiology. 2018;289:604-615.

[73] Nyström N, Hamilton A, Xia W, Liu S, Scholl T, Ronald J. Longitudinal Visualization of Viable Cancer Cell Intratumoral Distribution in Mouse Models Using Oatp1a1-Enhanced Magnetic Resonance Imaging. Invest Radiol. 2019;54:302-311.

Chapter 11

Radiopharmaceuticals in Modern Cancer Therapy

Aisyah Elliyanti

Abstract

Nuclear medicine plays a role in oncology. It uses tracers (radiopharmaceuticals) to study physiological processes and treat diseases. The radiopharmaceuticals can be formed as radionuclides alone or radionuclides labeled with other molecules as a drug, a protein, or a peptide. The radiopharmaceutical is introduced into the body and accumulates in the target tissue of interest for therapy or imaging purposes. It offers to study cancer biology in vivo to optimize cancer therapy. Another advantage of radiopharmaceutical therapy is a tumor-targeting agent that deposits lethal radiation at tumor sites. This review outlines radiopharmaceuticals agents in current cancer therapy.

Keywords: radionuclides, beta particles, alpha particles, auger electron, radioimmunotherapy, peptide receptor radionuclide therapy

1. Introduction

Usage of radiopharmaceuticals has increased in recent decades, mainly for the treatment of cancer diseases [1]. However, the oncology community is still unfamiliar with radiopharmaceutical therapy (RPT). Compared with all other systemic cancer treatment options, radiopharmaceuticals have an efficacy result with minimal toxicity [2]. The radiopharmaceutical therapy application introduces new tumor-targeting agent therapy, different from external radiotherapy (**Figure 1**). It quantifies radioactivity distribution in tumor sites and in vivo detection [2]. The advantages of RPT are: firstly, it is targeted into tumor, included metastasis sites. Secondly, the high linear energy transfer (LET) radionuclides are effectively killed the radioresistant hypoxic cells. Thirdly, relatively lower whole-body absorbed dose [3–5]. The therapy might be used as adjuvant therapy with or after other treatment options such as chemotherapy and surgery [6, 7]. In controlling the symptoms, shrink and stabilize the tumors for systemic metastatic cancer, where conventional radiotherapy or chemotherapy is impossible, RPT can be a choice, especially for patients who no longer respond to other treatments [2, 6].

The radiopharmaceuticals can be in the form of radionuclides alone or radionuclides labeled (radiolabeled) for imaging or therapy. They can be labeled with molecules such as a drug, a protein, or a peptide for the therapy. Physical and biochemical characteristics of radiopharmaceuticals/radionuclides should be considered for treatment purposes. The physical characters are included physical half-life, energy radiation(s), type of emissions, daughter product(s), production method, and radionuclide purity [6, 8]. The biochemical characteristic includes tissue targeting, radioactivity retention in the tumor, in vivo stability, toxicity and the

IntechOpen

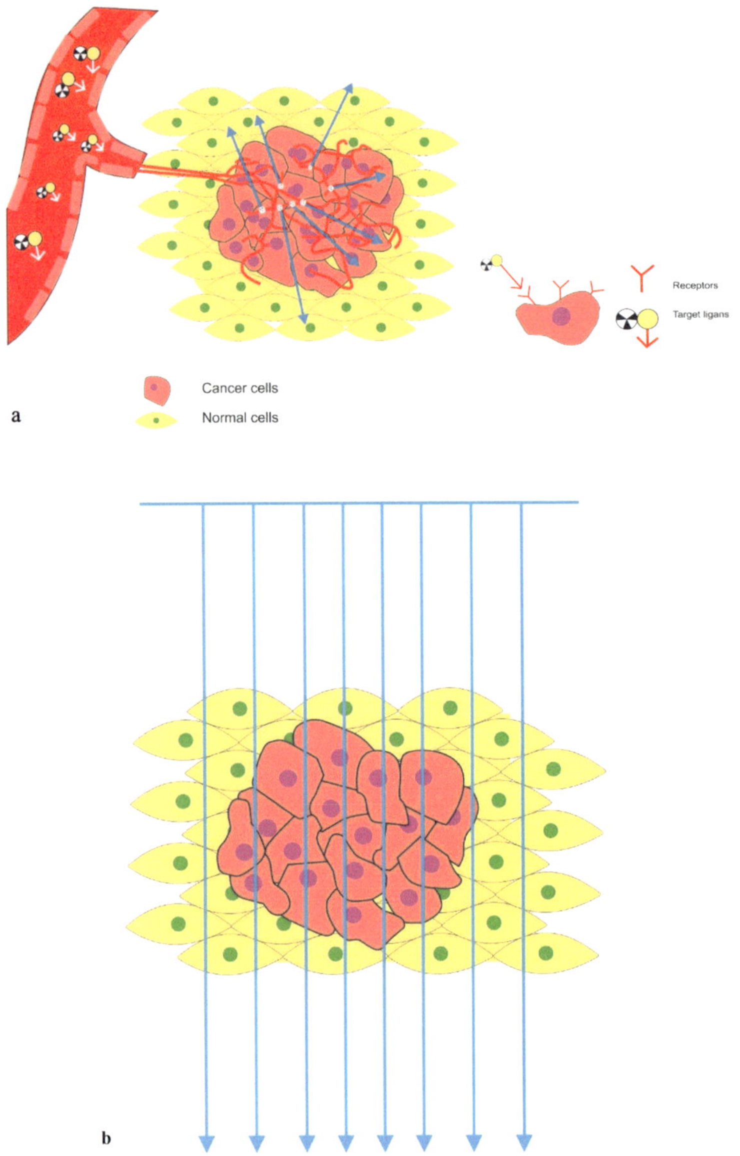

Figure 1.
Radiopharmaceutical therapy versus external radiotherapy. In RPT, radionuclide has administrated intravenous delivery to the targeted tumor. The tumor cells will receive an absorbed dose which is exponentially decreasing over the period. The dose is delivered per cell by emissions originating from cells is influenced by the range of the emissions. When the range of the emitted particle is much longer than the dimension of the cell, periphery tumor cells of tumor mass will receive absorbed dose and crossfire dose from other target cells, and it caused a crossfire dose to normal tissue. However, the response of the normal cell will differ from the tumor cell (a). In external radiotherapy, radiation delivers the same absorbed dose per cell regardless the number of cells (b).

effective half-life within the patient's body [2]. A convenience range of the physical half-life of radionuclide is between 6 hours and seven days [9]. A very short physical half-life has a limitation due to the delivery time, and a long half-life of radiopharmaceuticals will expose the surrounding environment to more time radiation. The physical half-life should not too long, but it should have sufficient retention time. So, the radiation can be delivered to the tumor efficiently [1]. On the other hand, when the biological half-life is too short, the radionuclide will be discharged with significantly high activity. Therefore, for efficient radiation delivery for therapy purposes, a balanced optimal biological and physical half-life should be considered, besides the type of tumor, method of administration, and uptake mechanism [1, 6]. Radionuclides radiations as alpha (α)-particle (50–230 keV/μm) and beta (β)-particle (0.2 keV/μm), and Äuger electrons (4–26 keV/μm) are used for therapy purposes [1, 3, 6, 10, 11]. These particles allow ionization per travel length, and they are fully deposited within a small range of tissue. The distance traveled, and the energy deposited in cells is vital that lead the most efficient route for cell destruction is the direct interaction of ionization events with DNA.

Some β-emitter radionuclides also decay γ-particle, which is used for imaging. Radionuclides that emit α or β-particles are preferred for the treatment of bulky solid tumors, and radionuclides that emit Äuger electrons are considered for the treatment of tiny clusters of cancer cells or small tumor deposits because of their high-level cytotoxicity and short-range biological effectiveness [3]. The other factor that needs to be considered is the daughter product of the radionuclides. If the daughter product is unstable, it should be short-life and may decay within hours into a stable product, and un-stable daughter nuclide will contribute to the amount of absorbed dose. Radiopharmaceuticals' biochemical characteristics are selective tumor target concentrations and have optimal retention time in the tumor and avoid uptake in the normal cells [6, 9]. Depending on the tumor uptake mechanism, either by bone deposition, protein binding, or metabolic uptake, the ratio concentration of radionuclides on the tumor to normal tissues should be as optimal as possible [6]. The other factors that have to be considered are the radionuclides particles' size, low toxicity, specific gravity for optimal flow and distribution, and clearance rate [6, 12–16].

Iodine-131 (^{131}I) was one of the first radionuclides used for therapy in clinical oncology, especially for thyroid cancer patients. Phosphorous-32 (^{32}P), strontium-89 (^{89}Sr), and yttrium-90 (^{90}Y) also have been used for the treatment of benign and malignant diseases [6, 17, 18]. Various alpha- and beta-radiation-emitting isotopes are used lately. Most of them are labeled with peptides and antibodies for specific tumor targeting, where radiopharmaceuticals are used as vehicles to deliver ionizing radiation to the tumor tissue. This review discusses radiopharmaceuticals are used for therapy and their application in the modern era of cancer therapy.

2. Radionuclides

The growth in nuclear medicine has been stimulated by introducing several new radionuclides and radiopharmaceuticals. They have been used to treat benign and malignant tumors. Types of radiation that are relevant to RPT are electrons and α-particles. Electron emissions are classified by energy and by the type of decay; Auger electrons, beta (β)-particles are related to RPT [2]. Currently, β particle emitters radionuclides are mostly used for therapy purposes. However, they have a limitation of radiobiological properties. An alpha particle emitting as a new generation radionuclides is being developed, with advantages in high energy and a short path length, which show higher efficacy [19]. Below we discuss the physical differences between a beta particle, Auger electrons, and an alpha particle.

2.1 Beta particles

Beta particles are produced in the beta decay process, wherein an unstable nucleus, a neutron, is converted to a proton, creating an energetic electron (beta particle) [2, 19]. They are the most frequently used for RPT agents and widely available. Many of them also emit photon energy that is easily imaged. Beta particles are negatively charged and have a relatively long path length from 0.0 to 12 mm.

They have low linear energy transfer (LET) of approximately 0.2 keV/μm, and more particles are required for a similar absorbed dose as alpha particles (**Figure 2**). For high energy beta, like ^{90}Y and ^{188}Re, which they energy 2.28 Mev and 2.21 MeV respectively (**Table 1**), they can cause crossfire doses to neighbor cells. So, they are preferable for higher volume solid tumors, poorly perfuse tumors, and less suited for targeting micro-metastases [3, 8, 23]. For the small tumor, low-energy β-rays such as lutetium-177 (^{177}Lu) would be more β-emitting efficient [8].

The most familiar and frequent beta particle used is iodine-131 (^{131}I) for hyperthyroidism and thyroid cancers therapy [20, 24, 25]. Subsequently, samarium-153, lutetium-177, yttrium-90 and have been introduced over the last 40 years (**Table 1**) [2]. Several other β-emitting radionuclides have been investigated or considered. However, those agents have not widely adopted, related to several reasons: limited availability, complex radiochemistry process, or the absence of a commercial products [26]. A variety of reasons for the shift to different radionuclides of the different β-particle emitters used over time. For example, an early evaluation of changing to different radionuclides was based on the tumor to non-tumor-absorbed dose ratio [2]. ^{90}Y has a high-energy β-particle, and it is widely available like ^{131}Iodine. It was used in colloidal form, mainly for rheumatoid treatment [27, 28]. ^{90}Y labeled antibodies initially focused on ovarian cancer, followed by hematological cancers and radiopeptide therapy [2, 29, 30]. ^{90}Y is a popular radionuclide for RPT because of the clinical impact of ^{90}Y-impregnated microspheres used for hepatic metastases therapy [31–33]. Lutetium-177 becomes

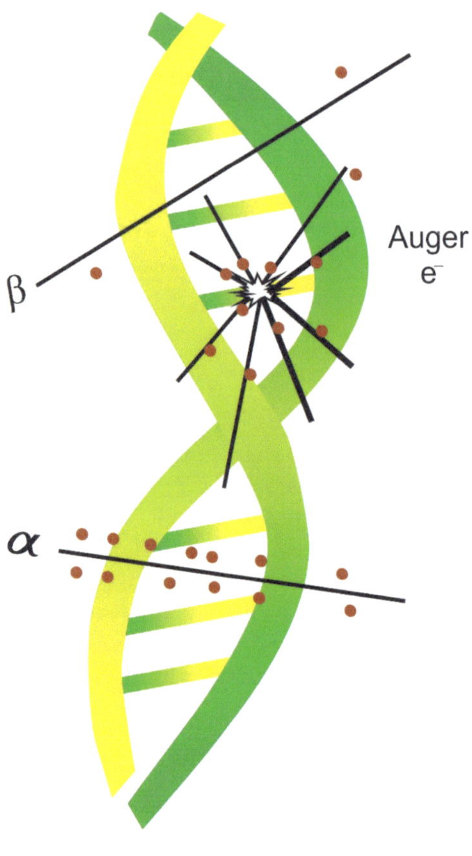

Figure 2.
Linear energy transfer alpha and beta particles and auger electron on DNA. Alpha particles have high LET (~80 keV/μm) compared with the low LET (~0.2 keV/μm) of beta particles, and auger electron intermediate LET 4–26 keV/μM. Thus, alpha particles result in more double-strand breaks in DNA.

Radionuclides	Mode of decay	Physical half-life	Energy (KeV)	Indication
^{223}Ra	α	11.44 d	5979.2	Bone pain palliation
^{211}At	α (41.8.9) EC(58.2)	7.21 h	5870–7450	Clinical trials in glioblastoma, ovarian cancer, blood-borne cancers
^{212}Bi	α (35.9) $β^-$ (97.8)	60.55 mins	6051–8785	Clinical trials in prostate cancer, ovarian cancer, pancreatic cancer, neuroendocrine tumor.
^{213}Bi	α (2.2) $β^-$ (64.1)	46.61 mins	5875–8376	Clinical trials in acute myeloid leukemia (AML), prostate cancer, lymphoma, melanoma, glioblastoma, neuroendocrine tumor and bladder cancer.
^{225}Ac	α	10 d	5732–5830	Clinical trial in AML, breast cancer, ovarian cancer, prostate cancer, glioblastoma, neoroblastoma.
^{227}Th	α	18.68 d	5709–6038	Clinical trial in AML, NHL, breast cancer, ovarian cancer.
^{131}I	$β^-$	8.02 d	606	Hyperthyroidism, thyroid cancer, Radioimmunotherapy (RIT) for non-Hodgkin's limphoma (NHL) and neuroblastoma, pheochromocytoma, carcinoid, medullary thyroid cancer
^{32}P	$β^-$	14.26 d	1710	Polycythemia vera, keloid, cystic craniopharyngioma.
^{89}Sr	$β^-$	50.53 d	1496	Bone pain palliation
^{90}Y	$β^-$	64.10 d	2280	Liver metastasis, hepatocellular carcinoma, RIT for NHL, neuroendocrine tumor
^{153}Sm	$β^-$	46.50 h	808.2	Bone pain palliation, synovitis
^{169}Er	$β^-$	9.4 0d	350	Synovitis
^{177}Lu	$β^-$	6.73 d	497.8	Synovitis and RIT for various cancer
^{186}Re	EC,$β^-$	3.72 d	1069.5	Bone pain palliation, arthritis Bone pain
^{188}Re	$β^-$	17.00 h	2120.4	Bone pain palliation, RIT for various cancer, rheumatoid arthritis

Table 1.
Characteristics of alpha and beta emitters radionuclides for therapy [6, 8, 20–22].

popular because it emits photons in the 100–200-keV optimal imaging range and has a β-particle energy between ^{131}I and ^{90}Y, which is appropriate for therapy, particularly for small tumors [2, 8]. All these factors, along with a half-life that is compatible with the pharmacokinetics of both antibodies and peptides. It is a reactor production and widely available, with relatively straightforward conjugation chemistry [2]. Samarium-153 (^{153}Sm) is a β-emitting radionuclide that is used for palliative treatment in breast and prostate cancer with bone metastases, and other primary cancers [34, 35]. Radiopharmaceuticals therapy agent that uses the ethylenediamine-tetra-methylene-phosphonic acid (EDTMP) chelator, binding samarium-153 through six ligands (four phosphate groups and two amines) is FDA approved. ^{153}Sm alternative formulation as ^{153}Sm-DOTMP (1,4,7, 10-tetraazacyclododecanetetramethylenephosphonic acid), which is thought to have a more favorable chelant-to-metal ratio [2].

2.2 Auger electrons

Auger electrons are generated from suborbital transitions. They are typically very short-range emissions, of the order of 1–1000 nm, depending on their emission energy. Auger electron is intermediate (4–26 keV/μM) of LET [3, 22, 23]. These emissions could be highly cytotoxic if the RPT drug localizes within the cell nucleus [36, 37]. Bromine-77, indium-111, iodine-123, and iodine-125 are the most commonly used Auger electron emitters. In vitro studies had shown highly effective and specific tumor cell killing when they labeled with targeting vehicles that can localize these subcellular-range radiations close to cellular DNA [38, 39]. Human studies using locoregional administration showed promise regarding tumor cell incorporation of the Auger emitters [2]. However, Auger electron-emitter RPT has not been widely adopted yet. Besides, auger electron agents must be incorporated into the DNA, and their unfavorable pharmacokinetics might be the reasons for the lack of efficacy. Technological developments that could overcome those factors will interest RPT development [2].

2.3 Alpha particle

Alpha particles have a similar structure to a ^{4}He nucleus without surrounding electrons (sometimes denoted as He^{2+}) [19]. They are produced in alpha decay and emitted from the nucleus of a radioactive atom [2, 40]. Alpha particles have higher energy (4–9 MeV) and travel in tissue over a few cell diameters. Thus, the particle range is equivalent to the thickness of 1–3 cell widths (40–100 μm) [1, 2, 40]. They have high LET (~100 keV/μm) throughout their range and three times greater at the end of the path range (the Bragg peak) [19, 40]. Intracellular accumulation of the alpha particle effectively creates double-strand breaks (DSBs) in DNA [2, 40]. The cytotoxicity of α-particles is thus considered much higher than that of β-particles (**Figure 2**). Another advantage of α-particles compared with β-particles is the short distance traveled by the ionization products, reducing the damage to healthy surrounding cells. Moreover, the effect is not dependent on dose and oxygen concentration during any cell cycle (**Table 2**) [1].

Targeted alpha therapy (TAT) is an attractive therapeutic option for multiple micro-metastases. It has many advantages, such as easy administration, the ability

	Alpha particle	Beta particle
Type of particle	^{4}He nucleus	Energetic electron
Particle energy	4–9 MeV	50–2,300 keV
Particle path length	40–100 μm	0.05–12 mm
Linear energy transfer	~80 keV/μm	~0.2 keV/μm
Hypoxic tumors	Effective	Less effective
Toxicity	effective in creating double strand breaks (DSBs) in DNA	high dose rates (tumor survival rates close to linear exponential) low dose rates (single-strand breaks (repairable) with shouldering of the dose–response curve
Bystander effect	Yes	Yes
Tumor cross-fire	Low	Yes
Tumor size	Micro/small	Solid high tumor volume

Table 2.
Physics and biology characteristic of alpha and beta particles [2, 19, 40, 41].

to treat multiple lesions simultaneously, and the possibility of combining with other therapeutic approaches, and primarily for cancer treatment. By attaching an α-particles to a biological molecule with targeting capabilities, such as a monoclonal antibody (mAb), with the help of a bi-specific chelating agent or bonding it to a disease-targeting vector, and the vector used as a targeting agent. In this way, RPT selectively delivers a high radiation dose directly to the target, with generally limited toxicity to the surrounding normal tissues. Advances in understanding tumor biology, together with progress in mAb technology, chemical labeling techniques, and other related disciplines, provide significant advances in developing of new clinical applications of α-particles radionuclides in novel therapeutic agents [1, 2, 42].

The α-particles are used for RPT over 40 years included as bismuth-212 (^{212}Bi), bismuth-213 (^{213}Bi) and astatine-211 (^{211}At), actinium-225 (^{225}Ac), radium-223 (^{223}Ra) and thorium-227 (^{227}Th) as shown in **Table 1** [2]. ^{223}RaCl2 is the first alpha-emitting radiopharmaceutical for prostate and breast cancer patients' bone pain palliation [2, 3, 8, 19, 40]. The energetic α-particles emitted by ^{223}Ra can generate irreparable DNA DSBs in the adjacent osteoblasts and osteoclasts, leading to their death. The results in detrimental effects on the neighboring cells, inhibit abnormal bone formation, both at a cellular level and a signaling level, ultimately negatively affect tumor growth [2]. ^{223}Ra is being studied in combination with other cytotoxic agents such as docetaxel (DORA trial), poly(ADP-ribose) polymerase inhibitors (olaparib), and new androgen axis inhibitors as enzalutamide and abiraterone citrate. It is also being explored in combination with immuno-oncology agents such as pembrolizumab and in combination with external-beam radiotherapy [2].

Bismuth-213 (^{213}Bi) and astatine-211 (^{211}At) labeled monoclonal antibodies in patients with leukemia and brain tumors, respectively [3, 22]. Moreover, ^{225}Ac and ^{213}Bi labeled somatostatin receptor (SSR) are preclinical and clinical trials [1, 19, 40]. ^{213}Bi has a short half-life and can be produced from the generator, and because of that, it is required on-site labeling to produce TAT compound. The short half-life of ^{213}Bi has some advantages as higher dose rates given over a short period are more effective than low dose rates given over a longer period [19, 40]. Studies reported that ^{213}Bi had been labeled with DOTA peptides in preclinical and clinical trials with >99% purity [1, 19].

Furthermore, also there is a growing interest in using ^{255}Ac as a therapeutic alpha particle source. It is produced via the neutron transmutation of ^{226}Ra or decay of ^{233}U [19]. The type of production caused ^{225}Ac has a lack the capacity of clinical use of labeled peptide. So, production via a high-energy proton accelerator at multiple sites will overcome ^{225}Ac labeled to treat neuroendocrine tumors. It has been labeled with PSMA with a radiochemical purity of >98% to treat prostate cancer [19]. ^{225}Ac labeled antibodies are being tested in advanced myeloid malignancy [8]. ^{225}Ac shows a potential appealing radionuclide for TAT, and post-therapy imaging of ^{225}Ac is possible, although images are also suboptimal 19, 40, 41].

The results of clinical trials using TAT indicate that this treatment strategy presents a promising alternative for targeted therapy of cancer [22]. Lately, it has been gaining popularity that TAT to be a successful treatment in prostate cancer in patients refractory to ^{177}Lu prostate-specific membrane antigen (PSMA) [19]. Therefore, alpha-emitters and Auger electron emitters (^{77}Br, ^{111}In, ^{123}I, ^{125}I) are getting more attention for targeted therapy lately. Auger electron and alpha-emitter are intermediate (4–26 keV/μM) and high (50–230 keV/μM) of LET radiation respectively. They deliver the radiation dose within the short range of the tissue (~ tens microns) have an actual tumor cell killing if they can be conjugated with suitable ligands that effectively targeted micro-metastasis therapy [3, 22, 23].

3. The concept of therapy

Various alpha- and beta-radiation-emitting isotopes for therapy are mostly labeled with peptides or antibodies for specific tumor targeting, which are used only as vehicles to deliver ionizing radiation to the tumor tissue. The vehicle concentrates radioactivity at the tumor tissue expressing specific tissue elements and avoiding concentrating at normal cells [2, 7, 10]. Different radioligands are being developed and investigated for uniquely targeting molecular receptors or intracellular components that currently lead to planning personal patient-tailored therapy [43]. Radionuclides are coupled to ligands that recognize and bind the tumor-associated molecules, ensuring the precise targeting of cancerous cells that can be used for therapeutic approaches and live-monitoring of treatment efficacy [43].

4. Radioimmunotherapy (RIT)

Radioimmunotherapy (RIT) is targeting therapy using radionuclide labeled with specific mAbs directed against tumor antigens [6, 8]. The antibody is primarily a delivery vehicle of radiation to tumors sites. Besides therapy, radionuclide combines with mAbs has been used for imaging. The imaging provides specific non-invasive information regarding the expression, location, and modulation of targets. The therapeutic effect of RIT is achieved by tissue absorption of the energies from continuous radiation emitted from the radionuclides tagged to mAbs. More specific bound between antibody and tumor antigen increase the dose delivered to tumor cells and, at the same time, reduce the dose to normal cells [6]. RIT has been evaluated in clinical trials across the full spectrum of malignancies [8].

The type of radioactive combines with mAb depends on emission characteristics, the radiolabeling chemistry, and the malignancy of cells targeted [8]. Beta and alpha emitter particles are labeled with mAbs. However, alpha emitters have limitations in practice due to mostly very short half-life (**Table 1**) [41]. For optimal therapy, the residence time of RIT ranges from a few days to weeks, which reach optimal tumor-to-background ratios 2–4 days post-injection. Radionuclides labeled mAbs bind several antigens and receptors expressed on the surface of tumor cells. They include CD20, prostate-specific membrane antigen (PSMA), human epidermal growth factor receptor 2+ (HER2+), mucin 1 (MUC1), epidermal growth factor receptor (EGFR), tumor necrosis factor (TNF), vascular endothelial growth factor (VEGF), and et cetera [8].

Radioimmunoconjugates targeting CD20 have been approved to treat non-Hodkin's lymphoma (^{90}Y-ibritumomab tiuxetan and ^{131}I-tositumomab) [6, 8]. Both radiolabeled mAbs are more efficacious at inducing remissions than the respective unlabeled molecules and are also more effective than earlier courses of chemotherapy in these patients [8]. Other potentials of RIT include lung, pancreatic, stomach, ovarian, breast, colorectal cancers, leukemia, high-grade brain glioma [6]. On the other hand, the application of RIT for solid tumors has been less successful than in patients with malignant lymphoma. Several problems have to be addressed to its efficacy:

1. Higher solid tumor volume indicates lower radiosensitivity compare to small volume tumors usually.

2. The delivery of therapeutic radionuclide to solid tumors might be less effective. It can be by poor perfusion, elevated intra-tumoral hydrostatic pressure, and heterogeneous radionuclide uptake by tumor cells.

3. Furthermore, ^{223}Ra-chloride showed that these limitations could be successfully circumvented in patients with castration-resistant prostate cancer and bone metastases. RIT therapy may become an effective treatment modality for disseminated solid tumors in the future [8].

5. Peptide receptor radionuclide therapy (PRRT)

Several radionuclides have been used for peptide therapy in neuroendocrine tumor (NET) patients. The expression of peptide receptors on various tumor cells, including NETs, was significantly higher than normal tissues or cells [25]. Over the last decade, such receptors have become recognized targets for molecular imaging and therapy because they are expressed on the cell surface. Upon binding a ligand, the receptor-ligand complex is internalized. Radiolabeled peptide ligands are known to be used for imaging and somatostatin receptor therapy (SSTR) [25].

Peptide receptor radionuclide therapy (PRRT) has been known to be an effective systemic treatment of patients with advanced, metastatic, or inoperable, slowly progressing NETs with high somatostatin receptor expression. The principles behind PRRT efficacy are the somatostatin receptor ligand that binds the specific receptor (SSTR1–5). Particularly, SSTR2 overexpressed on the surface of neuroendocrine tumor cells. The high energy of β-particle (^{90}Y or ^{177}Lu) labeled to a somatostatin receptor (SSTR) ligand caused cell death through direct or indirect DNA damage of target cells (self-dose) or neighboring cells (crossfire effect) [42]. The binding of the radiopharmaceutical to the targeted cells will be indispensable when using Auger emitters. Beta-particles become more effective in damaging and killing target cells that radiopharmaceutical is bound to and several cells around the target. It is the so-called "crossfire" effect. Lower tissue penetration of ^{177}Lu favors the use in small-sized tumors, whereas, in larger tumors, ^{90}Y might be a better choice [25]. ^{117}Lu or ^{90}Y labeled DOTATATE (DOTA, Tyr(3)-octreotate) was the most widely used peptide. It is a higher SSTR2 affinity compared to DOTATOC (DOTA, D-Phe1, Tyr (3)-octreotide) and DOTANOC (DOTA, 1-Nal(3)-octreotide) [43].

Furthermore, targeted peptide receptor alpha therapy with ^{213}Bi/^{225}Ac has been clinically tested to treat brain tumors, neuroendocrine tumors, and prostate cancer. ^{213}Bi and ^{225}Ac-DOTA chelated peptides developed for peptide receptor radiotherapies, such as DOTA-Substance P targeting the neurokinin-1 receptor and the widely used somatostatin-analogs (e.g., DO-TATOC, DOTATATE). The complexation efficiency, in vitro and in vivo stability of the radiopeptides is high [1, 44]. However, these promising results still need to be confirmed in further studies with therapeutic activities ^{213}Bi and ^{225}Ac.

6. Prostate-specific membrane antigen (PSMA)-targeting ligands

After promising results with ^{131}I-labeled prostate-specific membrane antigen (PSMA) ligands for prostate cancer therapy, it was introduced ^{177}Lu-PSMA by the German Cancer Research Center in 2015 [45]. PSMA is known as folate hydrolase 1 (FOLH1) or glutamate carboxypeptidase II (GCP II) and is overexpressed on the membrane of prostate cancer cells [45–47]. It remains high even after multiple lines of therapy [45, 46]. Metastatic castration-resistant prostate cancer (mCRPC) patients who shown ineffective by chemotherapy, radioligand therapy targeting the PSMA is a promising therapy approach [41, 45, 46]. First data showed that ^{177}Lu-PSMA is safe and effective in reducing tumor burden. It has been widely adopted in German and international sites, with likely more than a thousand therapy cycles performed [45].

PSMA targeting ligand using the beta emitter lutetium-177 [^{177}Lu]Lu-PSMA-617 or [^{177}Lu]Lu-PSMA-I&T) are currently being tested in phase III trials. It revealed encouraging data in several studies in mCRPC patients [46, 48, 49]. PSMA-targeting ligand using alpha emitters as actinium-225 may be advantageous compared to PSMA-targeting ligan with beta emitters. Clinical studies using ^{225}Ac-labeled PSMA-ligands ([^{225}Ac]Ac-PSMA-617 or [^{225}Ac]Ac-PSMA-I&T) have reported remarkable therapeutic results lately. However, it shows more substantial radiobiological effect of alpha particles on the organs at risk [46]. Combining alpha emitters in adjusted doses with beta emitters called 'tandem therapy' may reduce these significant adverse effects compared to using alpha emitters alone [46]. Furthermore, a novel alpha therapy approach with a thorium-227-labeled PSMA antibody shows strongly in vitro potency in several PSMA-positive cell lines and in vivo efficacy in xenograft models of prostate cancer [47]. These treatment approaches need more studies for effectiveness and limited toxicity.

7. Future prospective, challenges in radiopharmaceutical therapy

Radiopharmaceutical targeted therapy is a promising tumor treatment, particularly α-emitter, for effective and rapid cancer therapy due to the localized cell killing originated from high LET and short ranges of particles [8, 41]. Strategies to combine α-emitter with immunomodulators demonstrated higher tumor growth inhibition than α therapy alone [44].

Furthermore, intelligent drug delivery agents apart from peptides, small molecules, mAb, and mAb fragments can also achieve target-specific cancer therapy [41]. They are among the most searched cancer treatment issues due to their desired properties, including tumor-targeting uptake, bio-compatibility, reducing side-effects, and nonspecific uptake and distribution. So, the main problem of targeted radionuclide therapy, such as the radiation exposure effect in healthy tissues upon the emission of the particles, can be removed significantly. The number and variety of studies about the delivery of radionuclides particles by drug delivery agents are still limited. The studies will probably increase considerably in the future due to the need for effective, rapid, and personalized cancer therapy approaches.

Regarding supply issues of radionuclides also need to be address. Some main reactors in the world now are aging, which affect to constant and reliable supply globally [6]. In particular, for α-particle-emitting radionuclide (such as actinium-225), the supply is considered a potential obstacle for the growth of RPT. Some opinions suggest that the supply problems are transient technical issues that will be resolved with a more significant investment if RPT is adopted as a mainstream cancer therapy [2]. RPT is an effective cancer treatment, particularly when other standard therapeutic approaches have failed. However, even more than 40 years of clinical investigation, RPT has not become a part of cancer treatment in the same way as other therapy approaches. Even though 'targeted' cancer therapies are associated with clinical trial failure rates of 97%, but experience with RPT was ignored mainly or presented as a burdensome multidisciplinary endeavor [2, 50]. Additionally, public perception and fear of radioactivity and the perceived complexity of the treatment are challenges in developing and applying RPT.

8. Conclusions

Radiopharmaceutical therapy is a safe and effective targeted approach to treating many types of cancer. Compared to other systemic cancer treatment options, RPT has shown efficacy with minimal toxicity. Different types of radionuclides relevant to the purpose are β-emitters, Auger electrons, and α-emitters. However, the targeted α-emitter has potential advantages over β-emitter therapy due to the high energy and short path length of α emissions causing double-stranded breaks in DNA and the relative tolerance to cell cycle effects and hypoxic conditions. Radionuclides are coupled to ligands that recognize and bind the tumor-associated molecules, ensuring the precise targeting of cancerous cells that can be used for therapeutic approaches and live-monitoring of treatment efficacy. Different radioligands are developed for uniquely targeting molecular receptors or intracellular components that currently lead to planning personal patient-tailored therapy in modern cancer therapy management.

Author details

Aisyah Elliyanti[1,2]

1 Department of Medical Physics, Faculty of Medicine, Universitas Andalas, Padang, Indonesia

2 Department of Radiology, Division of Nuclear Medicine, Dr. M. Djamil Hospital, Padang, Indonesia

*Address all correspondence to: aelliyanti@med.unand.ac.id

References

[1] Ferrier MG, Radchenko V. An appendix of radionuclides used in targeted alpha therapy. J Med Imaging Radiat Sci. 2019 Dec;50(4 Suppl 1):S58-S65. DOI:10.1016/j.jmir.2019.06.051.

[2] Sgouros G, Bodei L, McDevitt MR, Nedrow JR. Radiopharmaceutical therapy in cancer: Clinical advances and challenges. Nat Rev Drug Discov. 2020; 19: 589-608.

[3] Kumar C, Shetake N, Desai S, Kumar A, Samuel G, et al. Relevance of radiobiological concepts in radionuclide therapy of cancer. Int J Radiat Biol. 2016; 92: 173-186.

[4] Wulbrand C, Seidl C, Gaertner FC, Bruchertseifer F, Morgenstern A, Essler M, Senekowitsch-Schmidtke R. Alpha-particle emitting 213Bi-anti-EGFR immunoconjugates eradicate tumor cells independent of oxygenation. PLoS One. 2013; 8:e64730.

[5] Calais PJ, Turner JH. Outpatient 131I-rituximab radoimmunotherapy for non-Hodgkin lymphoma: A study in safety. Clin Nucl Med. 2012; 37:732-737.

[6] Yeong CH, Cheng MH, Ng KH. Therapeutic radionuclides in nuclear medicine: Current and future prospects. J Zhejiang Univ Sci B. 2014;15: 845-863.

[7] Elliyanti A, Rustam R, Tofrizal T, Yenita Y, Susanto YDB. Evaluating the Natrium iodide Symporter expressions in thyroid Tumors. Open Access Maced J Med Sci. 2021; 9(B): 18-23.

[8] Kramer-Marek G, Capala J. The role of nuclear medicine in modern therapy of cancer. Tumour Biol. 2012 Jun;33(3): 629-640.

[9] Qaim SM, 2001.Therapeutic radionuclides and nuclear data. Radiochim. Acta. 2001; 89: 297-302.

[10] Widel M, et al. Bystander normal human fibroblasts reduce damage response in radiation targeted

[11] International Atomic Energy Agency. Radiation Biology: A Handbook for teachers and students. IAEA. 2010; pp. 23-26

[12] Elliyanti, A. An introduction to nuclear medicine in oncological molecular imaging. In Proceeding of AIP Conference Proceedings December 2019. Indonesia 2019. 020050-1-020050-4. DOI:10.1063/1.5135559

[13] Arslan, N., Emi, M., Alagoz, E., et al. Selective intraarterial radionuclide therapy with Yttrium-90 (Y-90) microspheres for hepatic neuroendocrine metastases: Initial experience at a single center. Vojnosanit. Pregl. 2011; 68: 341-348.

[14] Kucuk ON, Soydal C, Lacin S, et al. Selective intraarterial radionuclide therapy with yttrium-90 (Y-90) microspheres for unresectable primary and metastatic liver tumors. World J. Surg. Oncol. 2011; 9: 86.

[15] Houle S, Yip TK, Shepherd FA, et al. Hepatocellular carcinoma: Pilot trial of treatment with Y-90 microspheres. Radiology. 1989; 172: 857-860.

[16] Thamboo T, Tan KB, Wang SC, et al. Extrahepatic embolisation of Y-90 microspheres from selective internal radiation therapy (SIRT) of the liver. Pathology. 2003; 35: 351-353.

[17] Gabriel M. Radionuclide therapy beyond radioiodine. Wien Med Wochenschr. 2012;162:430-439.

[18] Hillegonds DJ, Franklin S, Shelton DK, Vijayakumar S, Vijayakumar V. The management of painful bone metastases with an

emphasis on radionuclide therapy. J Natl Med Assoc. 2007;99:785-794.

[19] Navalkissoor S, Grossman A. Targeted alpha particle therapy for neuroendocrine tumours: The next generation of peptide receptor radionuclide therapy. Neuroendocrinology. 2019;108:256-264.

[20] Elliyanti A, Radioiodine for Graves' Disease Therapy. In Gensure R, Editor. Graves' Disease: IntechOpen;2021. DOI:10.5772/intechopen.96949

[21] van der Doelen, MJ, et al. 'Clinical experience with PSMA-Actinium-225 (Ac-225) radioligand therapy (RLT) in end-stage metastatic castration-resistant prostate cancer (mCRPC) patients.', Journal of Clinical Oncology. 2018; 36(6_suppl): 344.

[22] McDevitt MR, Sgouros G, Sofou S. Targeted and nontargeted α-particle therapies. Annu Rev Biomed Eng. 2018; 20: 73-93.

[23] Pouget J, Navarro-Teulon I, Bardie's M, Chouin N, Cartron G, et al. clinical radioimmunotherapy – The role of radiobiology. Nat Rev Clin Oncol. 2011; 8: 720-734.

[24] Elliyanti A, Rusnita D, Afriani N, Susanto YD, Susilo VY, Setiyowati S, et al. Analysis natrium iodide symporter expression in breast cancer subtypes for radioiodine therapy response. Nucl Med Mol Imaging. 2020;54:35-42.

[25] Kendi AT, Moncayo VM, Nye JA, Galt JR, Halkar R, Schuster DM. Radionuclide therapies in molecular imaging and precision medicine. PET Clin. 2017;12:93-103.

[26] Barendsen GW, Vergroesen AJ. Irradiation of human cells in tissue culture with alpha-rays, beta-rays and x-rays [abstract]. Int J Radiat Biol Relat Stud Phys Chem Med. 1960; 2:441.

[27] Goodhead DT, Munson RJ, Thacker J, Cox R. Mutation and inactivation of cultured mammalian cells exposed to beams of accelerated heavy ions. IV. Biophysical interpretation. Int J Radiat Biol Relat Stud Phys Chem Med. 1980; 37:135-167.

[28] Munson RJ, Bance DA, Stretch A, Goodhead DT. Mutation and inactivation of cultured mammalian cells exposed to beams of accelerated heavy ions. I. Irradiation facilities and methods. Int J Radiat Biol Relat Stud Phys Chem Med. 1979; 36:127-136

[29] Kvinnsland Y, Stokke T, Aurlien E. Radioimmunotherapy with alpha-particle emitters: Microdosimetry of cells with a heterogeneous antigen expression and with various diameters of cells and nuclei. Radiat Res. 2001; 155:288-296.

[30] Neti PVSV, Howell RW. Log normal distribution of cellular uptake of radioactivity: Implications for biologic responses to radiopharmaceuticals. J Nucl Med. 2006; 47:1049-1058

[31] Bird RP, Rohrig N, Colvett RD, Geard CR, Marino SA. Inactivation of synchronized Chinese hamster V79 cells with charged-particle track segments. Radiat Res. 1980; 82:277-289.

[32] Todd P, Wood JCS, Walker JT, Weiss SJ. Lethal, potentially lethal, and nonlethal damage induction by heavy-ions in cultured human-cells. Radiat Res. 1985; 104(suppl):S5–S12.

[33] Roberts CJ, Goodhead DT. The effect of ^{238}Pu alpha-particles on the mouse fibroblast cell line C3H 10T1/2: Characterization of source and RBE for cell survival. Int J Radiat Biol Relat Stud Phys Chem Med. 1987; 52:871-882.

[34] Sartor, O. Overview of samarium Sm 153 lexidronam in the treatment of painful metastatic bone disease. Rev. Urol. 2004;6: S3–S12

[35] Anderson, P. M., Subbiah, V. and Rohren, E.In: Current Advances in Osteosarcoma. 291-304 (Springer International Publishing, 2014).

[36] Geerlings MW, Kaspersen FM, Apostolidis C, van der Hout R. The feasibility of ^{225}Ac as a source of alpha-particles in radioimmunotherapy. Nucl Med Commun. 1993; 14:121-125.

[37] Hultborn R, Andersson H, Back T, et al. Pharmacokinetics and dosimetry of ^{211}At-MX35 F(AB′) (2) in therapy of ovarian cancer: preliminary results from an ongoing phase I study [abstract]. Cancer Biother Radiopharm. 2006; 21: 395.

[38] Kennel SJ, Mirzadeh S, Eckelman WC, et al. Vascular-targeted radioimmunotherapy with the alpha-particle emitter ^{211}At. Radiat Res. 2002; 157:633-641.

[39] Chen P, Wang J, Hope K, Jin L, Dick J, Cameron R, Brandwein J, Minden M, Reilly RM. Nuclear localizing sequences promote nuclear translocation and enhance the radiotoxicity of the anti-CD33 monoclonal antibody HuM195 labeled with ^{111}In in human myeloid leukemia cells. J Nucl Med. 2006;47:827-836.

[40] Kassis AI. Therapeutic radionuclides: biophysical and radiobiologic principles. Semin Nucl Med. 2008;38(5):358-66. Doi:10.1053/j.semnuclmed.2008.05.002.

[41] Silindir-Gunay M, Karpuz M, Ozer AY. Targeted alpha therapy and Nanocarrier approach. Cancer Biother Radiopharm. 2020;35:446-458.

[42] Liberini V, Huellner MW, Grimaldi S, Finessi M, Thuillier P, Muni A, Pellerito RE, Papotti MG, Piovesan A, Arvat E, Deandreis D. The challenge of evaluating response to peptide receptor radionuclide therapy in Gastroenteropancreatic neuroendocrine Tumors: The present and the future. Diagnostics (Basel). 2020 Dec 12;10(12): 1083.

[43] Heesch A, Maurer J, Stickeler E, Beheshti M, Mottaghy FM, Morgenroth A. Development of radiotracers for breast Cancer-the tumor microenvironment as an emerging target. Cells. 2020 Oct 21; 9(10):2334.

[44] Morgenstern A, Bruchertseifer F. Development of Targeted Alpha Therapy from Bench to Bedside. J Med Imaging Radiat Sci. 2019;50(4S1):S18-S20.

[45] Fendler WP, Rahbar K, Herrmann K, Kratochwil C, Eiber M. ^{177}Lu-PSMA Radioligand Therapy for Prostate Cancer. J Nucl Med. 2017 Aug;58(8):1196-1200. DOI:10.2967/jnumed.117.191023. Epub 2017 Jun 29. Erratum in: J Nucl Med. 2018;59:346.

[46] Rosar F, Krause J, Bartholomä M, Maus S, Stemler T, Hierlmeier I, Linxweiler J, Ezziddin S, Khreish F. Efficacy and safety of [^{225}Ac] Ac-PSMA-617 augmented [^{177}Lu] Lu-PSMA-617 Radioligand therapy in patients with highly advanced mCRPC with poor prognosis. Pharmaceutics. 2021;13:722.

[47] Nevedomskaya E, Baumgart SJ, Haendler B. Recent advances in prostate Cancer treatment and drug discovery. Int J Mol Sci. 2018;19:1359.

[48] Fendler, W.P.; Reinhardt, S.; Ilhan, H.; Delker, A.; Böning, G.; Gildehaus, F.J.; Stief, C.; Bartenstein, P.; Gratzke, C.; Lehner, S.; et al. Preliminary experience with Dosimetry, response and patient reported outcome after 177Lu-PSMA-617 therapy for metastatic castration-resistant prostate Cancer. Oncotarge. 2017; 8: 3581-3590.

[49] Rasul, S.; Hacker, M.; Kretschmer-Chott, E.; Leisser, A.; Grubmüller, B.;

Kramer, G.; Shariat, S.; Wadsak, W.; Mitterhauser, M.; Hartenbach, M.; et al. Clinical outcome of standardized 177Lu-PSMA-617 therapy in metastatic prostate Cancer patients receiving 7400 MBq every 4 weeks. Eur. J. Nucl. Med. Mol. Imagin. 2020; 47; 713-720.

[50] Wong, C. H., Siah, K. W. and Lo, A. W. Estimation of clinical trial success rates and related parameters. Biostatistics. 2018; 20, 273-286.

Chapter 12

New Trends in Preparation, Bio Distribution, and Pharmacokinetics of Radiopharmaceuticals in Diagnosis and Research

Hasna Albander and Maisoon Ibrahim Aljalis

Abstract

Radiopharmaceuticals are radioactive compounds which have a bound radionuclide in their structure. It is used to direct the radionuclide to a location to be treated or to obtain images. Nuclear medicine is the science that in the charge of employing radiopharmaceuticals, which is very useful support for medicine assisting in several diagnoses and treatments for cancer. The main aim of this work is to shed lights on the main radionuclides and metal complexes which are used as radiopharmaceuticals. Radiopharmaceuticals are compounds of technetium (99mTc) is considered as the main metal complexes like sodium pertechnetate and methylenediphosphonate MDP99mTc and other compounds which used in nuclear medicine for diagnosis such as: (1) indium (111In); (2) thallium (201Tl); (3) gallium (67Ga, 68Ga); (4) iodine (123I and 131I); (5) chromium (51Cr); (6) sulfur (35S); (7) phosphorus (32P); (8) a18F. They are very important in the early diagnosis for several diseases such as cancer, kidney, cardiovascular, liver. Generally, technetium compounds are main radiopharmaceuticals, widely all over the word.

Keywords: therapy or diagnostic, radionuclide, compounds, stability, abnormal distribution, radionuclide reactor, a radioactive- reactor, therapeutic radiopharmaceutical precursor, technetium, radioisotopes-

1. Introduction

It is very effective to provide an introduction to this chapter of the field of nuclear medicine and how radioisotopes are used in nuclear medicine for both diagnostic and therapeutic applications. Radiopharmaceuticals are compounds that administered intravenously whether diagnostic or therapeutic applications [1]. Diagnostic applications in nuclear medicine use low activity tracer levels of generally gamma- or positron-emitting radioisotopes which are generally produced in nuclear reactors and accelerators. In other hands, therapeutic applications use particle-emitting radionuclides for induction of radio toxicity to kill cells in the intended tissue. It is also noted that in the form of radioactive sources, therapeutic radioisotopes are also used in other clinical specialties will be discussed in this chapter. As well as this chapter focuses on the description of radioactive materials which are used for nuclear medicine therapy and how they are produced.

IntechOpen

Improving the utilization of radiopharmaceuticals in the development of pharmaceutical drug delivery systems, the behavior of the tracers administered by various ways must be investigated. The main aim of radio pharmacology is to study the chemical properties of radiotracers and their interactions with living organisms. Radiopharmaceuticals are unique medicinal formulations containing radioisotopes which are used in major clinical areas for diagnosis and/or therapy. Radiopharmaceuticals is currently considered the cornerstone of nuclear medicine. That is why there is a requirement for new radiopharmaceuticals that could be utilized to explore more subtle mechanisms of body functions.

This part of chapter which presented in the symposium reflect current and future developments in diagnostic and therapeutic agents as it deals with (Tc-99 m), highlighting its continuing importance to nuclear medicine and the role of imaging as an important tool. The emerging interest in therapeutic radiopharmaceuticals based on beta emitting short lived isotopes such as Iodine (I-131).

It worth mentioning that The properties of bio distribution and pharmacokinetics play a major role in affecting and defining the efficacy and safety for the treatment with a medicine. Currently, several image guided modalities have been applied in nuclear medicine such as Single-Photon Emission Computed Tomography (SPECT), (SPECT/CT), Tomography Computed Tomography (PET/CT), and Positron Emission.

The use of radionuclides for medical applications has continued to grow at a very rapid pace. That is why, it is required to learn more about The use of radiotracers for nuclear medicine imaging as well as discussing in this part of chapter the different methods of preparation, bio distribution and pharmacokinetics of radio pharmaceuticals for diagnosis and research.

2. What is radiopharmaceutical?

Radiopharmaceuticals can be defined as a chemicals substances that contain radioactive atoms within its structure and suitable for administration to human used for either diagnose or treat diseases [2].

Radiopharmaceuticals can be categorized into:

1. Diagnostic radiopharmaceuticals are administered to a patient and enable physicians and researchers to see the biochemical activity of cells, to diagnose or stage disease

2. Therapeutic radiopharmaceuticals are administered to a patient to seek out and deliver cell-killing radiation to the site of disease.

3. Nuclear medicine and radiopharmaceuticals

Radiopharmaceuticals can be categorized into two groups:

1. First group includes radionuclides with radioactive decay period (half-life) less than 2 h

2. The group includes radionuclides with half life higher than 2.

Cameras in nuclear medicine are suitable for identifying radioactive particles. The type of camera can be defined by The type of radiation emitted:

1. SPECT cameras are used to detect nuclides that decay through direct emission of single gamma rays

2. PET cameras are able to detect the pair of gamma rays emitted after a decay of positron.

4. Nuclear stability

when the number of neutrons (N) and protons (P) are approximately equal it's called stable nuclei. The ratio of N/P is equal one when the elements become heavier, the ratio of neutrons (N) to protons (P) for nuclear stability increases from 1to 1.5. meanwhile the nucleuses has too high (Neutron rich) stability

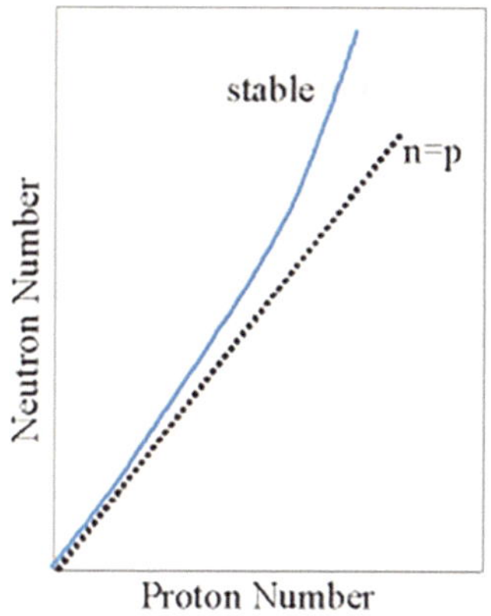

Figure 1.
Nuclear stability diagram.

decreases at the line of stability See **Figure 1**.If the N/P ratio is too low for stability, the radioactive decay take places in a manner that will be reduce the number of protons and increase the number of neutrons by the net conversion of proton to neutron.

5. Fundamentals of radioisotopes for radiopharmaceuticals

1. Radiopharmaceuticals are medicinal formulations involving radioisotopes which are safe for administration in humans with the purpose of diagnosis or for therapy.

2. Nuclear reactors have the ability to produce larger quantities of radioisotopes. Radioiodine (iodine-131), which was used as treatment of thyroid cancer, and still has the same importance but becomes the most efficacious method for the treatment of hyperthyroidism and thyroid cancer.

3. Preparing of radioisotopes is considered one of the most important and has the most priority among the several applications The medium flux and high flux research reactors are considered the most important source that used to produce radioisotopes for medical, and also industrial, applications and for producing isotopes in medical applications like molybdenum-99 (for production of technetium-99 m), iodine-131, phosphorus-32, chromium-51, strontium-89, samarium-153, rhenium-186 and lutetium-177.

4. Producing long lived radioisotopes use cyclotron in radiopharmaceuticals to prepare tracers for diagnostic imaging. Cyclotrons with high beam currents required For medium to high energy (20–70 MeV).

Most cyclotrons (~350) all over the world are used for the preparation of fluorine-18 for making radiolabelled glucose for medical imaging in the nuclear medicine.

6. Nuclear medicine techniques

Radioactive tracers is used by Diagnostic techniques in nuclear medicine that emit gamma radiation. The camera produces an image from the points at the radiation emission. The nuclear medicine techniques include

a. Single Photon Emission Computerized Tomography (SPECT)

b. Positron Emission Tomography (PET),

c. computed tomography-PET (PET-CT) (for better anatomical visualization)

d. micro-PET (with ultra-high resolution)

e. micro computerized axial tomography micro-CAT.

All above techniques are utilized to analyze biochemical dysfunctions with the purpose of showing early signs of the disease, their mechanisms and association with disease states.

7. Radiopharmaceuticals for diagnosis in human body

A large number of chemicals that are absorbed by specific organs have been identified by specialists. For examples Thyroid absorbs iodine while the brain absorbs glucose. To monitor blood flow to the brain, liver, lung, heart, and kidney diagnostic radiopharmaceuticals can be used for that purposes see **Figure 2**. Destroying or weakening cancer cells can be done by particulate radiation as well as beta radiation causes ([3], p. 7).

This can be concluded that each organs of the human body requires different Radiopharmaceuticals to be administrated to it for the purpose of diagnose or treatment. This depends on the absorption of this organ to this chemical.

We can summarize the difference between normal medicines and radiopharmaceuticals is that the normal medicine has therapeutic effect while the latter does not. Besides that, radiopharmaceuticals have a short half-life, because of their rapid decay. For this reason, radiopharmaceuticals must be prepared immediately before their administration. The preparation and use of

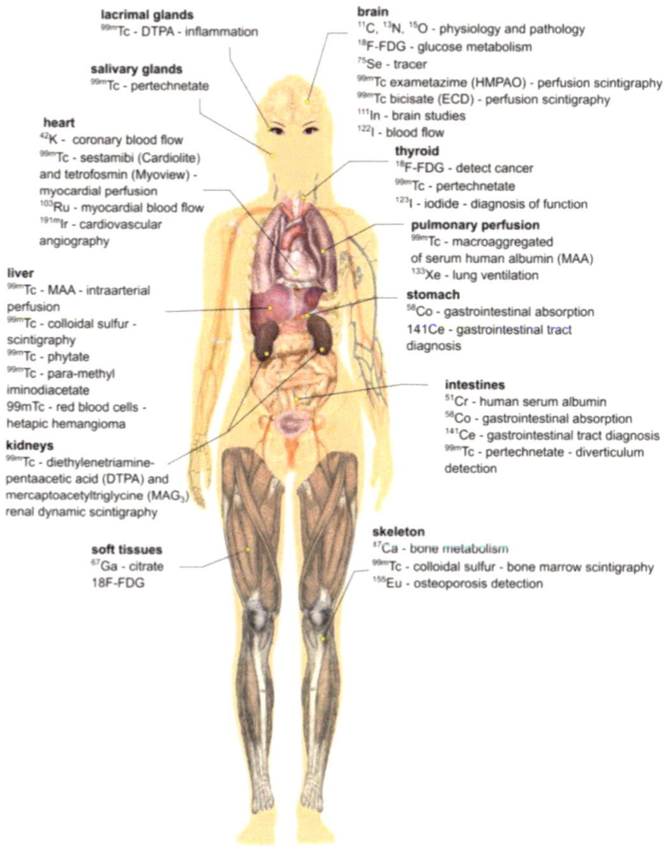

Figure 2.
Lists the radionuclides most commonly used for diagnosis and treatment of different organs of the human body.

radiopharmaceuticals with safety and expertise are therefore vital for operator and patient protection.

8. The Main characteristics for radiopharmaceuticals clinically useful for imaging

Firstly, we should discuss the characteristics for radiopharmaceuticals to help us understand how to deal with it during the chapter and these characteristics can be summarized in the below points:

1. The decay of the radionuclide should be in specific ranges of energy emissions (511 keV for positron emission tomography – PET and 100–200 keV for gamma cameras) and in sufficient quantity for tomography detection.

2. It should have particulate radiation beta emissions because it the radiation dose is increased in the patients.

3. The half-life should be for a minimal hours.

4. The radionuclides should not be mixed with other radionuclides of the same element or its stable radionuclides.

5. radiopharmaceuticals are supposed to have certain activity as well as the highest specific activity comes from carrier-f456ree radionuclides.

6. The radiopharmaceuticals are supposed not to have toxicity and do not manifest physiological impact.

7. The radiopharmaceutical should be available for instant usage and easy to compound and reach the target organ quickly and accurately.

9. Production of radionuclides

Generally

Most radionuclides are produced using two types of instruments:

9.1 In nuclear reactors

Through the fission, neutrons are generated of nuclear fuel or neutron-capture reactions on stable targets. These neutrons are then utilized to create neutron-rich radionuclides that typically decay through beta emission and are therefore appropriate for the aimed radiotherapy.

Meanwhile, Accelerators, in contrast, accelerate protons or other charged particles to induce nuclear reactions on target materials. During these reactions proton-rich radionuclides can be created that decay by positron emission and are therefore useful for imaging applications.

In the following lines, we are going to discuss the production of Radionuclides with more details.

The production of radiopharmaceuticals involves the handling of large quantities of radioactive substances and chemical processing. The radionuclides used to make radiopharmaceuticals are produced artificially, mainly in a cyclotron or in a nuclear reactor. The type of radionuclides produced in a cyclotron or in a reactor depends on the type of energy of the bombarding particles and the target material ([4], p. 5).

9.1.1 A-production of radionuclides in the cyclotron

The Cyclotrons are considered the most common type of accelerator which normally produce medical radionuclides through bombardment with charged particles. Its main usage is to accelerate charged particles in a circular fashion, cyclotrons used to take up less space than their linear counterparts.

The Cyclotrons typically accelerate charged particles to energies between 11 and 30 MeV, Despite the availability of the larger machines. Consequently, Cyclotrons can accelerate positive (e.g., protons, alpha particles) or negative (e.g., hydride ions) ions, but the majority of commercial machines manufactured today are negative ion.

The most important steps fundamentals of cyclotrons:

1. The radionuclides produced by the cyclotron are distinguished by a presence of fewer neutrons, and their nuclear stability is obtained through electron capture or positron emission.

2. A cyclotron is a charged particle (cation or an ion) accelerator that transfers high energy to these particles, accelerating them in circular orbits by means of alternating electromagnetic fields until they collide with a target, with the consequent nuclear reaction and the production of positron-emitting radio-

nuclides. The cyclotron was developed by with the purpose of accelerating particles such as protons or deuterons to achieve high levels of kinetic energy.

3. All cyclotrons are comprised of two electrodes in the form of semi-circular chambers (D) in which a vacuum is produced, and they are configured with the adjacent perimeter diameters in a uniform magnetic field. The Ds are coupled to a high-frequency electrical system that alternates about 107 times a second while the cyclotron is operating See **Figure 3**.

4. In each D, the ions are forced into a circular trajectory by means of an alternating magnetic field. When the ions complete a semi-circumference in the semi-period, the electrical field inverts polarity, causing acceleration of the ions in the electrical fields between the Ds, while also increasing the radius of their circular trajectory. This increase in acceleration involves an increase in kinetic energy See **Figure 4**.

5. continuously, this process is repeated, in semi-circular orbits that move in resonance with the oscillating field. In this way they gain energy continuously, describing a spiral trajectory until the periphery of the Ds is reached with the

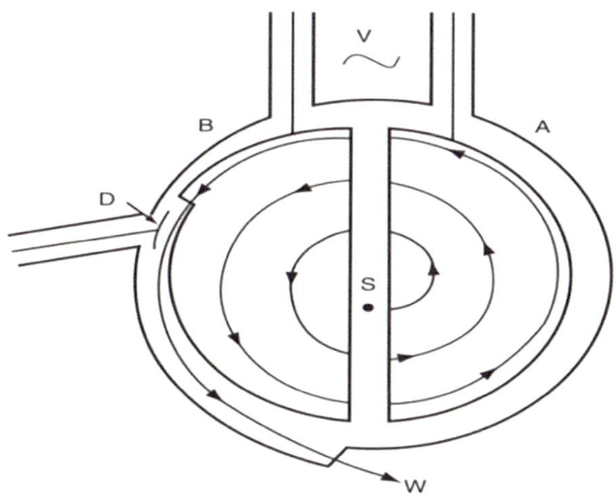

Figure 3.
Production processes in the cyclotron.

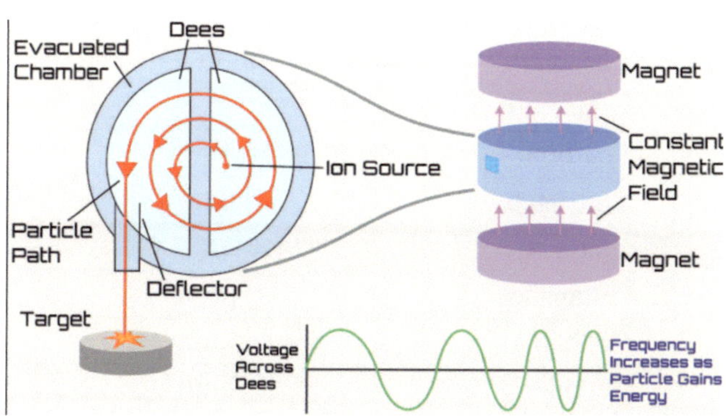

Figure 4.
The process of producing of radionuclides in cyclotron.

energy needed to escape from them and collide with the target, where the nuclear reactions will take place.

6. During nuclear reactions, The impacting particle can exit the nucleus after the interaction, and part of its energy is left in the nucleus, or it may be completely absorbed by the latter. In either case, a nucleus in an excited state is generated, and the excitation energy is released through the emission of nucleons (i.e., protons and neutrons). The emission of gamma radiation then occurs. Depending on the energy transmitted by the impacting particle, a random number of nucleons are emitted from the irradiated target, resulting in the formation of different nuclides. When the energy of the irradiating particle increases, more nucleons are generated and a greater variety of radionuclides are therefore produced. The radionuclides produced in a cyclotron are generally neutron-deficient and therefore decay with the emission of β + particles or through electron capture.

7. Radionuclides produced by the cyclotron and which are of interest in nuclear medicine comprise ([4], p.8):

Fluor-18: 18F - Carbon-11: 11C - Nitrogen-13: 13 N- Oxygen-15: 15O - Gallium-68: 68Ga - Scandium-44: 44Sc - Zirconium-89: 89Zr - Iodine-124: 124I See **Figure** 5.

9.1.2 Production of radionuclides in the nuclear reactor

The process of producing radionuclides in nuclear medicine generated in nuclear reactors has two kinds of nuclear reactions including an interaction with neutrons:

- **Neutron capture**
- **The fission of heavy elements.**

1. During **the neutron capture**, the target nucleus captures a thermal neutron, emitting gamma radiation to produce an isotope of the same element as the target nuclides. Some instances of radionuclides formed by this type of reaction are 131Te, 99Mo, 197Hg, 59Fe, 51Cr, etc.

2. Fission of heavy elements is categorized by the splitting of a heavy nucleus into two fragments of roughly the same mass, supplemented by the emission of two or three neutrons.

^{225}actinium	^{67}copper
^{211}astatine	^{67}gallium
^{213}bismuth	^{127}xenon
^{11}carbon	^{111}indium
^{13}nitrogen	^{123}iodine
^{15}oxygen	^{124}iodine
^{18}fluorine	^{81m}krypton
^{57}cobalt	^{82}rubidium
^{64}copper	^{201}thallium

Figure 5.
Selected radionuclides produced by cyclotrons.

Each fission reaction releases a considerable amount of energy that is take out through heat exchangers to provide electricity in nuclear energy plants. When a fissionable heavy element target is interleaved into the core of the reactor, the heavy nuclides absorb thermal neutrons and experience the so-called fission reaction. Some fissionable heavy elements with an atomic number over 90 are: 235U, 239Pu, 237Np, 233U 232To. On the other hand, many clinically suitable radionuclides for instance 131I, 99Mo 133Xe and 137Cs are attained from the fission of 235 U See **Figures 6** and 7.

The diagram illustrates the typical components found in radionuclide generator. It helps in the separation and elution of the daughter radionuclide and the parent radionuclide. This elution results in a product that is sterile and free of impurities thus making it immediately suitable for human injection See **Figure 8**.

9.1.3 What are the main purpose of the radionuclide reactors?

They are considered a source of radionuclides which used for the production of radiopharmaceuticals. The ^{99}Mo → ^{99m}Tc reactor often referred to as a technetium reactor is the most important radionuclide reactor for radiopharmaceutical preparation that is why it gets its importance. The reactor is capable of supplying short-lived radionuclides (short half-lives) over a time period much longer than this short half-life. It is also a unique equilibrium that is establishment between a long-lived

^{213}bismuth	^{59}iron	^{153}samarium
^{131}caesium	^{212}lead	^{75}selenium
^{137}caesium	^{177}lutetium	^{24}sodium
^{51}chromium	^{99}molybdenum	^{89}strontium
^{60}cobalt-60	^{103}palladium	^{99m}technetium
^{165}dysprosium	^{32}phosphorus	^{227}thorium
^{169}erbium	^{42}potassium	^{133}xenon
^{166}holmium	^{223}radium	^{169}ytterbium
^{131}iodine	^{186}rhenium	^{177}ytterbium
^{192}iridium	^{188}rhenium	^{90}yttrium

Figure 6.
Selected radionuclides produced by nuclear fission.

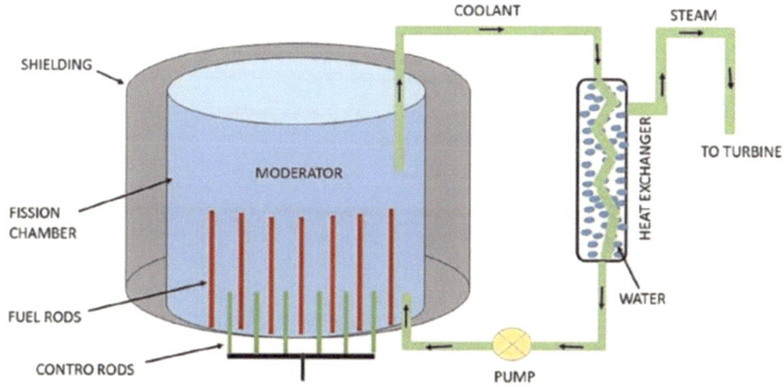

Figure 7.
Radionuclide reactors.

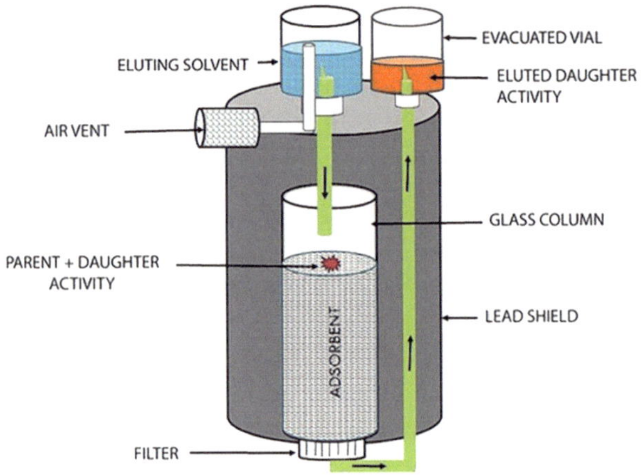

Figure 8.
Radionuclide generator.

Product
sodium iodide (^{123}I)
sodium iodide (^{131}I)
gallium citrate (^{67}Ga)
thallium chloride (^{201}Tl)
sodium chromate (^{51}Cr)
generator ^{99}Mo – ^{99m}Tc
sodium sulfate (^{35}S)
phosphoric acid (^{32}P)
sodium phosphate (^{32}P)
^{18}fluorodeoxyglucose (^{18}F-FDG)
EDTMP (^{153}Sm)
sodium fluoride (Na^{18}F)
^{111}indium (^{111}In)
dotatate (^{177}Lu)

Figure 9.
Products of Radiocludes.

"parent" radionuclide and its short-lived radioactive daughter. The second a ability to physically is the separation of the parent and daughter radionuclides to allow the daughter to be utilized for the preparation of short-lived radiopharmaceuticals. In the 99Mo → 99mTc reactor the parent is 99Mo with a half-life of 66 hours, which decays for producing the radioactive daughter 99mTc with a half-life of 6 hours. The separation of the parent and daughter is completed by simply washing the daughter from the reactor with sterile saline See **Figure 9** [5].

9.1.4 The Most common isotopes used in medicine

Several radioisotopes are produced by nuclear reactors and cyclotrons. As neutron-rich ones need to be made in reactors while neutron-depleted ones are made in cyclotrons, some examples of them as follows:

9.1.4.1 Cyclotron radioisotopes

- Carbon-11, Nitrogen-13, Oxygen-15, Fluorine-18: These positron emitters used in PET for studying brain physiology and pathology. They also have a significant role in cardiology. F-18 in FDG (fluorodeoxyglucose) is very important

- Iodine-123 (13 h): Increasingly used for diagnosis of thyroid function, it is a gamma emitter without the beta radiation of I-131.

- Thallium-201 (73 h): Used for diagnosis of coronary artery disease other heart conditions as well as it is used as substitute for technetium-99 in cardiac-stress tests.

9.1.4.2 Reactor radioisotopes

- **Iodine-131 (8 d)**: Widely used in treating thyroid cancer and in imaging the thyroid also in urinary tract obstruction it is also strong gamma emitter, but used for beta therapy.

- **Iridium-192 (74 d):** it is used as an internal radiotherapy source for treating cancer.

- **Lutetium-177 (6.7 d):** Lu-177, it emits just enough gamma for imaging while the beta radiation does the therapy on small (e.g., endocrine) tumors. Because its half-life is long enough to allow sophisticated preparation for use.

- **Molybdenum-99 (66 h)*:** generally, used as the 'parent' in a reactor to produce technetium-99 m.

- **Palladium-103 (17 d):** Mainly used to make brachytherapy permanent implant seeds for early stage prostate cancer. Emits soft x-rays.

- **Technetium-99 m (6 h):** Used in to image the skeleton and heart muscle in particular, but also for brain, thyroid, lungs (perfusion and ventilation), liver, spleen, kidney (structure and filtration rate), over 80% of scans of the nearly 25 million diagnostic nuclear medicine studies carried out annually are done with this single isotope. This percentage share is estimated to remain for the foreseeable future.

10. Radiopharmaceutical safety

It is required to have all the protective procedures towards the radiations in general and Pharmaceutical productions specifically Health and safety are an integral for protecting the patients, doctors, personnel and workers. The pharmacists are constantly being exposed to chemical and biological hazards which pose a serious threat to their health. Furthermore, during the production, lack of enough safety standards and non-compliance may cause negative impact in the long run. Therefore, it is important to have optimal health and safety practices while ensuring that all employees adhere to such regulations. Here are the tips to maintain improved health and safety standards in the pharmaceutical industry.

11. Health and Safety Standards in handling chemicals

In case transporting or handling pharmaceuticals inappropriately, they can be dangerous. The trained staff are able to prevent chemical releases which can cause explosions and fire. That is why to reduce and minimize the risk and ensure more safety, Classification of Chemicals should be done by an effective way of handling hazardous chemicals. This can be done by trained and professional staff.

In addition, the Classification of Chemicals is an effective method to identify the way of how the chemicals can have harmful effects. It also helps in labeling correctly and handled in a legally manner to avoid health risks. Exploding or releasing chemicals normally can be caused by high temperature, high pressure or oxidation. This problem can be processed by lowering the oxidation work scale and understanding the right flammable limits. Certainly pharmaceutical companies have the main role to reduce these risks [6].

12. Practice primary laboratory safety

In the pharmaceutical industry, basic safety has to be maintained in the laboratory as well as employees must be conscious to the basic health and safety practices and take preventive processes during work in a hazard environment. These procedures can be carried out to maintain health and safety at the laboratory such as [6]:

- Practice frequent cleaning
- particularly Never eat, drink or smoke inside the laboratory
- Making wearing suitable Personal Protective Equipment mandatory inside the laboratory
- Coveralls, eye gear, protective helmet, shoe covers, etc.

13. Conclusion

We can conclude that the Radionuclides which are used in nuclear medicine are considered mostly to be artificial ones. We learned that these are primarily produced in a cyclotron or a reactor. The type of radionuclide produced in a cyclotron or a reactor depends mainly on the irradiating particle, its energy, and the target nuclei. Generally, it is noted the facilities which having such equipment are limited and supply radionuclides to remote facilities that do not possess them. Nuclear medicine is the medical specialty that employs radiopharmaceuticals, has presented itself as a very useful assistant for medicine supporting in several diagnoses and treatments. The main aim of this work is to define the vital radionuclides and metal.

At the end, this chapter aims to be useful for all whom working in nuclear medicine and to be a guide for them. It is a guide to be used to shed some lights on radiopharmaceuticals and their uses, production and safety during handling [7].

Author details

Hasna Albander[1]* and Maisoon Ibrahim Aljalis[2]

1 Medical Physicist Department, Prince Sultan Military Medical City, Riyadh, Saudi Arabia

2 King Saud Medical City, Riyadh, Saudi Arabia

*Address all correspondence to: halbander@psmmc.med.sa

References

[1] Therapeutic Applications of Radiopharmaceuticals. Austria: IAEA; 2001

[2] Available from: https://www.nibib.nih.gov/science-education/science-topics/nuclear-medicine

[3] Radiopharmaceuticals for Diagnosis in Nuclear Medicine. Filipe Payolla. p. 7

[4] Trends in Radiopharmaceuticals (ISTR-2019). Austria: IAEA;

[5] Available from: https://world-nuclear.org/information-library/non-power-nuclear-applications/radioisotopes-research/radioisotopes-in-medicine.aspx

[6] Available from: https://lindstromgroup.com/in/article/maintaining-health-and-safety-in-the-pharmaceutical-industry/

[7] Radiopharmacology and pharmacokinetic evaluation of some radiopharmaceuticals, selcan Turker, A YEKETA; 2005. p. 1